Update in the Medical Management of the Long-Term Care Patient

Guest Editor

MIGUEL A. PANIAGUA, MD

CLINICS IN GERIATRIC MEDICINE

www.geriatric.theclinics.com

May 2011 • Volume 27 • Number 2

SAUNDERS an imprint of ELSEVIER, Inc.

W.B. SAUNDERS COMPANY
A Division of Elsevier Inc.

1600 John F. Kennedy Blvd., Suite 1800. Philadelphia, Pennsylvania 19103-2899

http://www.theclinics.com

CLINICS IN GERIATRIC MEDICINE Volume 27, Number 2
May 2011 ISSN 0749–0690, ISBN-13: 978-1-4557-0666-2

Editor: Yonah Korngold

Clinics in Geriatric Medicine (ISSN 0749-0690) is published quarterly by Elsevier Inc., 360 Park Avenue South, New York, NY 10010-1710. Months of issue are February, May, August, and November. Business and Editorial Offices: 1600 John F. Kennedy Blvd., Suite 1800, Philadelphia, PA 191023-2899. Periodicals postage paid at New York, NY, and additional mailing offices. Subscription prices is $241.00 per year (US individuals), $427.00 per year (US institutions), $167.00 per year (US student/resident), $314.00 per year (Canadian individuals), $532.00 per year (Canadian institutions), $333.00 per year (foreign individuals) and $532.00 per year (foreign institutions). Foreign air speed delivery is included in all *Clinics* subscription prices. All prices are subject to change without notice. POSTMASTER: Send address changes to *Clinics in Geriatric Medicine,* Elsevier Health Sciences Division, Subscription Customer Service, 3251 Riverport Lane, Maryland Heights, MO 63043. Telephone: 1-800-654-2452 (U.S. and Canada); 314-447-8871 (outside U.S. and Canada). Fax: 314-447-8029. E-mail: journalscustomer service-usa@elsevier.com (for print support) or journalsonlinesupport-usa@elsevier.com (for online support).

Reprints. For copies of 100 or more, of articles in this publication, please contact the Commercial Reprints Department, Elsevier Inc., 360 Park Avenue South, New York, New York 10010-1710. Tel.: (212) 633-3812; Fax: (212) 462-1935, email: reprints@elsevier.com.

Clinics in Geriatric Medicine is covered in *MEDLINE/PubMed (Index Medicus), EMBASE/Excerpta Medica, Current Contents/Clinical Medicine (CC/CM), and the Cumulative Index to Nursing & Allied Health Literature.*

Printed and bound by CPI Group (UK) Ltd, Croydon, CR0 4YY

Transferred to Digital Print 2011

Contributors

GUEST EDITOR

MIGUEL A. PANIAGUA, MD, FACP
Associate Professor, Division of Gerontology and Geriatric Medicine, Department of Internal Medicine; Director, Internal Medicine Residency Program, Saint Louis University School of Medicine, St Louis, Missouri

AUTHORS

LOUISE ARONSON, MD
Associate Professor, Division of Geriatrics, University of California at San Francisco, San Francisco, California

RACHELLE E. BERNACKI, MD, MS
Director of Quality Initiatives, Pain and Palliative Care Program, Dana Farber Cancer Institute, Harvard Medical School, Boston, Massachusetts

GWENDOLEN T. BUHR, MD, MHS
Assistant Professor of Medicine, Division of Geriatrics, Department of Medicine, Duke University Medical Center, Durham, North Carolina

ELIZABETH HERSKOVITS CASTILLO, MD, PhD
Director, Geriatric Medicine Program, MAHEC (Mountain AHEC), Asheville, North Carolina; Assistant Clinical Professor, Department of Family Medicine, University of North Carolina of Chapel Hill School of Medicine, Chapel Hill; Medical Director, Givens Estates (CCRC), Asheville, North Carolina

DIANE CHAU, MD, FACP
Chief, Division of Geriatric Medicine, Department of Medicine, University of Nevada School of Medicine; Veterans Affairs Community Living Center, Reno, Nevada

HUAI Y. CHENG, MD, MPH
Clinical Fellow, Department of Palliative Care and Rehabilitation Medicine, MD Anderson Cancer Center, Houston, Texas

AMY M. CORCORAN, MD
Assistant Professor of Clinical Medicine, Associate Program Director, Geriatric Fellowship, Palliative Medicine Fellowship, Division of Geriatric Medicine, Penn Medicine, Ralston-Penn Center, University of Pennsylvania, Philadelphia, Pennsylvania

JOHN W. CULBERSON, MD
Assistant Professor, Department of Medicine, Baylor College of Medicine; Extended Care Line, Michael E. DeBakey Veterans Affairs Medical Center, Houston, Texas

SANJAY DESAI, MD
Division of Pulmonary/Critical Care, Washington Hospital Center, Washington, DC

SHAWKAT DHANANI, MD, MPH
Clinical Professor, Geriatrics Veterans Affairs Greater LA Healthcare System, GRECC, Los Angeles, California

GEORGES EL HOYEK, MD
Geriatrics Fellow, PGY-4, Division of Geriatric Medicine, Department of Medicine, University of Nevada School of Medicine; Veterans Affairs Community Living Center, Reno, Nevada

DAVID ESPINO, MD
Division of Community Geriatrics, Department of Family and Community Medicine, University of Texas Health Science Center at San Antonio, San Antonio, Texas

MARGARET FINLEY, MD, CMD
Division of Community Geriatrics, Department of Family and Community Medicine, University of Texas Health Science Center at San Antonio, San Antonio, Texas

PETRA FLOCK, MD
Assistant Professor, Division of Geriatrics, University of Massachusetts Medical School, Worcester; Summit ElderCare, Charlton, Massachusetts

ANA TUYA FULTON, MD, FACP
Assistant Professor of Medicine, Division of Geriatrics, Department of Medicine, Warren Alpert Medical School of Brown University; Chief of Internal Medicine, Butler Hospital, Providence, Rhode Island

LIZA GENAO, MD
Advanced fellow in Geriatrics, Division of Geriatrics, Department of Medicine, Duke University Medical Center, Durham Veterans Affairs Medical Center, Durham, North Carolina

SUZANNE M. GILLESPIE, MD, CMD
Division of Geriatrics and Aging, School of Medicine and Dentistry, University of Rochester, Rochester, New York

MATTHEW J. GONZALES, MD
Fellow, Hospice and Palliative Medicine, Division of Hospital Medicine, Department of Medicine, University of California San Francisco, San Francisco, California

MONICA S. HORTON, MD, MSc
Assistant Professor, University of Texas Health Science Center; South Texas Veterans Health Care System, San Antonio, Texas

NAMIRAH JAMSHED, MD
Assistant Professor of Clinical Medicine, Georgetown University School of Medicine; Geriatric Division/Geriatric Education Director, Washington Hospital Center, Washington, DC

NAE-HWA KIM, MD
Resident PGY 2, Department of Internal Medicine, University of Nevada School of Medicine, Reno, Nevada

BEATRIZ KORC-GRODZICKI, MD, PhD
Associate Attending, Chief, Geriatrics Service, Department of Medicine, Memorial Sloan Kettering Cancer Center, New York, New York

THOMAS W. MEEKS, MD
Assistant Professor, Department of Psychiatry, Division of Geriatric Psychiatry, University of California, San Diego, California

S. LILIANA OAKES, MD, CMD
Division of Community Geriatrics, Department of Family and Community Medicine, University of Texas Health Science Center at San Antonio, San Antonio, Texas

MIGUEL A. PANIAGUA, MD, FACP
Associate Professor, Division of Gerontology and Geriatric Medicine, Department of Internal Medicine; Director, Internal Medicine Residency Program, Saint Louis University School of Medicine, St Louis, Missouri

NEELA K. PATEL, MD, MPH
Division of Community Geriatrics, Department of Family and Community Medicine, University of Texas Health Science Center at San Antonio, San Antonio, Texas

JENNIFER RHODES-KROPF, MD
Clinical Instructor of Medicine, Division of Geriatrics, Medical Director, Center Communities of Brookline, Hebrew SeniorLife, Beth Israel Deaconess Medical Center, Harvard University Medical School, Boston, Massachusetts

MIRIAM B. RODIN, MD, PhD
Associate Professor Geriatrics, Division of Geriatrics, Department of Internal Medicine, St Louis University Medical School, St Louis, Missouri

MATHEW RUSSELL, MD
Section of Geriatrics, Boston University Medical Center, Boston, Massachusetts

BRYAN STRUCK, MD
Associate Professor, Reynolds Department of Geriatric Medicine, University of Oklahoma Health Sciences Center; Geriatrics and Extended Care, Oklahoma City Veterans Affairs Medical Center, Oklahoma City, Oklahoma

GEORGE TALER, MD
Professor of Clinical Medicine, Georgetown University School of Medicine; Division of Geriatrics, Director Long Term Care, Washington Hospital Center, Washington, DC

JAMES A. WALLACE, MD
Co-Director, Specialized Oncologic Care and Research of the Elderly (SOCARE), University of Chicago – Ongology/Geriatrics, Chicago, Illinois

E. FOY WHITE-CHU, MD
Director of Wound Healing Center, Department of Medicine, Hebrew Senior Life, Roslindale; Instructor in Medicine, Division of Gerontology, Beth Israel Deaconess Medical Center, Harvard Medical School, Boston, Massachusetts

HEIDI K. WHITE, MD, MHS, MEd
Associate Professor of Medicine, Division of Geriatrics, Department of Medicine, Duke University Medical Center, Durham, North Carolina

ERIC WIDERA, MD
Director, Hospice and Palliative Care, Geriatrics and Extended Care, Department of Veterans Affairs Medical Center; Assistant Professor of Medicine, Division of Geriatrics, University of California San Francisco, San Francisco, California

CHRISTIAN WOODS, MD
Division of Pulmonary/Critical Care and Infectious Diseases, Washington Hospital Center, Washington, DC

YANPING YE, MD
Division of Community Geriatrics, Department of Family and Community Medicine, University of Texas Health Science Center at San Antonio, San Antonio, Texas

Contents

Preface: Update in the Medical Management of the Long-Term Care Patient **xiii**

Miguel A. Paniagua

Pneumonia in the Long-Term Resident **117**

Namirah Jamshed, Christian Woods, Sanjay Desai, Shawkat Dhanani, and George Taler

Pneumonia in the long-term resident is common. It is associated with high morbidity and mortality. However, diagnosis and management of pneumonia in long-term care residents is challenging. This article provides an overview of the epidemiology, pathophysiology, diagnostic challenges, and management recommendations for pneumonia in this setting.

Managing the Patient with Dementia in Long-Term Care **135**

Jennifer Rhodes-Kropf, Huai Cheng, Elizabeth Herskovits Castillo, and Ana Tuya Fulton

The majority of residents in a nursing home have some degree of dementia. The prevalence is commonly from 70% to 80% of residents. This article covers the following topics on caring for patients with dementia in long-term care: (1) the efficacy of cholinesterase inhibitors and memantine, (2) the optimal environment for maintenance of function in moderate dementia, (3) the treatment of depression and agitation, and (4) the evaluation and management of eating problems.

Palliative Care for Patients With Dementia in Long-Term Care **153**

Ana Tuya Fulton, Jennifer Rhodes-Kropf, Amy M. Corcoran, Diane Chau, and Elizabeth Herskovits Castillo

Seventy percent of people in the United States who have dementia die in the nursing home. This article addresses the following topics on palliative care for patients with dementia in long-term care: (1) transitions of care, (2) infections, other comorbidities, and decisions on hospitalization, (3) prognostication, (4) the evidence for and against tube feeding, (5) discussing goals of care with families/surrogate decision makers, (6) types of palliative care programs, (7) pain assessment and management, and (8) optimizing function and quality of life for residents with advanced dementia.

Medications in Long-Term Care: When Less is More **171**

Thomas W. Meeks, John W. Culberson, and Monica S. Horton

Attention has been drawn to the potential risks of several medications in the long-term care setting. Most of these medications deemed as inappropriate affect the central nervous system and are indicated only for select populations with specific conditions. Many of these drugs are prescribed without clear indications and continued indefinitely without critical decision-making about the potentially salutary effects of discontinuing medications. This article describes the increasing awareness of potentially inappropriate prescribing in the long-term care setting and reviews the rationale for why various types of medications are deemed inappropriate, with a focus on agents that affect central nervous system functioning.

Evidence-Based Medicine (EBM): What Long-Term Care Providers Need to Know **193**

Huai Y. Cheng

Evidence-based medicine (EBM) has been widely used in medicine for 2 decades. Recently, EBM has become a central part of reforming nursing homes and quality improvement. It is very important for long-term care providers to practice EBM. This article briefly introduces the concept of EBM; addresses some potential benefits, harms, and challenges of practicing EBM in long-term care settings; and promotes EBM and its appropriate use among long-term care providers.

Update on Teaching in the Long-Term Care Setting **199**

Gwendolen T. Buhr and Miguel A. Paniagua

Since the advent of the teaching nursing home, made formal in the 1980s, long-term care has been used to teach geriatric medicine. Despite this, national surveys have indicated a need for more training during residency to facilitate the appropriate care for the frail long-term care patient population. In addition to medical knowledge, the long-term care site is appropriate for teaching the Accreditation Council of Graduate Medical Education's core competencies of "practice-based learning and improvement," "interpersonal and communication skills," and "systems-based practice." Program planners should emphasize opportunities for students to demonstrate their skill in one of these competencies.

Nausea and Other Nonpain Symptoms in Long-Term Care **213**

Matthew J. Gonzales and Eric Widera

There is a need to improve the quality of end-of-life care in nursing homes by improving the timely assessment and management of various sources of suffering. Much of the research/discussion in this area has focused on the assessment and treatment of pain. This article reviews the frequency and management of nonpain symptoms in the long-term care setting, particularly focusing on patients at the end of life. Although the long-term care setting presents challenges to effective management, an approach for addressing these challenges is discussed and applied to 3 commonly encountered nonpain symptoms.

Urinary Tract Infections in Long-Term Care Residents **229**

Gwendolen T. Buhr, Liza Genao, and Heidi K. White

Urinary tract infection (UTI) is common in long-term care (LTC) residents; however, most infections are asymptomatic and do not require treatment. Differentiating asymptomatic from symptomatic UTI is challenging, because LTC residents typically have chronic genitourinary complaints, multiple comorbid illnesses, and communication barriers. Although consensus guidelines have been proposed to improve the accuracy of identifying symptomatic UTIs and minimize treatment of asymptomatic UTIs, diagnostic accuracy is not yet optimized. Strategies for prevention of UTI are unsatisfactory and require further study; nevertheless, there is some evidence for the efficacy of cranberry products and vaginal estrogen to prevent recurrent UTI in women.

Pressure Ulcers in Long-Term Care **241**

E. Foy White-Chu, Petra Flock, Bryan Struck, and Louise Aronson

Pressure ulcers are common, costly, and debilitating chronic wounds, which occur preferentially in people with advanced age, physical or cognitive impairments, and multiple comorbidities. Residents with pressure ulcers have decreased quality of life and increased morbidity and mortality, and facilities with high rates of pressure ulcers have higher costs and risks of litigation. Health professionals who practice in this setting should be well versed in pressure ulcer management. This article reviews the significance, risk factors, pathophysiology, prevention, diagnosis, and management of pressure ulcers in long-term care.

Transitional Care of the Long-Term Care Patient **259**

S. Liliana Oakes, Suzanne M. Gillespie, Yanping Ye, Margaret Finley, Mathew Russell, Neela K. Patel, and David Espino

This article reviews the literature on transitional care to and from the LTC environment, highlighting strategies to improve the quality of care transitions. Several factors are vital in the improvement of systems of care dealing with transitions. Key factors include communication with and among health care providers, effective medication reconciliation, advanced discharge planning, and timely use of palliative care.

Doing Dementia Better: Anthropological Insights **273**

Elizabeth Herskovits Castillo

Dementia, or neurodegenerative disease, is a disease category, and yet it is widely described in popular and professional media as a horror story. Patients with dementia and their families frequently report that they are less than pleased with their clinical encounters. This article reveals the deleterious impact that cultural assumptions about dementia have on the care provided, and, through an exploration of anthropological theories of personhood, suggests strategies for seeking improved quality of life through personhood-centered care.

Long-Term Care of the Aging Population with Intellectual and Developmental Disabilities **291**

Nae-Hwa Kim, Georges El Hoyek, and Diane Chau

The aging population with intellectual and developmental disabilities (I/DD) deserves appropriate health care and social support. This population poses unique medical and social challenges to the multidisciplinary team that provides care. In the past, long-term care (LTC) facilities played an essential role in the livelihood of this population. The likelihood that the geriatric LTC system must prepare for adequately caring for this population is high. This article conveys the need to prepare for the inclusion of the growing aging population with I/DD into long-term care with the general elderly population in the near future.

Cancer in Long-Term Care **301**

Beatriz Korc-Grodzicki, James A. Wallace, Miriam B. Rodin, and Rachelle E. Bernacki

This article describes the range of cancer patients in longterm care and provides a framework for clinical decision making. The benefits and burdens of providing standard therapy to a vulnerable population are discussed. To give more specific guidelines for advocates of treatment, skeptics, and others, the authors present best estimates of the current burden of cancer in the long-term care population and current screening guidelines that apply to the elderly under long-term care. Experience-based suggestions are offered for oncologists and clinicians involved in long-term care to help them respond to patient and family concerns about limitations of cancer care.

Index **329**

FORTHCOMING ISSUE

August 2011

Sarcopenia

Yves Rolland, MD, PhD, *Guest Editor*

RECENT ISSUES

February 2011

Frailty

Jeremy D. Walston, MD, *Guest Editor*

November 2010

Falls and Their Prevention

Laurence Z. Rubenstein, MD, MPH, and David A. Ganz, MD, PhD, *Guest Editors*

August 2010

Osteoarthritis

David J. Hunter, MBBS, PhD, *Guest Editor*

Preface
Update in the Medical Management of the Long-Term Care Patient

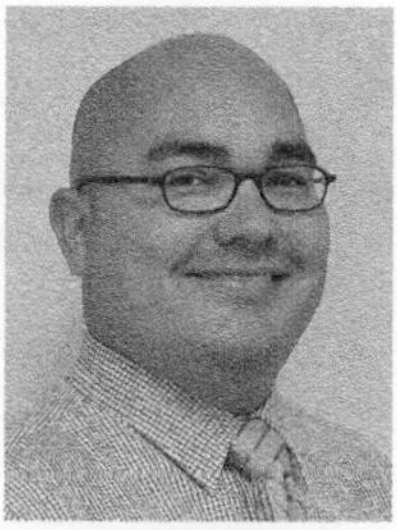

Miguel A. Paniagua, MD
Guest Editor

The word "doctor" has its origins in the Latin *doctoris*, which means *teacher*. Within the specialty of Geriatric Medicine, we are fortunate to have a means to specifically foster and support the careers of teachers who also care for one of our most vulnerable populations. In this issue of *Clinics in Geriatric Medicine*, we have deliberately sought out those teachers whose passions lie in the care of the frailest elders, and who have a shared passion to teach the next generation of health care professionals to do the same. Many of the authors in this issue of *Clinics in Geriatric Medicine* are, or have been in the past, recipients of Geriatric Academic Career Awards (GACA), which are administered by the US Department of Health and Human Services, Health Resources, and Services Administration's Bureau of Health Professions. This unique grant aims to increase the number of junior faculty at accredited schools of allopathic and osteopathic medicine and to promote the development of their careers as academic geriatricians who emphasize training in clinical geriatrics including the training of interdisciplinary teams of health professionals. The teachers in this issue have provided state-of-the-art reviews of a variety of timely issues that arise in the

Clin Geriatr Med 27 (2011) xiii–xiv
doi:10.1016/j.cger.2011.03.002 geriatric.theclinics.com

care of frail elders and which are pertinent for health care providers and practitioners across the spectrum of long-term care settings.

Miguel A. Paniagua, MD
Division of Gerontology and Geriatric
Department of Internal Medicine
Saint Louis University School of Medicine
Internal Medicine Residency Program
Fourteenth Floor, Desloge Tower
1402 South Grand Boulevard
St Louis, MO 63104, USA

E-mail address:
mpaniag1@slu.edu

Pneumonia in the Long-Term Resident

Namirah Jamshed, MD[a,b,*], Christian Woods, MD[c], Sanjay Desai, MD[d], Shawkat Dhanani, MD, MPH[e], George Taler, MD[a,f]

KEYWORDS

• Pneumonia • Nursing home • Long-term care • Aspiration

The population in the United States is aging. Successful management of chronic diseases has translated into increased life expectancy. The older population will more than double between 2002 and 2030, from 35.6 million to 71.5 million, and almost 1 in 5 people will be 65 years or older.[1] Currently, in the United States there are about 1.5 million residents of nursing homes (NHs).[2]

The number of infections occurring annually in long-term care facilities (LTCFs) or NHs is comparable with those occurring in hospitals. There is a higher incidence of pneumonia in LTCFs than in the community. Annual incidence in LTCFs ranges from 99 to 912 per 1000 persons in contrast with 12 per 1000 persons in the community.[3] Pneumonia is the second most common infection among older persons residing in LTCFs and is one of the most common reasons for transfer to hospital.[4,5] In addition, it is also the leading infectious cause of mortality in this setting.[3,6–11] Bacteremia, empyema, and meningitis are more likely to develop in patients with pneumonia.[12] With the growing elderly population, it is expected that about 40% of adults will reside in an LTCF in later life which would result in a higher prevalence of pneumonia and related complications.[13]

This article was support by funding from HRSA GACA-07.

[a] Georgetown University School of Medicine, Washington, DC, USA
[b] Washington Hospital Center, 110 Irving Street NW, East Building #3114, Washington, DC 20010, USA
[c] Division of Pulmonary/Critical Care and Infectious Diseases, Washington Hospital Center, Washington, DC, USA
[d] Division of Pulmonary/Critical Care, Washington Hospital Center, Washington, DC, USA
[e] Geriatrics VA Greater LA Healthcare System, GRECC, Los Angeles, CA, USA
[f] Division of Geriatrics, Washington Hospital Center, Washington, DC, USA
* Corresponding author. Washington Hospital Center, 110 Irving Street NW, East Building #3114, Washington, DC 20010.
E-mail address: namirah.jamshed@medstar.net

Clin Geriatr Med 27 (2011) 117–133
doi:10.1016/j.cger.2011.01.008 geriatric.theclinics.com
0749-0690/11/$ – see front matter

EPIDEMIOLOGY OF PNEUMONIA IN THE LTCF SETTING

Approximately 28% of Medicare beneficiaries hospitalized for pneumonia come from NHs.[14] In the United States, the 1-year incidence is estimated to range from 8% to 21%.[8,15,16]

Pneumonia causes significant morbidity and mortality in elderly people.[17–19] A recent prospective study analyzed 150 cases of pneumonia in a Spanish LTCF in a 10-year period and found the in-hospital and 30-day mortalities to be 8.7% and 20%, respectively.[20] A case-control study by Vergis and colleagues[21] found the mortality from pneumonia to be 23% at 14 days in residents of a Veterans Affairs LTCF. Mortality at 1 year was 75% compared with 40% for controls. Pneumonia was independently associated with mortality. Muder and colleagues[17] conducted a prospective study of 108 patients with pneumonia at another Veterans Affairs LTCF. The 14-day mortality in their sample was 19%. Mortality at 1 and 2 year was 59% and 75% respectively. Eighty-one patients were followed 30 days after the first episode of pneumonia. Forty-three percent of these subjects suffered a second episode of pneumonia, and 16% had had more than 1 subsequent episode. Patients in the NH units had a higher risk of a second episode. Thirty-seven percent of patients required hospitalization for diagnoses other than pneumonia during the year following the initial episode.[17] In addition, they found that an activities-of-daily-living (ADL) score of 16 or more carried a higher mortality than a score of 11 to 15. Functional status was a major factor in detrimental survival following an episode of pneumonia.[17]

Pneumonia is the leading cause of hospitalization for residents of LTCFs. Kruse and colleagues[22] prospectively compared mortality and cost for initial episodes of pneumonia treated in the NH versus the hospital. They identified 1406 episodes of lower respiratory tract infections in 36 NHs in central Missouri and St Louis between August 1995 and September 1998, of which 1033 episodes were analyzed for cost. The patients in the study were not randomized. The mean daily cost for initial NH treatment was $138 versus $419 for the hospital treatment. The total episode cost was $3789 for residents treated in the NH and $10,408 for those hospitalized. Higher hospital costs per episode have been reported previously. In addition, there was no mortality benefit for residents of LTCFs hospitalized for pneumonia[23]

Cause

Understanding the cause of pneumonia in LTCFs is important for understanding management guidelines. Pneumonia in the LTCF is usually of bacterial origin and is usually polymicrobial. In immunocompetent patients, it is rarely caused by viral or fungal pathogens.[24] Previous studies have identified the major pathogens responsible for pneumonia in the NH population to be *Streptococcus pneumoniae*, *Haemophilus influenzae*, *Moraxella catarrhalis*, and an increased occurrence of gram-negative organisms.[9,25–27] More recently, 2 studies from Spain found *S pneumoniae* to be the most common cause of pneumonia in the LTCF setting.[20,28] However, in the hospitalize patient, *Staphylococcus aureus* is emerging as the major pathogen.[29–31] El Solh and colleagues[32] studied the cause of pneumonia in the intensive care unit (ICU) setting for elderly patients aged 75 years and older from LTCFs. In their study, causative organisms were *S aureus* (29%), enteric gram-negative rods (15%), *S pneumoniae* (9%), and *Pseudomonas* species (4%). Methicillin-resistant *S aureus* (MRSA) was responsible for 6% of the pneumonia and all cases were identified in the patients from the NH setting. Based on accumulating data and the high incidence of infection caused by *S aureus*, it has emerged as the dominant organism in patients who are hospitalized with health-care-acquired pneumonia (HCAP). Patients residing in LTCFs are included in the category of HCAP as per the most recent American Thoracic Society (ATS) guidelines.[24] However, most data showing *S aureus* as the leading pathogen in HCAP is from hospitalized patients and the ICU setting.

Risk of Multidrug-resistant Infections in the NH Setting

Residents of LTCFs are at high risk of infection from multidrug-resistant (MDR) organisms.[25] In hospitalized patients, the risk of acquiring MDR organisms has been associated with length of stay, functional status, presence of wounds or pressure ulcers, advanced age, comorbid illness, and prior exposure to antibiotics.[33–41] Many of these risk factors are also present in residents of LTCFs. However, LTCFs may differ in patient populations and the number and nature of risk factors, which would influence the proportion of MDR organisms at each setting.

El Solh and colleagues[42] found drug-resistant organism in 19% of 183 NH residents admitted to the ICU for severe pneumonia. Patients with drug-resistant pathogens (DRP) had more comorbidities and a statistically significant worse functional status. Previous antibiotic exposure was also more common in this group, although not statistically significant. *S aureus* was identified as the most common pathogen (31%), followed by gram-negative bacilli (28%) and *S pneumoniae* (25%). Based on their data, they were able to develop a classification tree to predict DRP. The model had a sensitivity of 100% and a specificity of 53.5%. Prior antibiotic use and poor functional status defined by ADL score of more than or equal to 12.5 were the factors that had the most effect on risk. Patients with both factors had a 90% probability of infection with a DRP.

The prevalence of MRSA in LTCFs ranges from 10% to 30%. Colonization with MRSA is more common in NH, with up to 10% to 25% of all residents of NHs fostering the pathogen.[12] However, clinical infection is infrequent.[12] The risk of infection from *S aureus*, including MRSA, increases with impairments in ADL in patients in LTCFs.[32,41] Evidence shows that resident-to-resident contact plays little role in the transmission of MRSA in LTCFs, and that most infection is transmitted from health care workers to patients.[43] The best way to prevent spread of infection is for health care workers to engage in proper hand hygiene with antibacterial soap, which has been associated with a decreased risk of MRSA acquisition.[44]

Infection Control Issues in NH Care

Medicare-certified and Medicaid-certified LTCFs are required to have an infection control program, of which screening and prevention strategies are an integral part.[45] These programs should ensure that residents and staff of LTCFs receive appropriate immunizations. Currently, there is no evidence to support surveillance cultures or patient isolation in LTCFs, likely because of the low rates of patient-to-patient transmission. However, it is recommended to isolate patients with MRSA wound infections, or those with MRSA device-related infections that cannot be contained.[43]

Physiology of the Aging Respiratory System

There are age-related and exposure-related changes in the respiratory system, including that from tobacco use.[46] Three main structural changes occur in the aging lung. First, lung parenchyma changes, with subsequent loss of elastic recoil. Second, there is a reduction in chest wall compliance, resulting in stiffer lungs. Third, the respiratory muscles undergo aging. These changes result in a loss of alveolar surface area as alveoli and alveolar ducts enlarge, without much effect on the bronchi. This phenomenon has been called senile emphysema. As long as the older person is healthy, these changes are usually of no consequence. However, an acute infection would put extra burden on the aging respiratory system. In addition, chronic illnesses such as chronic obstructive pulmonary disease (COPD), congestive heart failure, and malnutrition are associated with harmful changes in respiratory muscle, structure, and function.[47–49] These age-related changes can also be exacerbated by deconditioning and medications such as corticosteroids.

Pathophysiology of Pneumonia in NH

Many factors play a role in risk of pneumonia in the elderly population. In addition to the structural changes that occur in an aging lung, there is an alteration in the immune system. Elderly people have an upper respiratory tract that is colonized with bacteria.[50] Colonization of the stomach is also more common in old age and can be exacerbated by antacids or H_2 blockers.[51] Older age, male sex, swallowing difficulties, and the inability to take oral medications have been found to be significant risk factors for pneumonia.[27] Older people with cerebrovascular accidents or other neurologic conditions, including those with cognitive impairment, have a higher risk of aspiration. If tracheal intubation or placement of a nasogastric tube is required for management of the patient's illness, the risk of aspiration would increase. Malnutrition and presence of chronic illness like diabetes and renal disease increase susceptibility to pneumonia as well. Because there is an age-related decline in immune function, the response of the immune system to preventive vaccination is reduced, which increases the patient's susceptibility to respiratory infections and pneumonia. Other studies indicate poor functional status, COPD, and tracheostomy as probable risk factors.[52–56] Potentially modifiable risk factors may include large-volume aspiration and administration of sedating medications.[21] One study found that gastroesophageal reflux disease caused more than one-third of aspiration pneumonia mortality.[57] Residents of LTCFs frequently have multiple medical comorbid diseases including diabetes, COPD, renal disease, malignancy, and malnutrition. Age-related changes, along with other factors, increase the risk of respiratory infections in older people in this setting.

Diagnostic Challenges in the NH

The diagnosis of pneumonia poses a significant challenge to the nursing staff and the clinicians in the LTCF environment. Acute changes in condition are most often found by the nursing staff. If the staff is not adequately trained in recognizing these changes, and no care plans are in place, pneumonia in patients with subtle and atypical signs or symptoms will likely be missed. The bedside assessment by the nursing staff is a critical component of diagnosing and managing infections in the LTCF because clinicians are infrequently present. Without written protocols to guide the staff in these diagnoses, assessments can be variable. Ideally, there would be a clear diagnosis to guide treatment to avoid adverse effects of treatment. However, this may not be possible in an LTCF because of lack of resources of laboratory and radiology access and difficulty of acquiring adequate sputum for Gram stain and culture in residents of LTCFs.

Treatment of pneumonia in an LTCF is expensive and provides poor reimbursement to the facility. There may be a financial incentive to transfer patients to the hospital for treatment.[58] A study by Konetzka and colleagues[58] found that both the type of facility (nonprofit vs for profit) and payer source influenced the rate of hospitalization.

Other challenges making diagnosis and treatment of pneumonia in LTCFs difficult include the inability to provide more frequent assessments in patients with pneumonia, limited laboratory access, lack of provision of potential intravenous hydration, and the relative paucity of licensed nurses available per shift.

Clinical Evaluation of the Patient in an LTCF

Elderly patients with pneumonia in LTCFs usually present with atypical signs and symptoms. About 25% of older patients may not exhibit fever in the presence of pneumonia and other infectious processes.[59] Marrie and colleagues[59] found that patients age 65 years and older are less likely to complain of fever, chills, myalgia, and pleuritic chest pain compared with their younger counterparts. Despite this, Mehr and colleagues[60] found that 92% of patients with pneumonia have at least 1 identifiable respiratory manifestation such as a cough, tachypnea, crackles, and absence of wheezing on auscultation.

Laboratory Evaluation

Blood cultures are rarely positive in patients with pneumonia and are not indicated unless patients are hospitalized or in ICUs. Blood culture yield is low when patients are treated in the LTCF setting. Many patients have nonproductive cough or are too weak to give an adequate sputum sample. Because of these barriers to the collection of sputum for Gram stain and culture, it is not recommended for initial evaluation. Suctioning to get a specimen can cause discomfort to the patient and does not have much overall benefit.[61] During the appropriate season, rapid antigen testing can help in the diagnosis of influenza and *respiratory syncytial virus* lower respiratory infections. In most NH patients with pneumonia, the causal agent is not identified.[62]

Chest radiograph is considered the gold standard for diagnosis of pneumonia in the LTCF setting. The advantages of having a chest radiograph is that it can define the presence of a new infiltrate, the severity of the disease, and the presence of complications.[63] However, the ability to perform chest radiographs across LTCFs is variable.[64] Many facilities have no access to radiology, and the diagnosis is made clinically. Therefore, it is important to have some guidance in the clinical diagnosis of pneumonia in facilities where such resources are not readily available.

Aspiration Pneumonia

The incidence of pneumonia as a result of aspiration is hard to determine. Aspiration is defined as the inhalation of oropharyngeal or gastric contents into the respiratory tract.[65] Tube feeding has been identified as a risk factor for aspiration.[66] Enteral feeding via gastrostomy or jejunostomy does not prevent aspiration of oral or gastric secretions.[65,67] Feeding tubes can reduce the lower esophageal sphincter pressure and increase risk of regurgitation of gastric contents into the esophagus and, potentially, the lungs. Caregivers and staff may neglect oral hygiene when nothing is being fed by mouth, which may increase risk of aspiration from the oropharyngeal cavity. Many older people are on medications that cause decreased salivary flow, such as diuretics, anticholinergics, anxiolytics, and antipsychotics. Reduction in salivary flow leads to a higher concentration of bacteria in the oropharynx.[68] Furthermore, the number of decayed teeth directly correlates with the incidence of aspiration pneumonia.[69,70] In addition, medications such as antipsychotics, benzodiazepines, anticholinergics, and histamine receptor blockers have been associated with an increased risk of aspiration.[17] Histamine receptor blockers are commonly prescribed in the hospitalized elderly for stress ulcer prevention. However, the patients are often continued on these unnecessarily when they get transferred back from the hospital to the LTCF.

Treatment

Advance care planning

Patients' desire for hospitalization and aggressive care should be assessed directly if possible. Chart review or prior discussions with the patient or their surrogate decision maker can help with this decision if documented or present. Patients who have clearly defined their directive for no hospitalization, or those who refuse, should be treated at the LTCF.[71] Patient autonomy is of utmost important for any residents of LTCFs. The goal of NH care is to provide the environment for such autonomy, to maximize residents' function, preserve dignity, and provide comfort. Goals of care should be a continuing discussion and reevaluated frequently. Patient preferences can be documented through advance directives, living wills, or even code status orders. It is important to identify a surrogate decision maker and to involve them in these discussions. The Physician Orders for Life-Sustaining Treatment (POLST) paradigm program was designed in the United States to ensure that the full range of patient treatment preferences is honored throughout the health care system. Evidence shows that patients with POLST are more likely to receive comfort care and less likely to be hospitalized.[72] POLST has also been found to be useful in hospice patients, but it has not been investigated in an LTCF setting.[72] The patient Self-determination Act requires that all residents of LTCFs be offered information on advance care planning.[73]

Location

In the elderly, hospitalization is associated with complications including deconditioning, pressure ulcer development, delirium, and nosocomial infections. Residents with mild to moderate symptoms of pneumonia (or with an advance care directive indicating a wish to not be hospitalized) can be treated in the LTCF setting. Zweig and colleagues[74] found that residents with pneumonia who had do-not-attempt-resuscitation orders were less likely to be hospitalized. Studies have not shown clear benefit in mortality from hospitalization if treatment can adequately be given in the LTCF.[16,75] The decision to treat in the LTCF may be affected by advance care planning, time of decompensation (ie, night time or weekends when physicians are less available), and severity of symptoms. Attempts have been made to identify pathways to help in making such decisions. Loeb and colleagues[76] conducted a clinical trial developing such a pathway. However, this pathway needs to be studied in sicker patients before it can be widely applied. The overall goal for residents of LTCFs should be to identify those with pneumonia early, to treat them in the LTCF more frequently, and to hospitalize those who desire transfer or who have more severe symptoms. However, there is not clear evidence as to when a patient with pneumonia in an LTCF should be transferred to an acute care hospital for management. It is estimated that the rate of hospitalization for pneumonia from LTCFs is 22% to 37%. In a recent study of treatment of pneumonia in LTCFs with oral antibiotics versus routine transfer to a hospital, patients were only treated at the LTCF if they had stable vital signs and could take oral antibiotics. Using these criteria, only 10% of patients were hospitalized when treated at the LTCF compared with 22% directly transferred to the hospital. In addition, there were fewer total hospital days and cost savings of at least $1000 per patient.[77] A retrospective analysis of acute cases of pneumonia in an NH setting by Fried and colleagues[78] studied survival rates in patients treated in LTCFs versus hospitals. The survival rates were comparable in patients treated either at the NH or in a hospital. In addition, patients treated in the NH had better preservation of function and less mortality in the 2 months following the episode compared with the hospital group. Advance care planning and challenges or limitations of the LTCF setting may play a role in this decision. Specialized NH is less likely to transfer patients to the hospital for management of pneumonia.[77] The pneumonia prediction rule frequently used for identifying low risk patients with community-acquired pneumonia is not valuable in the NH setting because it would place all patients in the highest risk group.[79] **Fig. 1** shows an algorithm for management of pneumonia in the LTCF setting.

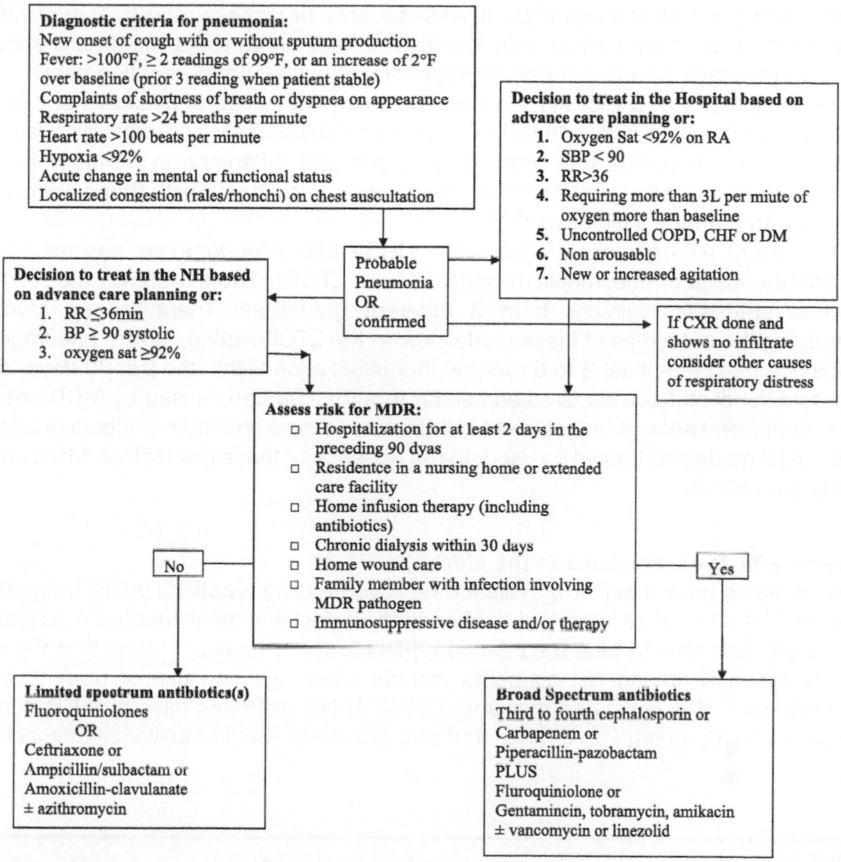
Diagnostic criteria for pneumonia:
New onset of cough with or without sputum production
Fever: >100°F, ≥ 2 readings of 99°F, or an increase of 2°F over baseline (prior 3 reading when patient stable)
Complaints of shortness of breath or dyspnea on appearance
Respiratory rate >24 breaths per minute
Heart rate >100 beats per minute
Hypoxia <92%
Acute change in mental or functional status
Localized congestion (rales/rhonchi) on chest auscultation
Decision to treat in the Hospital based on advance care planning or:
1. Oxygen Sat <92% on RA
2. SBP < 90
3. RR>36
4. Requiring more than 3L per miute of oxygen more than baseline
5. Uncontrolled COPD, CHF or DM
6. Non arousable
7. New or increased agitation
Probable Pneumonia OR confirmed
Decision to treat in the NH based on advance care planning or:
1. RR ≤36min
2. BP ≥ 90 systolic
3. oxygen sat ≥92%
If CXR done and shows no infiltrate consider other causes of respiratory distress
Assess risk for MDR:
Hospitalization for at least 2 days in the preceding 90 dyas
Residentce in a nursing home or extended care facility
Home infusion therapy (including antibiotics)
Chronic dialysis within 30 days
Home wound care
Family member with infection involving MDR pathogen
Immunosuppressive disease and/or therapy
No
Yes
Limited spectrum antibiotics(s)
Fluoroquiniolones
OR
Ceftriaxone or
Ampicillin/sulbactam or
Amoxicillin-clavulanate
± azithromycin
Broad Spectrum antibiotics
Third to fourth cephalosporin or
Carbapenem or
Piperacillin-pazobactam
PLUS
Fluroquinilone or
Gentamincin, tobramycin, amikacin
± vancomycin or linezolid

Fig. 1. Algorithm for management of pneumonia in LTCFs. (*Data from* Refs.[24,61,71,108])

Empiric antibiotic selection

Randomized control trials in the NH setting are limited. The 2005 ATS/*Infectious Diseases Society of America* (IDSA) guidelines for the treatment of pneumonia do not specifically address treatment of pneumonia in the LTCF setting. It places pneumonia in residents of LTCFs in the HCAP category. In 2000, members of the Society of Healthcare Epidemiology of America (SHEA) had formulated a minimum criteria for the initial treatment of clinically stable residents of LTCFs with signs of bacterial infection.[80] In the following year, the Hutt Kramer group published another guideline specifically for pneumonia.[71] More recent literature advocates broad-spectrum antibiotic treatment of patients in LTCFs with pneumonia. Three major guidelines provide specific antibiotic recommendations for patients with pneumonia who reside in LTCFs.[24,81,82]

Treatment guidelines for NH versus inpatient hospitals

Guidelines addressing the treatment of pneumonia in residents of LTCFs being treated in the facility have been formulated by the Canadian Infectious Diseases Society and IDSA.[82,83] These guidelines are based on the assumption that *S pneumoniae*, gram-negative enteric bacilli, and *H influenzae* are the dominant organisms. Determination of risk for MDR organisms should be based on the MDR prevalence at each facility, and the patient's comorbid illness, severity of disease, and history of MDR organisms. In a stable patient with low risk of MDR organisms, treatment should include antibiotics covering *S pneumoniae*, *H influenzae*, gram-negative bacilli, and *S aureus*. Acceptable choices include monotherapy with a fluoroquinolone, or a macrolide in combination with ceftriaxone, ampicillin/sulbactam, or amoxicillin/clavulanate. Evidence suggests that there is no significant difference in mortality in NH residents who are initially treated with an oral agent compared with those who were treated with parental antibiotics.[14,83]

The current ATS guidelines[24] consider MRSA and *Pseudomonas* species to be important causes of pneumonia in patients from LTCFs. **Table 1** shows the recommended antibiotic regimens from 3 different guidelines. There are no studies comparing the outcomes of these guidelines. In the LTCF setting, severe pneumonia, antibiotics use in the past 3 to 6 months, hospitalization within the last 90 days, and poor functional status were cited as risk factors for infection caused by MDR organisms. In the presence of any of these risk factors, broad-spectrum antibiotics based on the ATS guidelines should be used. In the absence of these risk factors, MDR pathogens are unlikely.

Adverse affects of antibiotics in the elderly

Older patients have a higher prevalence of adverse drug reactions (ADR) than other patients.[84] It is therefore important to choose the safest and most effective medication for the shortest time to treat the infection. Field and colleagues[85] found that the risk factors for ADR among NH residents include older age and use of more than 8 medications.[86] It is estimated that about 67% of NH residents have an ADR during a stay of 6 to 12 months.[87] Nursing staff and providers should familiarize themselves

Table 1
Antimicrobial treatment of pneumonia diagnosed in residents of LTCFs

Site of Therapy	IDSA	Canadian Infectious Disease Society	ATS
NH	Oral fluoroquinolone or amoxicillin/clavulanic acid plus a macrolide	Oral fluoroquinolone or amoxicillin/clavulanic acid plus a macrolide Second-generation oral cephalosporin plus a macrolide	None
Hospital	Parenteral third-generation cephalosporin or ampicillin sulbactam plus macrolide Parenteral fluoroquinolone alone	Parenteral fluoroquinolone alone Parenteral third-generation or fourth-generation cephalosporin plus macrolide	Antipseudomonal cephalosporin or antipseudomonal carbapenem or antipseudomonal penicillin plus antipseudomonal fluoroquinolone or aminoglycoside plus anti–methicillin-resistant *Staphylococcus* agents

Data from El-Solh AA. Nursing home-acquired pneumonia. Semin Respir Crit Care Med 2009;30:17.

with the common drug and drug-drug interactions. Because most antibiotics interact with warfarin, patients on warfarin should have their international normalized ratio checked more frequently with appropriate dosage reductions while on antibiotic therapy.

Timing and Treatment Duration

There are conflicting data regarding survival benefit in relation to timing of antibiotics administration.[88–90] In patients admitted to the ICU, evidence indicates that, if antibiotics are initiated within 8 hours of diagnosis, survival is improved.[91] There are no specific recommendations for timings in patients treated in the NH setting. However, the 2007 IDSA/ATS guidelines recommend that, for community-acquired pneumonia, initiation of antibiotic therapy should take place in the emergency department. The total duration of treatment recommended is 7 to 8 days for appropriately treated pneumonia that has clinically improved and is not caused by non–lactose-fermenting gram-negative bacteria such as *Pseudomonas*.[63] Currently, similar recommendations apply for residents of LTCFs treated for pneumonia in either hospital or NH settings.

Prognosis: implications for mortality

Poor functional status is not only a major predictor of worse outcomes for pneumonia in the NH,[17] but also a major consequence of the pneumonia itself. A large Swiss cohort study found that 22% of residents with 1 or more infections experienced functional decline, compared with 16% of residents without infections.[92] Researchers have attempted to develop tools to predict mortality in patients in LTCFs. The model developed by Mehr and colleagues[93] depends on blood work that is not routinely available in all NHs. Mylotte and colleagues[94] developed another prognostic model with more routinely available data in NHs, but the tool has not been validated. However, patients with severe functional impairment at baseline do worse than those with moderate impairment.[92]

Prevention

Aspiration precautions

Speech therapy does not prevent aspirations. Consequences of aspiration depend on (1) what is being aspirated, (2) how long a period of aspiration exists, (3) how much is aspirated at one time, and (4) the patient's immune status.[95] In 189 elders of an LTCF, followed for 4 years, Longmore and colleagues[96] found that the risks for developing pneumonia were dependent on feeding, oral care, number of decayed teeth, tube feeding, multiple medical diagnoses, number of medications, and smoking. Dysphagia was an important risk factor, but only in the presence of other risk factors. In addition, dependence on others for feeding was also an important risk factor. A great emphasis has been placed on the importance of aspiration of food and fluids. The reimbursement for aspiration pneumonia is higher than bacterial pneumonia, which has caused an increase in health care costs as Medicare diagnosis for this entity has increased in recent years, despite it being a difficult diagnosis to make.[97] Although prevention of aspiration is not the most hazardous variable that needs to be controlled, much significance is given to its management.[95]

Oral Hygiene

Residents of LTCFs have higher oral colonization by respiratory pathogens compared with nonresidents.[96] A recent study by El Solh and colleagues[98] linked pneumonia to dental plaque colonization with respiratory pathogens. Neglected oral health can have undesired consequences. However, few dentists see patients in LTCFs. Current data suggest that oral hygiene is important in patients residing in LTCFs, not only to reduce gingival pathogens but also because proper tooth brushing and professional care by a dental hygienist or a dentist can lead to a reduction in pneumonia rates.[69,99] Topical antiseptic agents such as chlorhexidine gluconate and 10% povidone-iodine have been shown to decrease the number of gingival pathogens.[99]

Vaccines

Immunization with influenza vaccine in institutionalized patients is associated with 56% efficacy in preventing respiratory illness, 53% efficacy in preventing pneumonia, 50% efficacy in preventing hospitalization, and 68% efficacy in preventing death.[100] Although a more recent analysis of persons aged 85 years and older shows that mortality after the early 1980s remained unchanged despite coverage, observational studies show benefit.[101–104] Vaccination of health care workers has also shown benefit in preventing influenza. In one study, vaccination of health care workers was associated with a reduction in total LTCF patient mortality from 17% to 10%.[105] A study by Carman and colleagues[101] showed mortality benefit for elderly people when their health care workers had been vaccinated for influenza.

Four systematic reviews studied the benefit of pneumococcal vaccine in elderly people.[102–104,106] Only 1 study specifically addressed residents of LTCFs. Currently, based on efficacy in observational studies, the United States and Canadian advisory committees strongly recommend its use, because of its cost-effectiveness and favorable safety profile.

A recent study conducted in LTCFs in 14 states showed that the vaccination rates for influenza and pneumococcus were 59% and 35% respectively.[107] Further analysis showed that presence of cognitive deficits and psychiatric illness was associated with receipt of immunizations. Standing orders also increase immunization coverage. A survey conducted in Washington state, showed that the odds of a resident receiving a pneumococcal vaccine in an NH having standing orders or other written guidelines was about 2.5 times greater than for residents in NH facilities without any guidelines.[108]

Palliative and end-of-life care for patients with pneumonia in the NH

Pneumonia is a common consequence of chronic conditions that lead to terminal illness. These conditions include dementia, malignancies, neurodegenerative disorders, respiratory conditions, and rheumatologic conditions.[109–112] Management of pneumonia in patients in NHs with progressive terminal illnesses (such as dementia) and an advance care directive indicating non-aggressive care should follow the principles of palliative medicine. For the dying patient, focus should be on managing symptoms such as dyspnea, respiratory congestion, secretions, agitation, delirium, and pain. Family or surrogate decision maker concerns should be addressed in the context of any prior advance care documentations. It is important to recognize pneumonia at the end of life, when antibiotics may have minimal affect on life expectancy or quality of life. Antibiotics could be used as palliative agents to relieve symptoms, but their use at the end is questionable. Recently, Givens and colleagues[113] studied survival and comfort after treatment of pneumonia in advance dementia. They prospectively analyzed data from 323 residents of NHs in a period of 6 years. Each resident was followed for 18 months or until death. They found that all antimicrobial treatments, regardless of route, improved survival compared with no treatment. However, residents who did receive antibiotics had worse comfort scores than those who were untreated. When discussing management of pneumonia as an end-of-life event, it is important to discuss with the family the possible harms of aggressive intervention.

SUMMARY

Pneumonia is common in residents of LTCFs. Rates of pneumonia acquired in NHs are comparable with rates of hospital-acquired pneumonia. In addition, pneumonia is a leading cause of mortality and morbidity in LTCFs. *S aureus* is emerging as the leading pathogen in residents who have severe pneumonia. In addition, consideration of the risk factors for MDR pathogens, and those who are hospitalized, especially in the ICU, should be considered. Aspiration pneumonia is a common cause, and better oral care and hygiene has emerged as a possible preventive care measure for residents of NHs. Management of pneumonia should be based on severity of symptoms, patient or surrogate decision maker preferences, and on MDR pathogen risk in the facility. Patients with less-severe symptoms and the desire to forgo hospitalization can be treated at the LTCF. It is also important to recognize pneumonia as a terminal event in many residents of NHs. As such, the management goals should be individualized based on advance directives, and should include discussing the risks and benefits of cure-oriented management.

REFERENCES

1. Centers for Disease Control and Prevention (CDC). Trends in aging-United States and worldwide. MMWR Morb Mortal Wkly Rep 2003;52(6):101–4, 106.
2. Bercovitz A, Decker FH, Jones A, et al. End-of-life care in nursing homes: 2004 National Nursing Home Survey. Natl Health Stat Report 2008;9:1–23.
3. Muder RR. Pneumonia in residents of long-term care facilities: epidemiology, etiology, management, and prevention. Am J Med 1998;105(4):319–30.
4. Reza Shariatzadeh M, Huang JQ, Marrie TJ. Differences in the features of aspiration pneumonia according to site of acquisition: community or continuing care facility. J Am Geriatr Soc 2006;54(2):296–302.
5. Kerr HD, Byrd JC. Nursing home patients transferred by ambulance to a VA emergency department. J Am Geriatr Soc 1991;39(2):132–6.
6. Gross JS, Neufeld RR, Libow LS, et al. Autopsy study of the elderly institutionalized patient. Review of 234 autopsies. Arch Intern Med 1988;148(1):173–6.
7. Gloth FM 3rd, Burton JR. Autopsies and death certificates in the chronic care setting. J Am Geriatr Soc 1990;38(2):151–5.
8. Sund-Levander M, Ortqvist A, Grodzinsky E, et al. Morbidity, mortality and clinical presentation of nursing home-acquired pneumonia in a Swedish population. Scand J Infect Dis 2003;35(5):306–10.
9. Mylotte JM. Nursing home-acquired pneumonia. Clin Infect Dis 2002;35(10): 1205–11.
10. Furman CD, Rayner AV, Tobin EP. Pneumonia in older residents of long-term care facilities. Am Fam Physician 2004;70(8):1495–500.
11. Drinka PJ, Crnich CJ. Pneumonia in the nursing home. J Am Med Dir Assoc 2005;6(5):342–50.
12. Yoshikawa TT, Norman DC. Approach to fever and infection in the nursing home. J Am Geriatr Soc 1996;44(1):74–82.
13. Richards C. Infections in residents of long-term care facilities: an agenda for research. Report of an expert panel. J Am Geriatr Soc 2002;50(3):570–6.
14. Naughton BJ, Mylotte JM. Treatment guideline for nursing home-acquired pneumonia based on community practice. J Am Geriatr Soc 2000;48(1):82–8.

15. Drinka PJ, Gauerke C, Voeks S, et al. Pneumonia in a nursing home. J Gen Intern Med 1994;9(11):650–2.
16. Thompson RS, Hall NK, Szpiech M. Hospitalization and mortality rates for nursing home-acquired pneumonia. J Fam Pract 1999;48(4):291–3.
17. Muder RR, Brennen C, Swenson DL, et al. Pneumonia in a long-term care facility. A prospective study of outcome. Arch Intern Med 1996;156(20):2365–70.
18. Jackson MM, Fierer J, Barrett-Connor E, et al. Intensive surveillance for infections in a three-year study of nursing home patients. Am J Epidemiol 1992; 135(6):685–96.
19. Farber BF, Brennen C, Puntereri AJ, et al. A prospective study of nosocomial infections in a chronic care facility. J Am Geriatr Soc 1984;32(7):499–502.
20. Polverino E, Dambrava P, Cilloniz C, et al. Nursing home-acquired pneumonia: a 10 year single-centre experience. Thorax 2010;65(4):354–9.
21. Vergis EN, Brennen C, Wagener M, et al. Pneumonia in long-term care: a prospective case-control study of risk factors and impact on survival. Arch Intern Med 2001;161(19):2378–81.
22. Kruse RL, Mehr DR, Boles KE, et al. Does hospitalization impact survival after lower respiratory infection in nursing home residents? Med Care 2004;42(9): 860–70.
23. Dempsey CL. Nursing home-acquired pneumonia: outcomes from a clinical process improvement program. Pharmacotherapy 1995;15(1 Pt 2):33S–8S.
24. American Thoracic Society, Infectious Diseases Society of America. Guidelines for the management of adults with hospital-acquired, ventilator-associated, and healthcare-associated pneumonia. Am J Respir Crit Care Med 2005;171(4): 388–416.
25. Marrie TJ, Blanchard W. A comparison of nursing home-acquired pneumonia patients with patients with community-acquired pneumonia and nursing home patients without pneumonia. J Am Geriatr Soc 1997;45(1):50–5.
26. Lim WS, Macfarlane JT. A prospective comparison of nursing home acquired pneumonia with community acquired pneumonia. Eur Respir J 2001;18(2): 362–8.
27. Loeb M, McGeer A, McArthur M, et al. Risk factors for pneumonia and other lower respiratory tract infections in elderly residents of long-term care facilities. Arch Intern Med 1999;159(17):2058–64.
28. Carratala J, Mykietiuk A, Fernandez-Sabe N, et al. Health care-associated pneumonia requiring hospital admission: epidemiology, antibiotic therapy, and clinical outcomes. Arch Intern Med 2007;167(13):1393–9.
29. Kollef MH, Shorr A, Tabak YP, et al. Epidemiology and outcomes of health-care-associated pneumonia: results from a large US database of culture-positive pneumonia. Chest 2005;128(6):3854–62.
30. Micek ST, Kollef KE, Reichley RM, et al. Health care-associated pneumonia and community-acquired pneumonia: a single-center experience. Antimicrob Agents Chemother 2007;51(10):3568–73.
31. Venditti M, Falcone M, Corrao S, et al. Outcomes of patients hospitalized with community-acquired, health care-associated, and hospital-acquired pneumonia. Ann Intern Med 2009;150(1):19–26.
32. El Solh AA, Sikka P, Ramadan F, et al. Etiology of severe pneumonia in the very elderly. Am J Respir Crit Care Med 2001;163(3 Pt 1):645–51.
33. MacArthur RD, Lehman MH, Currie-McCumber CA, et al. The epidemiology of gentamicin-resistant *Pseudomonas aeruginosa* on an intermediate care unit. Am J Epidemiol 1988;128(4):821–7.

34. Wingard E, Shlaes JH, Mortimer EA, et al. Colonization and cross-colonization of nursing home patients with trimethoprim-resistant gram-negative bacilli. Clin Infect Dis 1993;16(1):75–81.
35. Washio M, Nishisaka S, Kishikawa K, et al. Incidence of methicillin-resistant *Staphylococcus aureus* (MRSA) isolation in a skilled nursing home: a third report on the risk factors for the occurrence of MRSA infection in the elderly. J Epidemiol 1996;6(2):69–73.
36. Muder RR, Brennen C, Drenning SD, et al. Multiply antibiotic-resistant gram-negative bacilli in a long-term-care facility: a case-control study of patient risk factors and prior antibiotic use. Infect Control Hosp Epidemiol 1997;18(12): 809–13.
37. Terpenning MS, Bradley SF, Wan JY, et al. Colonization and infection with antibiotic-resistant bacteria in a long-term care facility. J Am Geriatr Soc 1994; 42(10):1062–9.
38. Gaynes RP, Weinstein RA, Chamberlin W, et al. Antibiotic-resistant flora in nursing home patients admitted to the hospital. Arch Intern Med 1985; 145(10):1804–7.
39. Trick WE, Weinstein RA, DeMarais PL, et al. Colonization of skilled-care facility residents with antimicrobial-resistant pathogens. J Am Geriatr Soc 2001;49(3):270–6.
40. Ewig S, Torres A, El-Ebiary M, et al. Bacterial colonization patterns in mechanically ventilated patients with traumatic and medical head injury. Incidence, risk factors, and association with ventilator-associated pneumonia. Am J Respir Crit Care Med 1999;159(1):188–98.
41. El Solh AA, Aquilina AT, Dhillon RS, et al. Impact of invasive strategy on management of antimicrobial treatment failure in institutionalized older people with severe pneumonia. Am J Respir Crit Care Med 2002;166(8):1038–43.
42. El Solh AA, Pietrantoni C, Bhat A, et al. Indicators of potentially drug-resistant bacteria in severe nursing home-acquired pneumonia. Clin Infect Dis 2004; 39(4):474–80.
43. McNeil SA, Mody L, Bradley SF. Methicillin-resistant *Staphylococcus aureus*. Management of asymptomatic colonization and outbreaks of infection in long-term care. Geriatrics 2002;57(6):16–8, 21–14, 27.
44. Loeb MB, Craven S, McGeer AJ, et al. Risk factors for resistance to antimicrobial agents among nursing home residents. Am J Epidemiol 2003;157(1):40–7.
45. Goldrick BA. Infection control programs in long-term-care facilities: structure and process. Infect Control Hosp Epidemiol 1999;20(11):764–9.
46. Griffith KA, Sherrill DL, Siegel EM, et al. Predictors of loss of lung function in the elderly: the Cardiovascular Health Study. Am J Respir Crit Care Med 2001; 163(1):61–8.
47. Enright PL, Kronmal RA, Manolio TA, et al. Respiratory muscle strength in the elderly. Correlates and reference values. Cardiovascular Health Study Research Group. Am J Respir Crit Care Med 1994;149(2 Pt 1):430–8.
48. Lindsay DC, Lovegrove CA, Dunn MJ, et al. Histological abnormalities of muscle from limb, thorax and diaphragm in chronic heart failure. Eur Heart J 1996;17(8): 1239–50.
49. Stubbings AK, Moore AJ, Dusmet M, et al. Physiological properties of human diaphragm muscle fibres and the effect of chronic obstructive pulmonary disease. J Physiol 2008;586(10):2637–50.
50. Valenti WM, Trudell RG, Bentley DW. Factors predisposing to oropharyngeal colonization with gram-negative bacilli in the aged. N Engl J Med 1978; 298(20):1108–11.

51. du Moulin GC, Paterson DG, Hedley-Whyte J, et al. Aspiration of gastric bacteria in antacid-treated patients: a frequent cause of postoperative colonisation of the airway. Lancet 1982;1(8266):242–5.
52. Beck-Sague C, Banerjee S, Jarvis WR. Infectious diseases and mortality among US nursing home residents. Am J Public Health 1993;83(12):1739–42.
53. Magaziner J, Tenney JH, DeForge B, et al. Prevalence and characteristics of nursing home-acquired infections in the aged. J Am Geriatr Soc 1991;39(11): 1071–8.
54. Jacobson C, Strausbaugh LJ. Incidence and impact of infection in a nursing home care unit. Am J Infect Control 1990;18(3):151–9.
55. Setia U, Serventi I, Lorenz P. Nosocomial infections among patients in a long-term care facility: spectrum, prevalence, and risk factors. Am J Infect Control 1985;13(2):57–62.
56. Maruyama T, Niederman MS, Kobayashi T, et al. A prospective comparison of nursing home-acquired pneumonia with hospital-acquired pneumonia in non-intubated elderly. Respir Med 2008;102(9):1287–95.
57. Rantanen TK, Salo JA. Gastroesophageal reflux disease as a cause of death: analysis of fatal cases under conservative treatment. Scand J Gastroenterol 1999;34(3):229–33.
58. Konetzka RT, Spector W, Shaffer T. Effects of nursing home ownership type and resident payer source on hospitalization for suspected pneumonia. Med Care 2004;42(10):1001–8.
59. Marrie TJ, Haldane EV, Faulkner RS, et al. Community-acquired pneumonia requiring hospitalization. Is it different in the elderly? J Am Geriatr Soc 1985; 33(10):671–80.
60. Mehr DR, Binder EF, Kruse RL, et al. Clinical findings associated with radiographic pneumonia in nursing home residents. J Fam Pract 2001;50(11):931–7.
61. Bentley DW, Bradley S, High K, et al. Practice guideline for evaluation of fever and infection in long-term care facilities. Clin Infect Dis 2000;31(3):640–53.
62. Restrepo MI, Anzueto A. The role of gram-negative bacteria in healthcare-associated pneumonia. Semin Respir Crit Care Med 2009;30(1):61–6.
63. Mandell LA, Wunderink RG, Anzueto A, et al. Infectious Diseases Society of America/American Thoracic Society consensus guidelines on the management of community-acquired pneumonia in adults. Clin Infect Dis 2007;44(Suppl 2): S27–72.
64. Bentley DW. Bacterial pneumonia in the elderly: clinical features, diagnosis, etiology, and treatment. Gerontology 1984;30(5):297–307.
65. Marik PE, Kaplan D. Aspiration pneumonia and dysphagia in the elderly. Chest 2003;124(1):328–36.
66. Oh E, Weintraub N, Dhanani S. Can we prevent aspiration pneumonia in the nursing home? J Am Med Dir Assoc 2005;6(Suppl 3):S76–80.
67. Croghan JE, Burke EM, Caplan S, et al. Pilot study of 12-month outcomes of nursing home patients with aspiration on videofluoroscopy. Dysphagia 1994; 9(3):141–6.
68. Palmer LB, Albulak K, Fields S, et al. Oral clearance and pathogenic oropharyngeal colonization in the elderly. Am J Respir Crit Care Med 2001;164(3):464–8.
69. Yoneyama T, Yoshida M, Ohrui T, et al. Oral care reduces pneumonia in older patients in nursing homes. J Am Geriatr Soc 2002;50(3):430–3.
70. Terpenning MS, Taylor GW, Lopatin DE, et al. Aspiration pneumonia: dental and oral risk factors in an older veteran population. J Am Geriatr Soc 2001;49(5): 557–63.

71. Hutt E, Kramer AM. Evidence-based guidelines for management of nursing home-acquired pneumonia. J Fam Pract 2002;51(8):709–16.
72. Hickman SE, Nelson CA, Moss AH, et al. Use of the Physician Orders for Life-Sustaining Treatment (POLST) paradigm program in the hospice setting. J Palliat Med 2009;12(2):133–41.
73. Cox DM, Sachs GA. Advance directives and the patient Self-determination Act. Clin Geriatr Med 1994;10(3):431–43.
74. Zweig SC, Kruse RL, Binder EF, et al. Effect of do-not-resuscitate orders on hospitalization of nursing home residents evaluated for lower respiratory infections. J Am Geriatr Soc 2004;52(1):51–8.
75. Degelau J, Guay D, Straub K, et al. Effectiveness of oral antibiotic treatment in nursing home-acquired pneumonia. J Am Geriatr Soc 1995;43(3):245–51.
76. Loeb M, Carusone SC, Goeree R, et al. Effect of a clinical pathway to reduce hospitalizations in nursing home residents with pneumonia: a randomized controlled trial. JAMA 2006;295(21):2503–10.
77. Intrator O, Castle NG, Mor V. Facility characteristics associated with hospitalization of nursing home residents: results of a national study. Med Care 1999;37(3): 228–37.
78. Fried TR, Gillick MR, Lipsitz LA. Whether to transfer? Factors associated with hospitalization and outcome of elderly long-term care patients with pneumonia. J Gen Intern Med 1995;10(5):246–50.
79. Fine MJ, Auble TE, Yealy DM, et al. A prediction rule to identify low-risk patients with community-acquired pneumonia. N Engl J Med 1997;336(4):243–50.
80. Loeb M. Pneumonia in older persons. Clin Infect Dis 2003;37(10):1335–9.
81. Mandell LA, Marrie TJ, Grossman RF, et al. Canadian guidelines for the initial management of community-acquired pneumonia: an evidence-based update by the Canadian Infectious Diseases Society and the Canadian Thoracic Society. The Canadian Community-Acquired Pneumonia Working Group. Clin Infect Dis 2000;31(2):383–421.
82. Mandell LA, Bartlett JG, Dowell SF, et al. Update of practice guidelines for the management of community-acquired pneumonia in immunocompetent adults. Clin Infect Dis 2003;37(11):1405–33.
83. Peterson PK, Stein D, Guay DR, et al. Prospective study of lower respiratory tract infections in an extended-care nursing home program: potential role of oral ciprofloxacin. Am J Med 1988;85(2):164–71.
84. Faulkner CM, Cox HL, Williamson JC. Unique aspects of antimicrobial use in older adults. Clin Infect Dis 2005;40(7):997–1004.
85. Field TS, Gurwitz JH, Avorn J, et al. Risk factors for adverse drug events among nursing home residents. Arch Intern Med 2001;161(13):1629–34.
86. Kaufman DW, Kelly JP, Rosenberg L, et al. Recent patterns of medication use in the ambulatory adult population of the United States: The Slone Survey. JAMA 2002;287(3):337–44.
87. Nguyen JK, Fouts MM, Kotabe SE, et al. Polypharmacy as a risk factor for adverse drug reactions in geriatric nursing home residents. Am J Geriatr Pharmacother 2006;4(1):36–41.
88. Houck PM, Bratzler DW, Nsa W, et al. Timing of antibiotic administration and outcomes for Medicare patients hospitalized with community-acquired pneumonia. Arch Intern Med 2004;164(6):637–44.
89. Marrie TJ, Wu L. Factors influencing in-hospital mortality in community-acquired pneumonia: a prospective study of patients not initially admitted to the ICU. Chest 2005;127(4):1260–70.

90. Benenson R, Magalski A, Cavanaugh S, et al. Effects of a pneumonia clinical pathway on time to antibiotic treatment, length of stay, and mortality. Acad Emerg Med 1999;6(12):1243–8.
91. Chroneou A, Zias N, Beamis JF Jr, et al. Healthcare-associated pneumonia: principles and emerging concepts on management. Expert Opin Pharmacother 2007;8(18):3117–31.
92. Bula CJ, Ghilardi G, Wietlisbach V, et al. Infections and functional impairment in nursing home residents: a reciprocal relationship. J Am Geriatr Soc 2004;52(5): 700–6.
93. Mehr DR, Binder EF, Kruse RL, et al. Predicting mortality in nursing home residents with lower respiratory tract infection: the Missouri LRI Study. JAMA 2001; 286(19):2427–36.
94. Mylotte JM, Naughton B, Saludades C, et al. Validation and application of the pneumonia prognosis index to nursing home residents with pneumonia. J Am Geriatr Soc 1998;46(12):1538–44.
95. Campbell-Taylor I. Oropharyngeal dysphagia in long-term care: misperceptions of treatment efficacy. J Am Med Dir Assoc 2008;9(7):523–31.
96. Langmore SE, Terpenning MS, Schork A, et al. Predictors of aspiration pneumonia: how important is dysphagia? Dysphagia 1998;13(2):69–81.
97. Baine WB, Yu W, Summe JP. Epidemiologic trends in the hospitalization of elderly Medicare patients for pneumonia, 1991-1998. Am J Public Health 2001;91(7):1121–3.
98. El-Solh AA, Pietrantoni C, Bhat A, et al. Colonization of dental plaques: a reservoir of respiratory pathogens for hospital-acquired pneumonia in institutionalized elders. Chest 2004;126(5):1575–82.
99. Shay K. Infectious complications of dental and periodontal diseases in the elderly population. Clin Infect Dis 2002;34(9):1215–23.
100. Gross PA, Hermogenes AW, Sacks HS, et al. The efficacy of influenza vaccine in elderly persons. A meta-analysis and review of the literature. Ann Intern Med 1995;123(7):518–27.
101. Carman WF, Elder AG, Wallace LA, et al. Effects of influenza vaccination of health-care workers on mortality of elderly people in long-term care: a randomised controlled trial. Lancet 2000;355(9198):93–7.
102. Fine MJ, Smith MA, Carson CA, et al. Efficacy of pneumococcal vaccination in adults. A meta-analysis of randomized controlled trials. Arch Intern Med 1994; 154(23):2666–77.
103. Hutchison BG, Oxman AD, Shannon HS, et al. Clinical effectiveness of pneumococcal vaccine. Meta-analysis. Can Fam Physician 1999;45:2381–93.
104. Moore RA, Wiffen PJ, Lipsky BA. Are the pneumococcal polysaccharide vaccines effective? Meta-analysis of the prospective trials. BMC Fam Pract 2000;1:1.
105. Potter J, Stott DJ, Roberts MA, et al. Influenza vaccination of health care workers in long-term-care hospitals reduces the mortality of elderly patients. J Infect Dis 1997;175(1):1–6.
106. Cornu C, Yzebe D, Leophonte P, et al. Efficacy of pneumococcal polysaccharide vaccine in immunocompetent adults: a meta-analysis of randomized trials. Vaccine 2001;19(32):4780–90.
107. Bardenheier B, Shefer A, McKibben L, et al. Characteristics of long-term-care facility residents associated with receipt of influenza and pneumococcal vaccinations. Infect Control Hosp Epidemiol 2004;25(11):946–54.
108. Carusone SC, Loeb M, Lohfeld L. A clinical pathway for treating pneumonia in the nursing home: part I: the nursing perspective. J Am Med Dir Assoc 2006;7(5):271–8.

109. Brandt HE, Ooms ME, Deliens L, et al. The last two days of life of nursing home patients–a nationwide study on causes of death and burdensome symptoms in the Netherlands. Palliat Med 2006;20(5):533–40.
110. Abdel-Karim IA, Sammel RB, Prange MA. Causes of death at autopsy in an inpatient hospice program. J Palliat Med 2007;10(4):894–8.
111. Chen JH, Lamberg JL, Chen YC, et al. Occurrence and treatment of suspected pneumonia in long-term care residents dying with advanced dementia. J Am Geriatr Soc 2006;54(2):290–5.
112. Mitchell SL, Teno JM, Kiely DK, et al. The clinical course of advanced dementia. N Engl J Med 2009;361(16):1529–38.
113. Givens JL, Jones RN, Shaffer ML, et al. Survival and comfort after treatment of pneumonia in advanced dementia. Arch Intern Med 2010;170(13):1102–7.

Managing the Patient with Dementia in Long-Term Care

Jennifer Rhodes-Kropf, MD[a,*], Huai Cheng, MD, MPH[b],
Elizabeth Herskovits Castillo, MD, PhD[c,d,e], Ana Tuya Fulton, MD[f]

KEYWORDS

- Dementia • Cholinesterase inhibitors • Memantine
- Environment • Function • Depression • Agitation
- Eating problems

The majority of residents in a nursing home have some degree of dementia. The prevalence is commonly from 70% to 80% of residents. This article covers the following topics on caring for patients with dementia in long-term care (LTC): (1) the efficacy of cholinesterase inhibitors and memantine, (2) the optimal environment for maintenance of function in moderate dementia, (3) the treatment of depression and agitation, and (4) the evaluation and management of eating problems.

THE EFFICACY OF CHOLINESTERASE INHIBITORS AND MEMANTINE FOR DEMENTIA

People with Alzheimer disease have reduced cerebral synthesis of choline acetyltransferase, which leads to a reduction in acetylcholine production and impaired cortical cholinergic function. Cholinesterase inhibitors increase cholinergic transmission by

---

This work was supported by Geriatric Academic Career Awards from the Health Resources and Services Administration.
The authors have nothing to disclose.
[a] Division of Geriatrics, Center Communities of Brookline, Hebrew SeniorLife and Beth Israel Deaconess Medical Center, Harvard University Medical School, 100 Centre Street, Boston, MA 02446, USA
[b] Department of Palliative Care and Rehabilitation Medicine, MD Anderson Cancer Center, 1515 Holcombe Boulevard, Unit 1414/FCT5.6057, Houston, TX 77030, USA
[c] Geriatric Medicine Program, MAHEC (Mountain AHEC), 118 WT Weaver Boulevard, Asheville, NC 28804, USA
[d] Department of Family Medicine, UNC Chapel Hill School of Medicine, 590 Manning Drive, Chapel Hill, NC 27599, USA
[e] Givens Estates (CCRC), 2360 Sweeten Creek Road, Asheville, NC 28803, USA
[f] Division of Geriatrics, Department of Medicine, Warren Alpert Medical School of Brown University, Butler Hospital, 345 Blackstone Boulevard, Center House Rear #207, Providence, RI 02906, USA
* Corresponding author.
E-mail address: jrhodeskropf@hsl.harvard.edu

Clin Geriatr Med 27 (2011) 135–152
doi:10.1016/j.cger.2011.01.001
geriatric.theclinics.com
0749-0690/11/$ – see front matter

inhibiting cholinesterase at the synaptic cleft. There are 4 cholinesterase inhibitors approved by the Food and Drug Administration: tacrine, rivastigmine, galantamine, and donepezil. Tacrine is rarely used because of hepatotoxicity.[1] Rivastigmine is rarely used because of excessive cholinergic effects that may produce nausea, vomiting, anorexia, and headaches.[2] Galantamine has similar (limited) efficacy to donepezil, but may have more gastrointestinal side effects. Consequently, donepezil is usually the preferred drug.

The efficacy of donepezil for mild to moderate cognitive impairment was demonstrated in a double-blind trial and a placebo-controlled trial.[3,4] The former used the 70-point Alzheimer Disease Assessment Scale with cognitive subscale (ADAS-cog) and the latter study used the Mini Mental Status Examination (MMSE). These studies showed statistically significant improvement of a few points on the 70-point ADAS-cog and 0.8 point difference on the MMSE. Many experts believe that this is of minimal clinical significance.

There have been two placebo-controlled trials in nursing homes that have evaluated the efficacy of donepezil. One study had 216 nursing home residents and the other 208. Different assessment instruments were used in these studies. Both studies demonstrated statistically significant differences in cognitive function between the intervention and control groups.[5,6] Again, these were very modest differences.

There is, however, additional evidence in all stages of dementia that suggests that the response to cholinesterase inhibitors may be variable, with a small proportion (up to 20%) who show a greater than average response ($\geq$7-point ADAS-cog improvement).[7,8] Thus it seems prudent to give donepezil to patients on a trial basis. If there is no improvement noted by the family and/or health care provider then the medication should be stopped. It is also advisable to stop donepezil when the person has very advanced dementia. If stopping the drug, then taper the medication over a 3-week period. Keep in mind that the medication is costly and that it is helpful to the patient to be on one less pill each day. Note that for an adequate trial, the patient needs to be titrated up to the research dose of 10 mg. The provider should evaluate the efficacy of the trial using several different cognitive assessment tests, as one alone is not enough to make a determination of medication efficacy. These tests could include, for example, the Montreal Cognitive Assessment instrument (MOCA), the MMSE, and the naming of as many grocery items or animals as possible in 1 minute (less than 16 in 1 minute is abnormal). It is obviously important that the same group of assessments should be used before and after the patient starts the medication.

Note that sometimes the condition of patients will worsen after stopping administration of the cholinesterase inhibitor.[9,10] If this occurs then it is best to resume the medication.

Donepezil was well tolerated in all of these studies. Gastrointestinal discomfort (diarrhea, nausea, and vomiting) were the most common side effects, so titrating to 10 mg over a few weeks is most helpful. There is also the potential risk of symptomatic bradycardia.[11,12] One study found that the incidence of hospitalization for syncope was 3.2 events per 100 person-years for patients on cholinesterase inhibitors (68% were taking donepezil).[12]

There is still real controversy regarding whether donepezil significantly improves outcomes such as the need for nursing home admission, the maintenance of daily living, and behavioral symptoms.[4,13–15] If there is any benefit, it is minimal.

The use of cholinesterase inhibitors is controversial in other dementias (vascular dementia, mixed dementia, Lewy Body dementia [LBD], and the dementia of Parkinson disease); however, there does seem to be cognitive improvement to a similar modest degree as shown in Alzheimer disease. Note that especially for some

Parkinson patients there can be a significant reduction in Parkinson-associated visual hallucinations. For LBD even greater improvement in cognition than in these other dementias may result.[7,14,16–18]

In contrast to the cholinergic agents, memantine seems to be neuroprotective.

Memantine is an *N*-methyl-D-aspartate (NMDA) receptor antagonist. Overstimulation of the NMDA receptor by glutamate is thought to contribute to neurodegenerative disorders.

Memantine seems to have a degree of benefit in patients with moderate to severe Alzheimer dementia (AD). A 28-week randomized trial in 252 patients with MMSE scores of 3 to 14 (mean approximately 8) at study inception found memantine was statistically significant in reducing decline on the following primary end point variables: Clinician's Interview-Based Impression of Change Plus Caregiver Input (mean difference between the groups of 0.3, where the greatest difference could have been 1, $P = .03$) and the Alzheimer's Disease Cooperative Study Activities of Daily Living Inventory modified for severe dementia (mean difference 2.1, where the greatest difference could have been 7, $P = .02$).[19]

However, for mild to moderate AD, a systematic review reported on 3 unpublished studies and found that memantine had a very small but statistically significant difference. The difference between groups was less than 1 point out of the 70-point ADAS-cog. Also, there was no effect on behavior or activities of daily living (ADL).[20]

Memantine may be of some benefit when used in conjunction with cholinesterase inhibitors, but similar to the studies already described, the following two studies showed benefit in the moderate to severe AD cohort and not in the mild to moderate AD cohort. Three hundred and twenty-two patients with moderate to severe AD (MMSE 5–14) underwent a 24-week placebo-controlled trial. The memantine and donepezil group resulted in significantly better outcomes than placebo plus donepezil on measures of cognition, ADL, global outcome, and behavior.[21] However, the second 24-week randomized trial, comprising 433 patients with mild to moderate AD, showed no significant difference between the group on cholinesterase inhibitor plus placebo and the group on cholinesterase inhibitor plus memantine.[22]

Hence, for moderate to advanced dementia many experts will prescribe memantine because it may be disease modifying, even when there is no clinical improvement.

As described herein, the benefit of pharmacologic therapy is limited; therefore it is particularly important to try to maximize the quality of the environment and social interactions, as described in the next section.

OPTIMAL ENVIRONMENT FOR MAINTENANCE OF FUNCTION IN MODERATE DEMENTIA

The function and quality of life of the person with dementia is contingent in many respects on their surroundings. Both the physical and interpersonal environment in the LTC setting will have an impact that enhances, or worsens, the patient's life.[23–25] So one may conclude that physicians and members of the elder-care team have both an opportunity and a responsibility to help preserve the capacities and pleasures of patients with dementia that goes well beyond medication. The architecture and physical plant, interior design, exterior landscaping, social atmosphere, and recreational palette[26–30] afforded to the patient are all important considerations. There is tremendous potential for the geriatrician to take a lead role with LTC staff and family, and perhaps even with the wider lay and medical communities.

In regard of dementia and the physical environment, lessons learned from the disability literature indicate that the "person-environment fit" must be analyzed and manipulated to maximize function and quality of life.[31–34] When the physical or built environment leads to loss of function, the result is an “excess disability”[35–37] that can be reversed by changing the built environment. For example, when ramps are introduced alongside stairs, or curb-cuts are placed into sidewalks, the mobility of those in wheelchairs is markedly improved. Similarly, when motion-detectors that trigger voice-over messages and sprinklers are placed at safe perimeters of the housing/landscape of an LTC facility, the doors may be unlocked and electronic anklets removed, enhancing daily quality of life for those at risk of wandering.[38,39]

Perceptual ability diminishes in the context of dementia. For example, the experience of color and light is altered[40–42]; consequently, modification of lighting in a room and hallway, as well as changes in flooring designs and materials, has a measurable impact on falls and injury rates.[36,43–45]

Furthermore, the brain’s ability to “filter” and manage multiple stimuli also diminishes with the progression of dementia.[38,46] Manipulating the physical and interpersonal environment to reduce the volume of perceptual stimuli can improve function and reduce patients’ fear and frustration. Fear and frustration are often communicated through so-called agitated behaviors.[47] The purposeful reduction of stimuli can be as simple as reducing the tableware and patterned cloths at mealtimes, culling collected tchotschkes on display, or carefully controlling the type and level of sounds in dementia-specialized LTC units.[40]

Through most of the trajectory of the natural history of dementia, people with dementia experience deficits in specific brain functions while other brain functions are preserved. Through careful observation and comprehensive cognitive testing, those domains which are impaired can be identified and strategies activated to compensate for the specific losses, preserving the function of many meaningful daily activities. A patient who has trouble with sequencing and organizing does not have to “lose” the ability to do laundry or to participate in cooking. Instead, the caregiving team can break down the organization and sequence of the desired activity and provide verbal or visual cues, such as little numbered signs with brief instructions that walk the patient step by step through the activity. Similarly, when a person with dementia demonstrates deficits in orientation or functions, careful manipulation of interior design—photographs with captions, personal reminiscence books, physical objects from the past that trigger specific memory pathways, calendars, clocks—maximize the presence of cues which anchor and orient the patient, diminish fear and frustration, and hence reduce so-called agitation behaviors. This approach reduces the tendency for the elder-care team to prescribe unnecessary (inappropriate) medications for chemical restraint.

DEMENTIA AND DEPRESSION

There is extensive literature on depression and agitation in patients with dementia in LTC. Research demonstrates that residents with dementia in LTC not only have multiple behavioral and psychological symptoms but also may be taking multiple psychotropic medications.[48–53] These symptoms can be difficult to treat[51,52] and have been associated with hospitalization, psychiatric medication use,[50,51] and poor quality of life.[54] In this article the authors review the evidence-based drug and nondrug interventions for dementia-associated depression, agitation, or both, to improve clinically important outcomes. Assessment of behavioral and psychological symptoms associated with dementia can be found elsewhere[55,56] and is not discussed here.

Depression was the most common psychological symptom associated with dementia among residents in LTC no matter what measurement of depression was used.[48,49] Twenty-nine percent of the residents with dementia in LTC had major depression; 19% and 34% for black and white residents, respectively. However, only 3% of black and 9% of white nursing home residents with dementia were diagnosed as probable major depression when the more strict DSM-IV (*Diagnostic and Statistical Manual of Mental Disorders* [Fourth Edition, Text Revised]) criteria were applied. The prevalence of depressive symptoms such as dysphoria or depressed mood varied from 8% to 74% among the residents with dementia. Twenty-two percent of the residents had crying episodes. Using Neuropsychiatric Inventory—Nursing Home Version,[53] a recent single large nursing home study of 59 dementia special care units revealed that 20% of 1322 dementia residents had depression. Unfortunately, depression without treatment tended to be persistent,[51,52] and was associated with hospitalization and psychiatric medication use other than antidepressants,[50,51] as well as poor quality of life.[54]

Without a doubt, the studies show that the treatment of depression associated with dementia in LTC is extremely important. The parameters used for this literature review are as follows: depression and nursing homes; limited to humans, English, meta-analysis, practice guidelines, reviews, and randomized controlled trials (RCT) in PubMed, Medline, and manual search. One consensus statement from the American Geriatric Society and American Association Geriatric psychiatry[57] and 2 review articles[56,58] on the treatment of depression associated with dementia among LTC residents were identified. It is recommended that depression can and should be treated. The authors' recommendations for the treatment of major depression with drug or nondrug therapy were based on a high level of evidence including RCTs. **Tables 1** and **2** summarize the RCTs for depression as the primary outcome and RCTs targeting depression and other behavioral symptoms.

DEMENTIA WITH AGITATION

In addition to depression, agitation is a very common psychological symptom associated with dementia in the LTC setting[48,49]; these studies found 28% to 53% of residents had agitation, 18% to 30% of residents had disinhibition, 31% to 67% of residents had irritability, 38% to 61% of residents had restlessness, and 32% to 51% of residents had aberrant motor behavior. A recent single large nursing home study of 59 dementia special care units, using the Cohen-Mansfield Agitation Inventory (CMAI), showed 85% of 1322 dementia residents had at least one symptom of agitation.[53]

Note that the concept of agitation is complex. Agitation is defined as distinct syndromes that include physically aggressive behaviors, physically nonaggressive behaviors, and verbally agitated behaviors.[67] Many instruments have been developed to assess agitation associated with dementia.[67–69] The CMAI is one of the most commonly used agitation assessment instruments. Multiple associated and potentially preventable risk factors for agitation in dementia have been identified. These risk factors include: pain, ADL dysfunction, cognitive impairment, depression, mental diseases other than schizophrenia and affective disorders, the use of physical restraints, psychosis, medical diseases such as sleep-disordered breathing, cardiovascular disease, antipsychotic and anxiolytic medications, the total number of drugs taken per day, physical environmental factors (eg, intrusion into the resident's own personal space such as bathing, toileting), and social environment (eg, the number of visitors or telephone calls per week, a lack of environmental stimuli, or an overwhelming influx of external stimuli such as television).[48,70–74] It is critically important that these risk factors be identified when assessing a patient with agitation and dementia. Wherever possible, these risk factors should be eliminated or prevented before drug therapy is started.

Agitation is associated with poor quality of life.[54] The treatment of the agitation that accompanies dementia has been widely studied. A literature search via PubMed,

Table 1
Randomized controlled trials of drug and nondrug treatment for patients with dementia and depression in LTC between 1968 and 2010[a]

Author,[Ref.] Year	Interventions	Sample Size (N)	Trial Length (wk)	Results	Notes
Drug Trial					
Magai et al,[59] 2000	Sertraline or placebo	31	8	Depressive symptoms were not improved	Possibly false negative because power was not calculated. Cornell Scale for Depression in Dementia, Gestalt Scale, Cohen-Mansfield Agitation Inventory, Aversive Feeding Behaviors Scale, and facial behaviors were used
Nondrug Trial					
Williams and Tappen,[60] 2008	Comprehensive exercise, supervised walking, or social conversation	42	16	Depression was reduced in all 3 groups	Quasi-experimental design with random assignment to treatment group. Raters were blinded. Cornell Scale for Depression in Dementia, Dementia Mood Assessment Scale, Alzheimer's Mood Scale, and Observed Affect Scale were used

[a] Not intended to retrieve all RCTs from all sources.

Table 2
Randomized controlled trials of drug and nondrug treatment for patients with dementia, depression, and agitation in demented nursing home residents between 1968 and 2010[a]

Author,[Refs.] Year	Interventions	Sample Size (N)	Trial Length	Results	Notes
Drug Trials					
Street et al,[61] 2000	Olanzapine or placebo	206	6 wk	Reduction of agitation, aggression, and psychosis	Power was not calculated. Participants must have any agitation/aggression, hallucination, or delusion
Tariot et al,[62] 1998	Carbamazepine or placebo	51	6 wk	Reduction of Brief Psychiatry Rating Scale, agitation and aggression	Power was not calculated. Brief Psychiatry Rating Scale was used
Coccaro et al,[63] 1990	Haloperidol or oxazepam or diphenhydramine	59	8 wk	Improvement of agitation and activities of daily living	Randomized double-blind comparison of 3 drugs without placebo. Brief Psychiatric Rating Scale and Alzheimer's Disease Assessment Scale were used
Nondrug Trials					
Testad et al,[64] 2010	Staff training or usual care	211	12 mo	Reduction of restraint use and severity of agitation	Power was not calculated. Single-blind randomized controlled trial. Cohen-Mansfield Agitation Inventory was used
Sloan et al,[65] 2004	Person-centered showering/bathing or usual care	73	Unclear	Reduction of agitation, aggression, and discomfort	Cross-over trial with random assignment. Care Recipient Behavior Assessment and modified Discomfort Scale for Dementia of the Alzheimer Type were used
McCallion et al,[66] 1999	Family visit education program or usual care	66	6 mo	Improved multiple outcomes such as depression and irritability	Participants displayed problem behaviors such as physical aggression, verbally abusive behaviors, disruptive vocalization, or motor restlessness. 2×3 single-blind, randomized control group design

[a] Not intended to retrieve all RCTs from all sources.

Medline, and manually has produced 5 review articles with or without meta-analysis on managing agitation associated with dementia in LTC, 1 RCT using agitation as primary outcome, and 1 RCT using agitation and other behavioral symptoms combined as outcomes, as summarized in **Tables 2** and **3**. Based on the literature review and their LTC practice experience, the authors recommend the following general approach for treating agitation associated with dementia in LTC. First, assess and remove potentially correctable risk factors as described above. For example, review medications and discontinue nonessential medications, preserve residents' privacy, and encourage visits and phone calls from family. Always attempt first nondrug intervention such as behavioral management, as supported by RCTs.

A short anecdote by the first author (J.R.-K.) illustrates the benefit of behavioral management.

> *I was on-call overnight in a nursing home and called to see a patient who had dementia and was very agitated. I walked into the patient's room and he was sitting upright in bed with 5 staff around him telling him loudly to calm down, with the overhead fluorescent light on. I asked the staff to leave the room, closed the window as it was too cool, covered him with a blanket, turned off the lights, spoke to him softly and reassuringly, and put on his favorite classical music station. He quickly went to sleep.*

Again, drug therapy should be the last means to relieve agitation in patients with dementia.

As already mentioned, pain can cause agitation and patients with cognitive impairment may not be able to verbalize that they are in pain. Pain is frequently overlooked as a cause of agitation.[70,88,89] However, RCTs on pain management for patients with dementia and agitation in the LTC setting is rare. The reader is referred to the article by Fulton and colleagues elsewhere in this issue on palliative care for patients with dementia in LTC. Note that many review articles and RCTs study together the often associated symptoms of depression, agitation, and other psychological symptoms for patients with dementia in LTC. The PubMed, Medline, and manual search located 2 guidelines,[57,90] 9 review articles with or without meta-analysis on managing psychotic and behavioral symptoms associated with dementia,[91–99] and the RCTs as summarized in **Table 2**.

In summary, depression and agitation associated with dementia in LTC are common and are associated with adverse outcomes. Depression and agitation should be treated appropriately, based on the evidence from RCTs and guidelines. Nondrug therapy should be the mainstay of the treatment. The potential benefit of drug therapy is appreciated and should be used cautiously.

EATING PROBLEMS ASSOCIATED WITH DEMENTIA

Difficulties with eating, maintaining weight, and loss of appetite are hallmarks of the later stages of dementia. It is almost a universal and expected complication of progressive dementia. Decisions surrounding feeding are often the most difficult, and emotional for families and caregivers to make. There is wide variation in practice among hospitals and physicians, and across the country, on the practice of feeding tube insertion. Despite evidence against the efficacy of feeding tubes, almost 30% of patients with advanced dementia have a feeding tube placed.[100] This high rate exists despite the evidence against the ability of feeding tubes to prolong life, reverse the effects of malnutrition, or to prevent the complications of aspiration. Despite the evidence that can help guide the choice, it is a decision that is wrought with emotional, cultural, and moral overlay for both physicians and family members of the patient, making it exceedingly difficult.

Eating problems associated with dementia include difficulty chewing and swallowing, pocketing or spitting, loss of appetite and interest in food, and an inability to sense hunger or thirst. Swallowing problems or dysphagia can often cause aspiration events and pneumonia (see the article by Fulton and colleagues elsewhere in this issue on palliation for residents with dementia, section on infections). It is helpful to be familiar with the commonly used term "failure to thrive." Failure to thrive describes a syndrome among older adults, with or without dementia, who demonstrate evident decline in weight and nutritional status. The Institute of Medicine defines failure to thrive late in life as a syndrome manifested by weight loss greater than 5%, decreased appetite, poor nutrition, and inactivity that can be accompanied by dehydration, depression, or impaired immune function.[101] Of importance, seniors with dementia commonly have concurrent depression, and this contributes to a decreased interest in food and reduced appetite.

A recent study reviewed the trajectory of patients with advanced dementia and identified that eating difficulties occurred in almost 86% of the study patients followed over an 18-month period.[102] This result affirms that eating difficulties are a common complication of dementia and an almost universal symptom of advanced dementia. Despite this, a workup to reveal underlying reversible causes is necessary for any patient presenting with feeding difficulty.

WORKUP AND EVALUATION OF EATING PROBLEMS IN DEMENTIA

Many older adults can present with nutritional concerns. Age-related changes can lead to decreased appetite through changes in the appearance, taste, smell, and even texture of food. As with all geriatric syndromes, presentation with failure to thrive or nutritional issues should begin with a complete history and physical, and a review of prescription and over-the-counter medications, or herbal supplements. Laboratory evaluation should include complete blood count with differential, fasting glucose, electrolytes, liver function tests, thyroid-stimulating hormone test, urinalysis, and albumin or prealbumin. Dental care should be updated as well as assessment for dysphagia or odynophagia.

Screening for possible dementia and/or depression should be performed. A particularly helpful screening instrument for seniors is the Geriatric Depression Scale (GDS). Depression can be missed in older adults because they do not complain of emotional or conventional symptoms of depression. Somatic or physical symptoms are more commonly reported, and changes in memory, attention, and activity can be mistaken for cognitive impairment, rather than depression.[101]

Also, as important in early dementia as the cause for poor nutrition and/or weight loss is poor oral intake because of poor access to food, simply forgetting to eat, or apraxia related to eating.[103] Discernment of this issue requires careful history taking and discussion with staff and family of the older adult. Of course, access to food and forgetting to eat are more common factors for seniors who still live independently in the community. Other causes of nutritional or feeding problems include malignancy, chronic infection (eg, abscess, tuberculosis, syphilis, human immunodeficiency virus [HIV]), congestive heart failure, chronic obstructive lung disease, and thyroid or other endocrine disease. In addition to the laboratory tests mentioned, and if the history and physical examination support, imaging for possible malignancy, HIV panel, and syphilis and tuberculosis screening should be included.

MANAGEMENT OPTIONS FOR EATING PROBLEMS IN DEMENTIA

Management options are broad and begin with targeted treatment of any underlying conditions such as dental problems or depression. In addition, universal measures

Table 3
Randomized controlled trials of drug and nondrug treatment for patients with dementia and agitation in LTC between 1968 and 2010[a]

Author,[Refs.] Year	Interventions	Sample Size (N)	Trial Length	Results	Notes
Drug Trials					
Tariot et al,[75] 2005	Divalproex sodium or placebo	153	8 wk	No difference	80% power with type I error of 5% was calculated. Primary outcome was Brief Psychiatric rating Scale Agitation factor
Finkel et al,[76] 1995	Thiothixene or placebo	33	17 wk	Significantly reduced agitated behaviors	Cross-over with random assignment
Nondrug Trials					
Cohen-Mansfield et al,[77] 2010	Standardized stimuli (live social, task, reading, self-identity, music, work, simulated social, manipulative) or no stimulation provided/usual care	110	3 wk	Significantly less physical agitation and less total agitation	Repeated-measure design with randomized assignment of conditions. Power was not calculated. Agitation Behaviors Mapping Instrument was used
Burns et al,[78] 2009	Right light or standard light	48	8 wk	Reducing agitation as measured by an actigraph, but not Cohen-Mansfield Agitation Inventory. Sleep was improved	80% power with a significant level of 5% was calculated. The primary outcome was Cohen-Mansfield Agitation Inventory
Wan-ki Lin et al,[79] 2007	Aromatherapy (*Lavandula angustifolia*) or sunflower inhalation	70	5 wk	Significantly reduced agitated behaviors	Cross-over randomized trial. 80% power with a significance level of 0.05 was calculated. Chinese version of Cohen-Mansfield Agitation Inventory and Neuropsychiatric Inventory was used

Cohen-Mansfield et al,[80] 2007	Systematic individualized intervention using the TREA (Treatment Routes for Exploring Agitation) decision tree protocol to uncover possible reasons for each participant and corresponding treatment was provided	167	10 d	Significant decreases in overall agitation	Power was calculated. Randomization unit was nursing home. Primary outcome was Agitation Behavior Mapping Instrument The TREA protocol can be very helpful in identifying the causes of agitation and taking action accordingly for individual patients
Garland et al,[81] 2007	Simulated family presence and preferred music or usual care	30	Unclear	Reduction of physical agitated behaviors	Randomized single blind trial
Sung et al,[82] 2006	Group music with movement or usual care	36	4 wk	Significantly reduced agitated behaviors	Power was not calculated. Cohen-Mansfield Agitation Inventory was used
Ancoli-Israel et al,[83] 2003	Morning bright light, morning dim red light, or evening bright light	92	15 d	No significant change in agitation	Power was not calculated. Cohen-Mansfield Agitation Inventory and Agitated Behavior Rating Scale were used
Ballard et al,[84] 2002	Aromatherapy with Melissa essential oil or placebo	72	4 wk	Significantly reduced agitated behaviors	Cohen-Mansfield Agitation Inventory and quality of life indices were used
Remington,[85] 2002	Calming music and hand massage or no intervention	68	1 h	Significantly reduced agitated behaviors	80% power with a significance level of 5% was calculated. Modified Cohen-Mansfield Agitation Inventory was used
Gerdner,[86] 2000	Individualized versus classical "relaxation" music	39	18 wk	Significantly reduced agitated behaviors	Power calculation was uncertain. Modified Cohen-Mansfield Agitation Inventory was used. Cross-over design with random assignment was used
Lyketsos et al,[87] 1999	Bright light or dim light exposure	15	9 wk	No improvement in agitated behaviors	Power was not calculated. Cross-over trial with random assignment. Behave-AD was used

[a] Not intended to retrieve all RCTs from all sources.

that can be added to the regimen for any patient with weight loss or failure to thrive are important. These measures include an increase in physical activity, resistive training, or endurance training, which can improve mood, outlook, and appetite.[101] Also, improving the environment at meal time, the appearance and taste of food, and the social aspect of eating can all increase intake in older adults. Speech and swallow therapists can suggest easier chewing and swallowing foods and textures. Changing meals to 5 smaller meals instead of the traditional 3 larger meals can help, as can making breakfast the larger meal of the day because older adults, especially those with dementia, tend to eat more in the morning.[101] Finger foods are also more appealing, as are foods that are either hot or cold rather than in between.[100] Supplements such as protein shakes, or meal replacement drinks augment caloric and protein intake; they are most helpful when used between meals. Offending medications that can affect taste (ie, hydrochlorothiazide, antihistamines, allopurinol, levodopa, lithium, carbamazepine) or olfaction (eg, lisinopril) should be discontinued if possible.[103,104] A large number of medications can cause anorexia, including antiepileptics, benzodiazepines, neuroleptics, opioids, and selective serotonin reuptake inhibitors.[101]

Medications that stimulate appetite can be tried. A common first-line choice is mirtazapine, an antagonist of the 5-HT_3 receptor, which at the lowest doses (7.5 or 15 mg daily) acts to increase appetite. It is also sedating, so if given at bedtime can help patients who suffer from both anorexia and insomnia. Appetite stimulants can be used if other options are unsuccessful. However, these agents have not been well studied in older adult populations.[103] Megestrol can be tried (800 mg in liquid formulation), but should be avoided in patients at risk for thromboembolic disease. Megestrol is a progesterone derivative that increases adipose tissue and appetite, but does not increase lean muscle mass.[104] The evidence base for megestrol is mixed; some randomized trials have demonstrated some clinical improvement in quality of life indicators, prealbumin levels, and cytokine measures, whereas others have shown no significant changes in nutritional indicators and have demonstrated adverse reactions, most commonly diarrhea and venous thromboembolism.[105,106]

SUMMARY

The management of patients with dementia in LTC is a real challenge. Dementia is a devastating illness for both patients and families. There is no cure, but clinicians can make decisions that will maintain patients' function as long as possible and optimize their quality of life. Unfortunately, cholinesterase inhibitors and memantine are of limited benefit. In the realm of "limited benefit," there may be the greatest benefit when memantine and donepezil are given together to patients with moderate to advanced dementia. There is evidence that the response to cholinesterase inhibitors is variable. Consequently, it is worth titrating donepezil to 10 mg and then adding memantine also by titration to 10 mg twice a day. It is important that a cognitive assessment is performed and the results recorded in the chart before medications are administered. If within a few months the family does not notice a difference and no difference is noted on another cognitive assessment, the medication should be tapered off over a few weeks. If the family then notices that there is a decline after the cessation of the medication, the medication should be resumed.

There is a high rate of depression and agitation associated with dementia. Fortunately, quality of life can be improved significantly with effective treatment. Nondrug therapy is preferable to drug therapy for the treatment of behavioral problems. Drugs should only be used after nondrug therapy is found to be ineffective. Selection of drug therapy should be based on evidence from RCTs and guidelines.

Eating problems are characteristic of the late stage of dementia. There should be an evaluation to search for contributing factors or reversible causes. Careful comfort hand feeding and the optimization of diet should be practiced. The next article in this issue by Fulton and colleagues reviews the data on the limitations and dangers involved in the use of feeding tubes, and discusses how the goals of care should be addressed with families.

REFERENCES

1. Watkins PB, Zimmerman HJ, Knapp MJ, et al. Hepatotoxic effects of tacrine administration in patients with Alzheimer's disease [see comments]. JAMA 1994;271:992.
2. Novartis Exelon labeling update reflects report of esophageal rupture. The Pink Sheet 2001;63:24.
3. Weyer G, Erzigkeit H, Kanowski S, et al. Alzheimer's disease assessment scale: reliability and validity in a multicenter clinical trial. Int Psychogeriatr 1997;9:123.
4. Courtney C, Farrell D, Gray R, et al. Long-term donepezil treatment in 565 patients with Alzheimer's disease (AD2000): randomised double-blind trial. Lancet 2004;363:2105.
5. Tariot PN, Cummings JL, Katz IR, et al. A randomized, double-blind, placebo-controlled study of the efficacy and safety of donepezil in patients with Alzheimer's disease in the nursing home setting. J Am Geriatr Soc 2001;49:1590.
6. Winblad B, Kilander L, Eriksson S, et al. Donepezil in patients with severe Alzheimer's disease: double-blind, parallel-group, placebo-controlled study. Lancet 2006;367:1057.
7. Langa KM, Foster NL, Larson EB. Mixed dementia: emerging concepts and therapeutic implications. JAMA 2004;292:2901.
8. Grossberg GT, Desai AK. Management of Alzheimer's disease. J Gerontol A Biol Sci Med Sci 2003;58:331.
9. Holmes C, Wilkinson D, Dean C, et al. The efficacy of donepezil in the treatment of neuropsychiatric symptoms in Alzheimer disease. Neurology 2004;63:214.
10. Rainer M, Mucke HA, Kruger-Rainer C, et al. Cognitive relapse after discontinuation of drug therapy in Alzheimer's disease: cholinesterase inhibitors versus nootropics. J Neural Transm 2001;108:1327.
11. Hernandez RK, Farwell W, Cantor MD, et al. Cholinesterase Inhibitors and incidence of bradycardia in patients with dementia in the veterans affairs New England healthcare system. J Am Geriatr Soc 2009;57(11):1997–2003.
12. Gill SS, Anderson GM, Fischer HD, et al. Syncope and its consequences in patients with dementia receiving cholinesterase inhibitors: a population-based cohort study. Arch Intern Med 2009;169:867.
13. Trinh NH, Hoblyn J, Mohanty S, et al. Efficacy of cholinesterase inhibitors in the treatment of neuropsychiatric symptoms and functional impairment in Alzheimer disease. A meta-analysis. JAMA 2003;289:210.
14. Schneider LS. AD2000: donepezil in Alzheimer's disease. Lancet 2004;363:2100.
15. Lopez OL, Becker JT, Wisniewski S, et al. Cholinesterase inhibitor treatment alters the natural history of Alzheimer's disease. J Neurol Neurosurg Psychiatry 2002;72:310.
16. Sandson TA. Metrifonate for Alzheimer's disease: is the next cholinesterase inhibitor better? [letter; comment]. Neurology 1999;52:675.
17. Erkinjuntti T, Roman G, Gauthier S, et al. Emerging therapies for vascular dementia and vascular cognitive impairment. Stroke 2004;35:1010.

18. McKeith I, Del Ser T, Spano P, et al. Efficacy of rivastigmine in dementia with Lewy bodies: a randomised, double-blind, placebo-controlled international study. Lancet 2000;356:2031.
19. Reisberg B, Doody R, Stoffler A, et al. Memantine in moderate-to-severe Alzheimer's disease. N Engl J Med 2003;348:1333.
20. McShane R, Areosa Sastre A, Minakaran N. Memantine for dementia. Cochrane Database Syst Rev 2006;2:CD003154.
21. Tariot PN, Farlow MR, Grossberg GT, et al. Memantine treatment in patients with moderate to severe Alzheimer disease already receiving donepezil: a randomized controlled trial. JAMA 2004;291:317.
22. Porsteinsson AP, Grossberg GT, Mintzer J, et al. Memantine treatment in patients with mild to moderate Alzheimer's disease already receiving a cholinesterase inhibitor: a randomized, double-blind, placebo-controlled trial. Curr Alzheimer Res 2008;5:83.
23. Day K, Carreon D, Stump C. The therapeutic design of environments for people with dementia: a review of the empirical research. Gerontologist 2000;40(4):397–416.
24. O' Connor D, Phinney A, Smith A, et al. Personhood in dementia care: developing a research agenda for broadening the vision. Dementia 2007;6(1):121–42.
25. Wahl HW, Fange A, Oswald F, et al. Home environment and disability-related outcomes in aging individuals: what is the empirical evidence? Gerontologist 2009;49(3):355–67.
26. Van Hoof J, Kort HS, van Waarde H, et al. Environmental interventions and the design of homes for older adults with dementia: an overview. Am J Alzheimers Dis Other Demen 2010;25(3):202–32.
27. Kramer AF, Bherer L, Colcombe SJ, et al. Environmental influences on cognitive and brain plasticity during aging. J Gerontol A Biol Sci Med Sci 2004;59(9): 940–57.
28. Kasl-Godley J, Gatz M. Psychosocial interventions for individuals with dementia: an integration of theory, therapy, m and a clinical understanding of dementia. Clin Psychol Rev 2000;20(6):755–82.
29. Teresi JA, Holmes D, Ory MG. The therapeutic design of environments for people with dementia: further reflections and recent findings from the National Institute on Aging collaborative studies of dementia Special Care Units. Gerontologist 2000;40(4):417–21.
30. Wood W, Harris S, Snider M, et al. Activity situations on an Alzheimer's disease special care unit and resident environmental interaction, time use, and affect. Am J Alzheimers Dis Other Demen 2005;20(2):105–18.
31. Verbrugge LM, Jette AM. The disablement process. Soc Sci Med 1994;38(1): 1–14.
32. Marquardt G, Schmieg P. Dementia-friendly architecture: environments that facilitate wayfinding in nursing homes. Am J Alzheimers Dis Other Demen 2009;24(4):333–40.
33. Brawley E. Alzheimer's disease: designing the physical environment. Am J Alzheimers Dis Other Demen 1992;7(1):3–8.
34. Iwarsson SA. Long-term perspective on person-environment fit and ADL dependence among older Swedish adults. Gerontologist 2005;45(3):327–36.
35. Letts L, Law M, Rigby P, et al. Person-environment assessments in occupational therapy. Am J Occup Ther 1994;48(7):608–18.
36. Iwarsson S, Horstmann V, Carlsson G, et al. Person-environment fit predicts falls in older adults better than the consideration of environmental hazards only. Clin Rehabil 2009;23(6):558–67.

37. Wahl HW, Oswarl D, Zimprich D. Everyday competence in visually impaired older adults: a case for person-environment perspectives. Gerontologist 1999; 39(2):140–9.
38. Kearns WD, Fozard JL. Technologies to manage wandering. Chapter 15. In: Nelson Audrey L, Algase Donna L, editors. Evidence-based protocols for managing wandering behaviors. New York (NY): Springer Publishing Co; 2007. p. 277–97.
39. Horvath KJ, Harvey RM, Trudeau SA. A home safety program for community based wanderers: outcomes from the Veterans Home Safety Project. Chapter 14. In: Nelson Audrey L, Algase Donna L, editors. Evidence-based protocols for managing wandering behaviors. New York (NY): Springer Publishing Co; 2007. p. 259–76.
40. Coste JK. Learning to speak Alzheimer's. New York (NY): Houghton Mifflin; 2003.
41. Hollinger LM, Buschmann MB. Factors influencing the perception of touch by elderly nursing home residents and their health caregivers. Int J Nurs Stud 1993;30(5):445–61.
42. Burns A, Jacoby R, Levy R. Psychiatric phenomena in Alzheimer's disease: disorders of perception. Br J Psychiatry 1990;157:76–81.
43. Eriksson S, Gustafson Y, Lundin-Olsson L. Characteristics associated with falls in patients with dementia in a psychogeriatric ward. Aging Clin Exp Res 2007; 19(2):97–103.
44. Shroyer JL. Recommendations for environmental design research correlating falls and the physical environment. Exp Aging Res 1994;20(4):303–9.
45. Ulfarsson J, Robinson BE. Preventing falls and fractures. J Fla Med Assoc 1994; 81(11):763–7.
46. Zeilel J, Hyde J, Levkoff S. Best Practices: an environment-behavior model for Alzheimer special care units. Am J Alzheimers Dis Other Demen 1994; 9:4–21.
47. Connell BR, Calkins MP. Environmental design. Chapter 16. In: Nelson Audrey L, Algase Donna L, editors. Evidence-based protocols for managing wandering behaviors. New York (NY): Springer Publishing Co; 2007. p. 301–36.
48. Zuidema S, Koopmans R, Verhey F. Prevalence and predictors of neuropsychiatric symptoms in cognitively impaired nursing home patients. J Geriatr Psychiatry Neurol 2007;20:41–9.
49. Seitz D, Purandare N, Conn D. Prevalence of psychiatric disorders among older adults in long-term care homes: a systematic review. Int Psychogeriatr 2010;4: 1–15.
50. Bartels SJ, Horn SD, Smout RJ, et al. Agitation and depression in frail nursing home elderly patient with dementia-treatment characteristics and service use. Am J Geriatr Psychiatry 2003;11:231–8.
51. Selboek G, Kirkevold Ø, Engedal K. The course of psychiatric and behavioral symptoms and the use of psychotropic medication in patients with dementia in Norwegian nursing homes—a 12 month follow-up study. Am J Geriatr Psychiatry 2008;16:528–36.
52. Ballard CG, Margallo-Lana M, Fossey J, et al. A 1-year follow-up study of behavioral and psychological symptoms in dementia among people in care environments. J Clin Psychiatry 2001;62:631–6.
53. Zuidema S, Dersksen E, Verhey F, et al. Prevalence and neuropsychiatric symptoms in a large sample of Dutch nursing home patients with dementia. Int J Geriatr Psychiatry 2007;22:632–8.

54. Wetzels RB, Zuidema SU, de Jonghe JF, et al. Determinants of quality of life in nursing home residents with dementia. Dement Geriatr Cogn Disord 2010;29:189–97.
55. Conn D, Thorpe L. Assessment of behavioural and psychological symptoms associated with dementia. Can J Neurol Sci 2007;34(Suppl 1):S67–71.
56. Snowden M, Sato K, Roy-Byrne P. Assessment and treatment of nursing home residents with depression or behavioral symptoms associated with dementia: a review of the literature. J Am Geriatr Soc 2003;51:1305–17.
57. American Geriatric Society and American Association Geriatric psychiatry. Consensus statement on improving the quality of mental health care in U.S nursing homes: management of depression and behavioral symptoms associated with dementia. J Am Geriatr Soc 2003;51(9):1287–98.
58. Peskind ER. Management of depression in long-term care of patients with Alzheimer's disease. J Am Med Dir Assoc 2003;4(Suppl 6):S141–5.
59. Magai C, Kennedy G, Cohen CI, et al. A controlled clinical trial of sertraline in the treatment of depression in nursing home patients with late-stage Alzheimer's disease. Am J Geriatr Psychiatry 2000;8:66–74.
60. Williams CL, Tappen RM. Exercise training for depressed older adults with Alzheimer's disease. Aging Ment Health 2008;12:72–80.
61. Street JS, Clark S, Gannon KS, et al. Olanzapine treatment of psychotic and behavioral symptoms in patients with Alzheimer disease in nursing care facilities—a double-blind, randomized, placebo-controlled trial. Arch Gen Psychiatry 2000;57:968–76.
62. Tariot PN, Erb R, Podgorski CA, et al. Efficacy and tolerability of carmazepine for agitation and aggression in dementia. Am J Psychiatry 1998;155:54–61.
63. Coccaro EF, Kramer E, Zemishlany Z, et al. Pharmacologic treatment of noncognitive behavioral disturbances in elderly demented patients. Am J Psychiatry 1990;147:1640–5.
64. Testad I, Ballard C, Bronnick K, et al. The effect of staff training on agitation and use of restraint in nursing home residents with dementia: a single-blind, randomized controlled trial. J Clin Psychiatry 2010;71:80–6.
65. Sloan PD, Hoeffer B, Mitchell CM, et al. Effect of person-centered showering and the towel bath on bathing-associated aggression, agitation, and discomfort in nursing home residents with dementia: a randomized, controlled trial. J Am Geriatr Soc 2004;52:1795–804.
66. McCallion P, Toseland RW, Freeman K. An evaluation of a family visit education program. J Am Geriatr Soc 1999;47:203–14.
67. Cohen-Mansfield J, Deutsch LH. Agitation: subtype and their mechanisms. Semin Clin Neuropsychiatry 1996;1:325–39.
68. Cohen-Mansfield J. Assessment of agitation. Int Psychogeriatr 1996;8:233–45.
69. Sommer OH, Kirkevold O, Cvancarova M, et al. Factor analysis of the brief agitation rating scale in a large sample of Norwegian nursing home patients. Dement Geriatr Cogn Disord 2010;29:55–60.
70. Gerdner LA. Evidence-based guideline: individualized music for elders with dementia. J Gerontol Nurs 2000;36:7–15.
71. Gehrman PR, Martin JL, Shochat T, et al. Sleep-disordered breathing and agitation in institutionalized adults with Alzheimer disease. Am J Geriatr Psychiatry 2003;11:426–33.
72. Menon AS, Gruber-Baldini AL, Hebel JR, et al. Relationship between aggressive behaviors and depression among nursing home residents with dementia. Int J Geriatr Psychiatry 2001;16:139–46.

73. Cohen-Mansfield J, Billig N, Lipson S, et al. Medical correlates of agitation in nursing home residents. Gerontology 1990;36:150–8.
74. Sloan PD, Mitchell CM, Preisser JS, et al. Environmental correlates of resident agitation in Alzheimer's disease special care units. J Am Geriatr Soc 1998;46: 862–9.
75. Tariot PN, Raman R, Jakimovich L, et al. Divalproex sodium in nursing home residents with possible or probable Alzheimer disease complicated by agitation: a randomized, controlled trial. Am J Geriatr Psychiatry 2005;13:942–9.
76. Finkel SI, Lyons JS, Anderson RL, et al. A randomized, placebo-controlled trial of thiothixene in agitated, demented nursing home patients. Int J Geriatr Psychiatry 1995;10:129–36.
77. Cohen-Mansfield J, Marx MS, Dakbeel-Ali M, et al. Can agitated behavior of nursing home residents with dementia be prevented with standardized stimuli? J Am Geriatr Soc 2010;58:1459–64.
78. Burns A, Allen H, Tomenson B, et al. Bright light therapy for agitation in dementia: a randomized controlled trial. Int Psychogeriatr 2009;21:711–21.
79. Wan-ki Lin P, Chan WC, Fung-leung Ng B, et al. Efficacy of aromatherapy (*Lavandula angustifolia*) as an intervention for agitated behaviors in Chinese older persons with dementia: a cross-over randomized trial. Int J Geriatr Psychiatry 2007;22:405–10.
80. Cohen-Mansfield J, Libin A, Mark MS. Nonpharmacological treatment of agitation: a controlled trial of systematic individualized intervention. J Gerontol A Biol Sci Med Sci 2007;62A:908–16.
81. Garland K, Beer E, Eppingstall B, et al. A comparison of two treatments of agitated behaviors in nursing home residents with dementia: simulated family presence and preferred music. Am J Geriatr Psychiatry 2007;15:514–21.
82. Sung HC, Chang SM, Lee WL, et al. The effects of group music movement intervention on agitated behaviours of institutionalized elders with dementia in Taiwan. Complement Ther Med 2006;14:113–9.
83. Ancoli-Israel S, Martin JL, Gebrman P, et al. Effect of light on agitation in institutionalized patients with severe Alzheimer disease. Am J Geriatr Psychiatry 2003; 11:194–203.
84. Ballard CG, O'Brien JT, Reichelt K, et al. Aromatherapy as a safe and effective treatment for the management of agitation in server dementia: the results of a double-blind, placebo-controlled trial with Melissa. J Clin Psychiatry 2002; 63:553–8.
85. Remington R. Calming music and hand massage with agitated elderly. Nurs Res 2002;51:317–23.
86. Gerdner LA. Effects of individualized versus classical "relaxation" music on the frequency of agitation in elderly persons with Alzheimer's disease and related disorders. Int Psychogeriatr 2000;12:49–65.
87. Lyketsos CG, Veiel LL, Baker A, et al. A randomized, controlled trial of bright light therapy for agitated behaviors in dementia patients residing in long-term care. Int J Geriatr Psychiatry 1999;14:520–5.
88. Closs SJ, Barr B, Briggs M. Cognitive status and analgesic provision in nursing home residents. Br J Gen Pract 2004;54:919–21.
89. Nagaard HA, Jarland M. Are nursing home patients with dementia diagnosis at increased risk for inadequate pain treatment? Int J Geriatr Psychiatry 2005;20: 730–7.
90. Locca JF, Bula CJ, Zumbach S, et al. Pharmacological treatment of behavioral and psychological symptoms of dementia (BPSD) in nursing homes: development of

practice recommendations in a Swiss canton. J Am Med Dir Assoc 2008;9: 439–48.
91. Class CA, Schneiderder L, Farlow MR. Optimal management of behavioral disorders associated with dementia. Drugs Aging 1997;10:95–106.
92. Cohen-Mansfield J. Nonpharmacologic interventions for inappropriate behaviors in dementia. J Geriatr Psychiatry Neurol 2001;9:361–81.
93. Cohen-Mansfield J. Nonpharmacologic interventions for psychotic symptoms in dementia. J Geriatr Psychiatry Neurol 2003;16:219–24.
94. Bharani N, Snowden M. Evidence-based interventions for nursing home residents with dementia-related behavioral symptoms. Psychiatr Clin North Am 2005;28:985–1005.
95. De Deyn PP, Katz IR, rodaty H, et al. Management of agitation, aggression, and psychosis associated with dementia: a pooled analysis including three randomized, placebo-controlled double-blind trials in nursing home residents treated with risperidone. Clin Neurol Neurosurg 2005;107:497–508.
96. Ayalon L, Gum AM, Feliciano L, et al. Effectiveness of nonpharmacological interventions for the management of neuropsychiatric symptoms in patients with dementia: a systematic review. Arch Intern Med 2006;166:2182–8.
97. Daiello LA. Atypical antipsychotics for the treatment of dementia-related behaviors: an update. Med Health R I 2007;90:191–4.
98. Rodda J, Morgan S, Walker Z. Are cholinesterase inhibitors effective in the management of the behavioral and psychological symptoms of dementia in Alzheimer's disease? A systematic review of randomized, placebo-controlled trials of donepezil, rivastigmine and galantamine. Int Psychogeriatr 2009;21: 813–24.
99. Lai CK, Yeung JH, Mok V, et al. Special care units for dementia individuals with behavioral problems. Cochrane Database Syst Rev 2009;4:CD006470. DOI: 10.1002/14651858.CD006470.pub2.
100. Li I. Feeding tubes in patients with severe dementia. Am Fam Physician 2002; 65(8):1605–10.
101. Robertson RG, Montagnini M. Geriatric failure to thrive. Am Fam Physician 2004; 70(2):343–50.
102. Mitchell SL, Teno JM, Kiely DK, et al. The clinical course of advanced dementia. N Engl J Med 2009;361:1529–38.
103. Rehman HU. Involuntary weight loss in the elderly. Clin Geriatr 2005;13(7): 37–47.
104. Farrell T, Tuya A. Nutrition in the older adult. Med Health R I 2008;91(2):65–6.
105. Yeh S, Wu SY, Levine DM, et al. Quality of life and stimulation of weight gain after treatment with megestrol acetate: correlation between cytokine levels and nutritional status, appetite in geriatric patients with wasting syndrome. J Nutr Health Aging 2000;4(4):246–51.
106. Reuben DB, Hirsch SH, Zhou K, et al. The effects of megestrol acetate suspension for elderly patients with reduced appetite after hospitalization: a phase II randomized clinical trial. J Am Geriatr Soc 2005;53(6):970–5.

Palliative Care for Patients With Dementia in Long-Term Care

Ana Tuya Fulton, MD[a], Jennifer Rhodes-Kropf, MD[b,*], Amy M. Corcoran, MD[c,d], Diane Chau, MD[e,f], Elizabeth Herskovits Castillo, MD, PhD[g,h,i]

KEYWORDS

- Palliative care • Dementia • Long-term care • Tube feeding
- Pain • Transitions • Prognostication • Quality of life

Seventy percent of people in this country who have dementia die in the nursing home.[1] This article addresses the following topics on palliative care for patients with dementia in long-term care (LTC): (1) transitions of care, (2) infections, other comorbidities, and decisions on hospitalization, (3) prognostication, (4) the evidence for tube feeding or no tube feeding, (5) discussing goals of care with families/surrogate decision makers,

This work was supported by Geriatric Academic Career Awards from the Health Resources and Services Administration.
The authors have nothing to disclose.
[a] Division of Geriatrics, Department of Medicine, Warren Alpert Medical School of Brown University, Butler Hospital, 345 Blackstone Boulevard, Center House Rear #207, Providence, RI 02906, USA
[b] Division of Geriatrics, Hebrew SeniorLife and Beth Israel Deaconess Medical Center, Harvard University Medical School, Center Communities of Brookline, 100 Centre Street, Boston, MA 02446, USA
[c] Geriatric Fellowship, Division of Geriatric Medicine, Penn Medicine, Ralston-Penn Center, University of Pennsylvania, 3615 Chestnut Street, Philadelphia, PA 19104-2676, USA
[d] Palliative Medicine Fellowship, Division of Geriatric Medicine, Penn Medicine, Ralston-Penn Center, University of Pennsylvania, 3615 Chestnut Street, Philadelphia, PA 19104-2676, USA
[e] Division of Geriatric medicine, Department of Medicine, University of Nevada School of Medicine, 1000 Locust Street, MS 18, Reno, NV 89502, USA
[f] VA Community Living Center, Reno, NV, USA
[g] Geriatric Medicine Program, MAHEC (Mountain AHEC), 118 WT Weaver Boulevard, Asheville, NC 28804, USA
[h] Department of Family Medicine, UNC Chapel Hill School of Medicine, 590 Manning Drive, Chapel Hill, NC 27599, USA
[i] Givens Estates (CCRC), 2360 Sweeten Creek Road, Asheville, NC 28803, USA
* Corresponding author.
E-mail address: jrhodeskropf@hsl.harvard.edu

Clin Geriatr Med 27 (2011) 153–170
doi:10.1016/j.cger.2011.01.002 geriatric.theclinics.com

(6) types of palliative care programs, (7) pain assessment and management, and (8) optimizing function and quality of life for residents with advanced dementia.

TRANSITIONS OF CARE

Transition of care is an emerging area of research, and an important quality improvement effort to reduce rehospitalization rates and the iatrogenic complications of health care. Transitions are the actions involved in coordination of care for patients as they move through the various settings in the health care system, and these play a major role in patient outcomes.[2–4] Increasing literature describes the challenges related to transitions, and characterizes points of high risk for patients. Interventions have been studied, published, and extrapolated successfully. However, only a smaller portion of this literature is focused on transitions involving patients with dementia. Patients with dementia are among the highest risk group during transitions of care because of high rates of comorbidity, inability to participate in or understand the care transition process, and reliance on caregivers to navigate the transitions for them.

Studies examining the needs of patients and caregivers of patients with dementia note a need for smoother, more controlled, well-coordinated transitions.[3] Patients with dementia have more complicated clinical and psychosocial situations. The complications of dementia, including memory, function, mood, and behavior, negatively impact transitions for both patient and caregiver.[5] Patients with dementia have difficulty comprehending diagnoses, understanding treatment options and interventions, and coordinating appointments and recommendations among physicians and specialists.[5]

The caregiver faces unique challenges beyond these caused by the nature of the illness. For example, patients with dementia have more difficulty adhering to medication regimens and changes in dietary recommendations. Caregivers are often forced to act as the "police" and are constantly placed in the difficult position of enforcing restrictions (eg, thickened liquids) and medication adherence. Caregivers are challenged with not only caring for a loved one with a terminal illness but also enforcing unpleasant prescriptions that are difficult for the person to comprehend. The behavioral disturbances of dementia can further complicate this function, and occasionally put caregivers at risk of physical harm.

In addition, dealing with the loss of a spouse, parent, or friend from dementia can be devastating because of the loss of personality, memory, and behavior that accompanies advancing dementia. The difficulties presented by wandering, agitation, paranoia, hallucinations, and sleep disturbances are foremost for many families struggling with dementia. Existing evidence suggests that caregivers of patients with dementia are among the most stressed, both physically and emotionally.[6] Transition and caregiver support that acknowledges these symptoms is highly valuable to caregivers.

Once a patient moves into a nursing home, the family caregiver is relieved of some of the mentioned stresses. However, one must also appreciate and "debrief"/discuss the stress the nursing home staff experiences caring for residents with dementia in long-term care. Results from work focused on transitions for patients with dementia show an increased need during the 1- to 2-week period after hospital discharge.[5] This interval was the period of highest vulnerability for both patients and caregivers. Unlike in transitions with noncognitively impaired adults, caregivers continued to report the need for support up to 6 weeks after the hospital discharge.[5] Transitional interventions for dementia patients may need to be longer and should be specifically designed to target this group of patients.

Although models and interventions have been researched and tested, further investigation is needed specifically focusing on patients with dementia. Most interventions have been tested in patients transitioning back to home from acute care hospitals. More work is needed to assist in transitions to long-term care, especially for patients with dementia. Ways to improve transitions in and out of the hospital to decrease adverse events in long-term care overall, not specific to patients with dementia, are discussed by Oakes and colleagues elsewhere in this issue.

INFECTIONS, OTHER COMORBIDITIES, AND DECISIONS ON HOSPITALIZATION

Treating infections and comorbidities as much as possible on-site is now known to be the best course of action to avoid the "hazards of hospitalization" for older patients in the long-term care facility, and this is especially for those with dementia. Residents with dementia who are admitted to the hospital are more likely to develop delirium, functional incontinence, pressure sores, and infections, and to suffer from inadequate pain control and become deconditioned. Most nursing homes are able to obtain laboratory tests and radiographs on site, and are able to place lines for intravenous treatments. When in-house radiographs are not possible, arrangements can usually be made for these to be performed elsewhere and then the patient can return to the nursing home.

Long-term care providers should be familiar with the recent research by Mitchell and colleagues[7] prospectively documenting the clinical course of advanced dementia. From 2003 to 2009, data were prospectively gathered from 323 nursing home residents with advanced dementia and their health care proxies for 18 months in 22 facilities. Over 18 months, 55% of residents died. During this period the probability of a febrile episode was 53%, pneumonia 41%, and the development of an eating problem 86%. The 6-month mortality rate was 45% for residents who had a febrile episode, 47% for those with pneumonia, and 39% for those with an eating problem. Uncomfortable symptoms were common, including pain (39%) and dyspnea (46%). In the last 3 months of life, 41% of residents experienced at least one burdensome intervention (emergency room visit, hospitalization, parenteral therapy, or tube feeding).

Providers should share these findings on the natural history of advanced dementia with families when discussing goals of care. Discussing goals of care with patients and families helps them decide on the degree to which therapeutic rather than solely palliative care should be pursued. These conversations are best conducted when the resident's health is stable and not in moments of acute crisis; this allows patients to be involved in the decision-making process, and both patients and families can think about these decisions with less stress. Subsequently, when a resident develops an infection or exacerbation of a comorbidity, the provider will talk to the family again, but everyone will be better informed of the options. Furthermore, and particularly for patients with advanced dementia, the family may want a "do not hospitalize" order. Discussing goals of care with families of patients with dementia is addressed further.

Infections, especially pneumonia, are common among patients with advanced dementia.[8] A recent study rigorously evaluated the impact of antimicrobial treatment for pneumonia in long-term care residents with advanced dementia. As in the study by Mitchell and colleagues,[7] the data was obtained from the Choices, Attitudes, and Strategies for Care of Advanced Dementia at the End-of-Life (CASCADE) study funded by the National Institutes of Health. Givens and colleagues[8] evaluated the benefit of antimicrobial agents for pneumonia on two treatment goals: survival and comfort for residents when given an antimicrobial agent of any formulation (eg, intravenous, oral, intramuscular) versus no antimicrobial agent. From 2003 to 2009, data were prospectively gathered from 323 nursing home residents with advanced dementia in 22 facilities. Residents were followed for as long as 18 months or until death. The comfort level was assessed using the Symptom Management at End-of-Life in Dementia scale among residents who did not die in the 90 days after the suspected pneumonia episode. Antimicrobial agents were prescribed 91% of the time for episodes of pneumonia in the cohort. Survival was improved in the residents prescribed antibiotics of all formulations; however, comfort was not improved and more aggressive care was shown to possibly be associated with greater discomfort.

Givens and colleagues[8] suggest that if the most important goal for a resident with advanced dementia is to prolong survival, then the antibiotic may extend survival by as much as 9 months after suspected pneumonia. However, an oral agent would be best to prescribe because no difference in survival was seen among the formulations, and oral treatment is less burdensome to the patient and less costly. In contrast, if the primary goal of care is comfort, or the provider of family believes that an additional few months of life with advanced dementia will not take importance over the burdens of antibiotic treatment, then antibiotics should be withheld and palliative care should be given.

This type of analysis should also be used when evaluating where and to what extent diagnostic workups and therapeutic interventions rather than simply palliative care should be pursued when patients with more advanced dementia have other illnesses. Medical interventions must always be evaluated with an awareness that hospitalization has associated risks, and procedures may create real discomfort in frail and cognitively impaired patients. Sometimes less treatment and more comfort is a wise goal.

PROGNOSTICATION IN DEMENTIA

Prognostication is often difficult and inherently inaccurate, and the best a clinician can do is to use currently available scores in estimating survival. The goal of prognostication is often to identify patients appropriate for hospice entry or supportive care. If a clinician can improve their prediction of decline to determine appropriate levels of support, earlier discussions about advanced care planning are beneficial.

In practical use, prognostication in dementia could be viewed as rates of functional decline and the impact of comorbidities on the rate of decline. Many inherent variables make dementia prognostication challenging, including different patient characteristics, differing comorbidities, different classification systems for dementia severity, inaccurate classification of dementia type, and different methods used to predict decline.

Furthermore, depending on the clinical skill and knowledge of the clinician, the classification of severity may vary. Knowledge of the types of dementia, their natural history, and the functional scales may improve the consistency of rating severity.

The natural history of most dementia types is marked by a decline in cognition and function. Alzheimer dementia makes up the bulk of clinical cases. Other dementia types include vascular dementia, mixed dementia (Alzheimer and vascular dementia), dementia with Lewy bodies, Parkinson-related dementia, and frontal-temporal dementia. Although the early presentation of these dementias may vary greatly, their advanced stages are similar in appearance because of the severity of functional impairments that coexist in the various types. For instance, dementia with Lewy bodies may present early with impaired attention, visual hallucinations, and periods of confusion when compared with the onset of Alzheimer dementia, which presents with predominantly memory impairment. However, at the end of the disease course, both will manifest immobility and persons will be nonverbal and dependent on others to perform all activities of daily living.

Although every type of dementia varies in its progression in rate and type of decline, most dementias progress through clinically visible stages of functional deterioration. A commonly used scale to mark the Alzheimer stages of decline is the 7-step Functional Assessment Staging Test, or FAST 7 (**Table 1**). The FAST scale does not provide a time frame until death, but a nonambulatory FAST 7C is commonly considered consistent with a prognosis of less than 6 months and eligibility for hospice if the patient also exhibits one or more specific dementia-related comorbidities, such as aspiration pneumonia, infections such as urinary tract infection or sepsis, multiple stage 3 or 4 pressure ulcers, persistent fevers, or weight loss greater than 10% within 6 months. Although this scale lacks large randomized trial validation for accuracy, it is used by many hospice organizations.

In a 1997 study, Luchins and colleagues[9] examined the correlation between the survival time on enrollment in the hospice program and death or the end of the study using the FAST scale. Most patients (n = 47) survived a median of 6.9 months. However, 41% of the patients progressed outside of the FAST 7 system (ie, their survival was not predictable using the FAST functional measures in a stepwise decline through the stages).

In a similar study by Hanrahan and colleagues,[10] 45 patients were enrolled in hospice using the FAST 7 system. These investigators examined the efficacy of FAST in identifying patients with dementia who were appropriate for hospice. The survival time was measured using FAST, and the mean survival for those at enrollment reaching 7C was 4.1 months. Most died within 6 months.

Additional scales are commonly used in dementia prognostication, including the Mortality Risk Index (MRI),[11] which was developed using data from the MDS (Minimum Data Set) to generate a 12-point plus system to predict risk of death within 6 months. Having an MRI score of 12 or greater estimates the risk of mortality at 6 months to be 70% (**Table 2**). The MRI score was obtained using the MDS of patients who were newly admitted to a nursing home, and may not be replicable in home care or established long-term care patients with dementia.[12]

In another model to estimate for death within 6 months, points are assigned when risk factors are identified. The total number of points is then translated into a percent risk of death within 6 months that would be useful for prognostication and discussing goals of care/quality of life issues with families (**Table 3**).

Table 1
FAST 7 and general terminology

Stages	Clinical Function	General Terms in Dementia
1	No difficulties	Normal
2	Subjective forgetfulness	Mild
3	Decreased job functioning and organizational capacity	Moderate
4	Difficulty with complex tasks and instrumental ADLs	Moderate
5	Requires supervision with ADLs	Moderate-to-severe
6	Impaired ADLs, with incontinence	Severe
7	A. Ability to speak limited to six words B. Ability to speak limited to single word C. Loss of ambulation D. Inability to sit E. Inability to smile F. Inability to hold head up	Severe-to-terminal

Abbreviation: ADL, activity of daily living.

Table 2
MRI scores

Points	Risk Factors
1.9	Complete dependence with ADLs
1.9	Male gender
1.7	Cancer
1.6	Congestive heart failure
1.6	Oxygen therapy needed within 14 days
1.5	Shortness of breath
1.5	<25% of food eaten at most meals
1.5	Unstable medical condition
1.5	Bowel incontinence
1.5	Bedfast
1.4	Age >83 y
1.4	Not awake most of the day

Abbreviation: ADL, activity of daily living.

Although both scales are useful, general tenets of prognostication and decline for diseases overall are applicable in dementia. Thus, disease conditions that decline slowly, such as dementia, will continue to decline slowly unless another disease condition accelerates the decline, such as pneumonia.

Other performance scales have not been validated in dementia but are clinically used in dementia prognostication because many patients in advanced states have comorbid conditions that make a more general scale useful. One scale is the Karnofsky performance scale, in which 100% is considered normal function and 0% is moribund. A score of 40% to 50% is generally acceptable for supportive care, although the patients still may not meet Medicare criteria for eligibility for hospice coverage.

EVIDENCE FOR AND AGAINST TUBE FEEDING

The feeding difficulties associated with dementia often lead to consideration of feeding tubes and their role in advanced dementia. Whether to insert a feeding tube is often the most difficult decision caregivers must make despite robust evidence supporting withholding tube-feeds in older adults with advanced dementia. Families and physicians agonize over the right decision regarding feeding in advanced cases of dementia. When feeding difficulties begin, patients are in the final stages of the disease trajectory and most have months to a year of life remaining. The evidence

Table 3
Risk estimate of death within 6 months (using MRI)

Score	Risk %
0	8.9
1–2	10.8
3–5	23.2
6–8	40.4
9–11	57.0
≥12	70.0

is presented and debated, but the decision remains an emotional one for physicians, family, and loved ones. To not do everything possible to save the patient's life is often incompatible to the logical or moral framework of a loving caregiver, and the apprehension that the patient is starving to death can be difficult to shake.

The evidence supporting the decisions made about feeding tube insertion consists mostly of retrospective analyses, observational studies, and review articles, because randomized controlled trials with well-defined control groups are challenging and difficult to perform. Several key questions should inform health care providers in making this decision: (1) what are the risks and benefits of a feeding tube? (2) are alternatives available? (3) what is legally and ethically sound? and (4) what decision is cohesive with the family's moral or cultural framework?

As described in the section above, in the 18-month prospective study of 323 nursing home residents with advanced dementia, Mitchell and colleagues[7] showed that the probability of pneumonia during the study period was 41%, and that of an eating problem was as high as 85.8%. Even higher was the probability of developing an eating problem in the last 3 months of life, which occurred in 90.4% of the patients. The 6-month mortality for residents with an eating problem was 39%.

This prospective study dramatically confirmed that advanced dementia is a terminal illness, and once complications such as aspiration pneumonia or eating difficulties begin, the person is in the final stages and in the last few months of life.[7] Sadly, the study also confirmed that patients with dementia are not being referred to hospice care in the same proportions as those with other terminal diseases. Only 29% of the patients who died during the study period received hospice referrals, and most of those referrals occurred between 0 and 90 days of death, despite a high rate of symptoms of discomfort such as pain and dyspnea.

Given the evident high rate of feeding difficulty and its marked association with the end of life for patients with advanced dementia, feeding tube discussions become more critical. Feeding tubes have a place in the care of some patients, as both short- and long-term solutions. In certain groups, such as patients undergoing treatment for head and neck cancers or for those with amyotrophic lateral sclerosis (ALS), a feeding tube can prevent malnutrition and its complications and can prolong life. However, these benefits have not been found in the systematic review of the literature among patients with dementia. In 1999, in the first systematic review of the evidence, Finucane and colleagues[13] noted that feeding tube insertion in a person with advanced dementia did not prolong survival. The review also did not show that feeding tube insertion led to improved quality of life, the prevention of aspiration pneumonia, or the improved healing of pressure ulcers.[12] This landmark review presented strong evidence that tube feeding in patients with advanced dementia does not lead to the expected desired outcomes.[13,14]

Additionally, Finucane and colleagues[13] focused on evaluating the prevention of aspiration pneumonia, treatment or reversal of the consequences of malnutrition, and overall survival rate. They showed that tube feeding did not prevent aspiration pneumonia. Aspiration of oral secretions continued, as did reflux aspiration from the tube feeding material. Three case-control studies described in the review showed higher risk of aspiration pneumonia and death in tube-fed patients. In addition, studies included in the systematic review showed that jejunostomy was not associated with lower risk than gastrostomy.[13]

The review also evaluated markers of malnutrition, which did not improve with tube feeding. Weight loss and muscle wasting persisted despite appropriate calorie and protein intake.[13] Evidence suggests that the underlying effects of the chronic disease, chronic immobility, and ongoing inflammation cancel out the artificial nutrition.[14]

In addition to their failure to prevent aspiration or the complications of malnutrition, feeding tubes have associated complications and risks. Despite being an endoscopic procedure, it is invasive and has the attendant risks for infection and mortality that accompany all invasive procedures. More commonly, the tubes cause morbidity from leakage, discomfort, and occasional blocking or displacement that requires an emergency room or an outpatient visit to correct. In addition, there is a risk of needing chemical or physical restraints to prevent the patient from pulling out the tube,[14] which can lead to pressure ulcers, sedation or delirium, and other complications. Finally, the survival of patients with feeding tubes was found to be reduced compared with those who were hand-fed.[13,14]

Two large studies discussed by Finucane and colleagues[13] showed that the median survival of tube-fed patients was reduced. In the first study, the median survival of tube-fed patients was 7.5 months, and in the second, 63% of patients had died 1 year after placement of a feeding tube. However, the studies showed that carefully hand-fed patients had similar survival rates, rather than lower as initially expected. In one study, patients with dementia who required assistance eating were compared with similar nondemented counterparts in a long-term care facility. The study followed patients for 2 years and showed that patients in the hand-fed program had similar survival to those who fed themselves.[13] The systematic literature review by Li[14] reached similar conclusions. This finding is not surprising given the trajectory of advanced dementia. As elaborated by Mitchell and colleagues,[7] once feeding difficulties develop, patients are at the end of life; interventions will not alter or reverse the disease trajectory.

A frequent argument for tube feeding is that patients will be more comfortable because they will not sense hunger or thirst. However, the evidence does not support this, and in fact reviews have found that tube feeding is associated with nausea and more discomfort because of the need for restraints, leaking, skin irritation, and decreased social interaction after tube placement.[13] The concern for suffering from hunger and thirst is a common one mentioned by families considering tube feeding. Studies that have interviewed terminally ill patients still capable of reporting their symptoms show that "comfort feeding," although it does not provide adequate nutrition, was able to eliminate any feelings of hunger or thirst. Comfort feeding, or hand-feeding, involves giving patients small amounts of food, ice chips, sips of liquids, or mouth swabs.[14] This alternative is more aligned with comfort, allows social interaction, and avoids the complications of tube feeding.

Despite this evidence, and position statements of organizations such as the American Geriatrics Society, tube feeding of with patients advanced dementia continues. The reasons for this are broad, and several researchers have attempted to elaborate. First and foremost is continued misunderstanding among decision makers and physicians about the disease trajectory of advanced dementia and the effects of tube feeding. Second is the misapprehension among nursing home staff and providers that they will be cited for weight loss and failure to treat. However, newer studies show that a large number, almost two-thirds, of feeding tubes are placed in acute care hospitals.[15] Therefore, efforts are needed to guide decision making in acute care settings among providers. Third are the fears of caregivers that they are not caring for their loved one by not providing artificial feeding. Cultural and moral standards often impede families from being able to withhold artificial support. Providers must explain to families that careful hand feeding fills patients' needs without subjecting them to invasive and unbeneficial artificial feeding.[16]

Finally, cost and reimbursement barriers exist that may explain some of the continued use of feeding tubes, especially in light of the noted state and regional variations. Mitchell and colleagues[17] found that the costs to a nursing home for a non–tube-fed patient were significantly higher than those for patients with feeding tubes. Despite the higher cost of staffing to spend the time and effort required to hand-feed, these patients have a much lower reimbursement rate than those with feeding tubes. Revisions in reimbursement patterns will need to follow the clinical push to promote hand-feeding.

In summary, eating difficulties are an almost universal complication of advanced dementia, and are harbingers of the end of life. The care of patients with advanced dementia should include the involvement of hospice and the move toward comfort feeding, which should encompass supportive mouth care at the end of life and careful hand-feeding before that to make the last few months of life comfortable and help families feel that their loved ones are cared for until the end. Dissociating feeding tubes from "caring" and nutritional support in the minds of families is as important as providing financial support to nursing homes and other care settings to pay for staff dedicated to performing the time-consuming process of hand-feeding.

DISCUSSING GOALS OF CARE WITH FAMILIES/SURROGATE DECISION MAKERS

Older adults who have viewed a video depiction of advanced dementia and have heard a verbal description of disease progression are more likely to opt for comfort-focused goals of care.[18] Similar methods have been found helpful for discussing this with surrogate decision makers.[7,19] This process is somewhat controversial, because some practitioners feel that a video may unfairly bias toward a more palliative focus rather than more medically intensive interventions.

Of importance, is the most recent study by Mitchell and colleagues,[7] on the "Clinical Course of Advanced Dementia." These investigators determined that residents whose proxies had an understanding of the poor prognosis and clinical complications expected in advanced dementia were much less likely to have burdensome interventions in the last 3 months of life than were residents whose proxies did not have this understanding. The earlier section on infections and comorbidities provides the specific prognosis data from the study.

Clinicians may find it helpful to consider the different types of goal-setting depending on the given situation (**Box 1**). Difficult goals of care discussions often occur while a long-term care resident is hospitalized, often leading to changes in goals. It is important for clinicians to send the appropriate documentation of changes in advance directives (ie, do not hospitalize) and goals of care to the long-term care community, and communicate them verbally to the nursing staff or staff physician.

TYPES OF PALLIATIVE CARE PROGRAMS

The Center to Advance Palliative Care (CAPC) indentifies four models of successful integration of palliative medicine into nursing homes: (1) hospice care, (2) palliative care consultation service, (3) hospice-based consultation service, and (4) nursing home services integrated palliative care.[20]

Hospice care has been shown to improve the palliative care of residents in long-term care facilities. Specifically, hospice enrollees have their pain assessed and treated more regularly, fewer hospitalizations, and less tube feeding, intravenous fluids, and need for physical restraints at the end-of-life.[24,25] Families of patients who were not enrolled in hospice felt their loved ones who died in long-term care facilities had unmet symptom burden (particularly dyspnea), not enough communication with physicians, and a lack of adequate emotional support and resident respect.[26]

Box 1
Framework for advance care planning in long-term care

Goal-based discussions

Maximizing comfort

Maintaining function

Prolonging life

Future treatment-based options

Hospitalizations

Antibiotics

Nutrition/hydration (ie, feeding tube or intravenous fluids)

Dialysis

Code discussions

Do not resuscitate (cardiopulmonary resuscitation or cardioversion)

Do not intubate (ventilatory support)

Full code

Approach to discussion

Clarify clinical situation

Establish primary goal

Present treatment options (benefits/burdens of each)

Weigh options against values/preferences

Provide ongoing decision-making support

Data from Refs.[21–23]

Although hospice seems to benefit those who die in long-term care communities, residents and their families who are in a nursing home for a Medicare-financed subacute rehabilitation stay have potential financial burdens; the Hospice Medicare Benefit will not pay for room and board in the long-term care community for routine level of care, which “disincentives” patients on a subacute rehabilitation unit from enrolling in hospice. Note that Medicaid will pay for room and board, and in most states the Medicare Hospice Benefit will also.

PAIN ASSESSMENT AND MANAGEMENT

Undertreated or untreated pain is recognized as a widespread problem in long-term care communities.[26] Furthermore, pain in many long-term care residents with dementia may go unrecognized because of their cognitive impairment.[27] Thus, in addition to the other areas described in studies mentioned earlier, pain management also often improves with hospice involvement in the long-term care setting. For example, many studies have shown that long-term care residents enrolled in hospice have a formal pain assessment and prescription for an opioid compared with those who are not enrolled.[28–30]

Assessment tools based on nonverbal signs and symptoms of discomfort were developed and implemented to help detect pain in cognitively impaired residents, such as Pain Assessment in Advanced Dementia (**Fig. 1**)[31] and Checklist of Nonverbal Pain Indicators (**Fig. 2**).[32] Other nonspecific signs and symptoms that may suggest

Items[a]	0	1	2	Score
Breathing independent of vocalization	Normal	Occasional labored breathing. Short period of hyperventilation.	Noisy labored breathing. Long period of hyperventilation. Cheyne-Stokes respirations.	
Negative vocalization	None	Occasional moan or groan. Low-level speech with a negative or disapproving quality.	Repeated troubled calling out. Loud moaning or groaning. Crying.	
Facial expression	Smiling or inexpressive	Sad. Frightened. Frown.	Facial grimacing.	
Body language	Relaxed	Tense. Distressed pacing. Fidgeting.	Rigid. Fists clenched. Knees pulled up. Pulling or pushing away. Striking out.	
Consolability	No need to console	Distracted or reassured by voice or touch.	Unable to console, distract or reassure.	
			Total[b]	

[a]Five-item observational tool (see the description of each item below).

[b]Total scores range from 0 to 10 (based on a scale of 0 to 2 for five items), with a higher score indicating more severe pain (0="no pain" to 10="severe pain").

Fig. 1. Assessment in Advanced Dementia (PAINAD) Scale. (*Adapted from* Warden V, Hurley AC, Volicer L. Development and psychometric evaluation of the pain assessment in advanced dementia (PAINAD) scale. J Am Med Dir Assoc 2003;4:14; with permission.)

Instructions: Observe the patient for the following behaviors both at rest and during movement.

Behavior	With Movement	At Rest
1. Vocal complaints: nonverbal (Sighs, gasps, moans, groans, cries)		
2. Facial Grimaces/Winces (Furrowed brow, narrowed eyes, clenched teeth, tightened lips, jaw drop, distorted expressions)		
3. Bracing (Clutching or holding onto furniture, equipment, or affected area during movement)		
4. Restlessness (Constant or intermittent shifting of position, rocking, intermittent or constant hand motions, inability to keep still)		
5. Rubbing (Massaging affected area)		
6. Vocal complaints: verbal (Words expressing discomfort or pain [e.g., "ouch," "that hurts"]; cursing during movement; exclamations of protest [e.g., "stop," "that's enough"])		
Subtotal Scores		
Total Score		

Scoring:

Score a 0 if the behavior was not observed. Score a 1 if the behavior occurred even briefly during activity or at rest. The total number of indicators is summed for the behaviors observed at rest, with movement, and overall. There are no clear cutoff scores to indicate severity of pain; instead, the presence of any of the behaviors may be indicative of pain, warranting further investigation, treatment, and monitoring by the practitioner.

Sources:

- Feldt KS. The checklist of nonverbal pain indicators (CNPI). *Pain Manag Nurs.* 2000 Mar;1(1):13-21.
- Horgas AL. Assessing pain in persons with dementia. In: Boltz M, series ed. *Try This: Best Practices in Nursing Care for Hospitalized Older Adults with Dementia.* 2003 Fall;1(2). The Hartford Institute for Geriatric Nursing. www.hartfordign.org

Fig. 2. Checklist of Nonverbal Pain Indicators. *From* Feldt KS. The checklist of nonverbal pain indicators (CNPI). Pain Manag Nurs 2000 Mar;1(1):13–21. Horgas AL. Assessing pain in persons with dementia. In: Boltz M, series ed. Try This: Best Practices in Nursing Care for Hospitalized Older Adults with Dementia. 2003 Fall;1(2). The Hartford Institute for Geriatric Nursing. www.hartfordign.org.

pain include loss of function, gait change, resisting personal care, rubbing, restlessness, behavior change, sleep disturbances, and repetitive vocalizations.[33] When using these nonverbal tools, it is very important to pick the tool that best suits the individual long-term care resident and then reuse the same tool for follow-up assessments.

Attempting to figure out the underlying cause of pain through history and physical examination may be difficult in patients with advanced dementia, and therefore choosing the appropriate pain medication may be complicated. Acetaminophen continues to be a great therapy for pain in older adults, either alone or as an adjuvant (http://www.americangeriatrics.org/files/documents/2009_Guideline.pdf).[34] Douzjian and colleagues[35] performed an empiric trial of scheduled Tylenol, 1 g every 8 hours, and saw a decrease in the number of behavioral symptoms in 63% of patients and a discontinuation of psychotropics in 75%.

Opioids are another effective medication for pain relief, but practitioners must keep in mind the advice for geriatric prescribing: "start low and go slow." For opioid-naïve older adults, it is best to start half the smallest dose (**Table 4**) and closely monitor for side effects (eg, somnolence, confusion). When ordering opioids, other considerations include constipation prophylaxis, alert charting, holding parameters, and nonopioid adjuvants (**Table 5**). For those with dementia who are unable to communicate verbally but show other signs that there may be untreated pain, an "opioid trial" may also be effective. One small crossover trial of long-term care residents older than 85 years with advanced dementia and severe agitation despite psychotropic drugs gave 25 nursing home residents either long-acting oxycodone, 10 mg every 12 hours, or long-acting morphine, 20 mg daily. Results showed a decrease in agitated behavior according to the Cohen-Mansfield Agitation Inventory Instrument.[36]

OPTIMIZING FUNCTION AND QUALITY OF LIFE FOR RESIDENTS WITH ADVANCED DEMENTIA

Physicians who understand the harm that can be caused by unintentionally "malignant social interaction"[37–39] can make a major contribution to the creation of beneficial interpersonal environments in long-term care facilities. The manner in which professional and lay-people perceive, frame, and interact with persons with dementia can either greatly enhance function and quality of life or cause great damage.[39,40] Residents with dementia must not be framed as "the living undead" or as people who no longer have a self.[42,43]

Recent dementia-related research shows that residents with dementia often have a wide range of preserved functions.[44–49] These findings should encourage physicians to develop effective interventions. For example, recognition of the changed perceptual experience and impact of sensory stimulation in dementia has led to the development of individualized sensory stimulation therapies and sensory-based group activities

Table 4
Opioid-naïve starting doses

Opioid	Suggested Starting Dose
Morphine	2.5–5 mg PO or SL
Oxycodone	2.5–5 mg PO or SL
Hydromorphone	0.5–1 mg PO or SL

Abbreviations: PO, by mouth; SL, sublingual.

Adapted from LTC Physician Information Tool Kit Series. Palliative care in the long-term care setting. American Medical Directors Association. William D. Smucker MD CMD, Project Chair. 2007.

Table 5
Opioid ordering pearls to consider

Constipation prophylaxis	Stimulant (ie, senna) +/− osmotic agent
Alert charting	"Notify practitioner for pain >5/10 (depending on scale used in your community)" "Notify practitioner if prn opioid used 2x/12 h or 3x/24 h"
Consider holding parameters (if appropriate)	RR <10/min Pulse oximetry <92% on RA Acute change in mental status (eg, more sedated, confused)
Consider adjuvant (if appropriate)	Acetaminophen Nonsteroidal anti-inflammatory drugs Other (eg, anticonvulsants, steroids)

Abbreviations: RR, respiratory rate; RA, room air; prn, as needed.
Adapted from LTC Physician Information Tool Kit Series. Palliative Care in the Long-Term Care Setting. American Medical Directors Association. William D. Smucker MD CMD, Project Chair. 2007.

that enhance function[50–53] and diminish behavioral problems,[54–56] and thus reduce the need for potentially harmful chemical restraints. Similarly, the authors have found that behavioral interventions and altered recreational activities improve function, quality of life, and decrease distress.[57–61] Physicians can build a social/interpersonal environment that maximizes staff/caregiver acquisition of strategies for responding in meaningful effective, nonpharmaceutical ways to fearful, angry, irritable patients with dementia who communicate their distress through "difficult" or "agitated" behaviors.

Perhaps most exciting is the ongoing research and clinical work in the domain of communication. Improved understanding of the deficits and capabilities for communication with persons with dementia can be harnessed to improve function and quality of life in long-term care.

Alzheimer dementia is characterized by verbal losses that impair linear conversational ability, yet the potential for meaningful communication persists.[62–65] Focused training of the family and the long-term care team can enhance communication.[66–68] Even more exciting is the increased awareness of the capacity and drive for self-expression in the face of moderate to advanced dementia. In the past, dense verbal losses seemed to suggest that individuals with dementia had nothing to express, but this is now known not to be true. The use of dementia story circles and dance troupes,[69–73] indicates that people with dementia retain a sense of narrative meaning and a desire to communicate through stories, with preserved capacities in humor and metaphoric/poetic sensibility.[74] With this awareness, long-term care physicians can provide a higher quality of dementia care through prioritizing the need to offer story-telling, dance, art, and musical activities, which put patients in the active creative position rather than the passive recipient mode.

The long-term care team for patients with dementia will need to elevate the role of the recreation therapy department and seek essential allies in the community. Exploring examples such as these shows that improvements in function and quality of life in dementia can be achieved through adjustments in the built and social environments.

SUMMARY

Dementia is a terminal disease. Even though it cannot be cured, palliative care can make an important contribution to the comfort of patients and reduce the inevitable stress felt by their families. It is helpful to introduce the concept of palliative medicine in the earlier stages of the disease before an acute crisis. Infections and comorbidities should be treated in the long-term care facility as much as possible to minimize the inevitable risks involved in the transition between institutions and the "hazards of hospitalization." These risks are especially prevalent among long-term care residents with cognitive impairment. Practitioners can use the advance care planning framework described in this article to guide discussion of the goals of care with families and provide a framework for future discussions of disease management with families.

Discussion should be guided by the understanding of the natural history of advanced dementia as shown through the research by Mitchell and colleagues.[7] They found that most (55%) long-term care residents with advanced dementia die within 18 months of admission. During this period, the probability of a febrile episode was 53%, pneumonia 41%, and development of an eating problem 86%. The 6-month mortality rate was 45% for residents who had a febrile episode, 47% for those with pneumonia, and 39% for those with an eating problem. Feeding tubes are not recommended for persons with advanced dementia; they do not decrease the risk of aspiration pneumonia and likely increase the risk of pneumonia because more food is entering the stomach and contributing to aspiration than when the patient eats what the body dictates. Even though feeding tubes may keep patients alive for a few months longer, their quality of life is severely limited and often fraught with secondary complications.

Prognostication for dementia is inherently difficult because the disease course often has "ups and downs" of acute illnesses such as urinary tract infections and pneumonia. An imperfect but commonly used scale to mark the Alzheimer's stages of decline is the FAST 7 scale. The FAST scale does not provide a time frame until death, but it is commonly accepted that a nonambulatory FAST 7C is commonly considered consistent with a prognosis of less than 6 months and eligibility for hospice if the patient also exhibits one or more specific dementia-related comorbidities. Other prognostication tools include the MRI and Karnofsky performance scale. Note that although different types of dementia vary in their rates of decline, most dementias progress through the same clinically visible stages of functional deterioration.

Introducing a palliative care program to one's facility is challenging in these fiscally difficult times, but fortunately The Center for Advancement of Palliative Care (CAPC) has a program that is very helpful in justifying the financial commitment to palliative care. Four models for the successful integration of palliative medicine into nursing homes programs are available: (1) hospice care, (2) palliative care consultation service, (3) hospice-based consultation service, and (4) nursing home services integrated palliative care.

To meet the palliative care needs of residents with dementia in long-term care facilities who are experiencing pain but have a limited ability to communicate verbally, it is helpful to chose one of the described pain assessment instruments. This instrument should be used by all staff in a regular and consistent manner. Practitioners should remember that agitated behavior is often a consequence of underlying untreated pain. Pain should first be treated with a maximum dose acetaminophen and then oxycodone, if necessary.

Lastly, for residents with advanced dementia, it is important for practitioners to work with staff and recreational therapies to foster an environment that is as comforting and compassionate as possible. The environment should be designed to maximize comfort to all of the patient's senses.

REFERENCES

1. Mitchell SL, Teno JM, Miller SC, et al. A national study of the location of death for older persons with dementia. J Am Geriatr Soc 2005;53(2):299–305.

2. Coleman EA, Parry C, Chalmers S, et al. The care transitions intervention: results of a randomized controlled trial. Arch Intern Med 2006;166:1822–8.
3. Epstein-Lubow G, Fulton AT, Gardner R, et al. Post-hospital transitions: special considerations for individuals with dementia. Med Health R I 2010;93(4):124–7.
4. Cummings SM. Adequacy of discharge plans and re-hospitalization among hospitalized dementia patients. Health Soc Work 1999;24:249–59.
5. Naylor MD, Stephens C, Bowles KH, et al. Cognitively impaired older adults: from hospital to home. Am J Nurs 2005;105:52–61.
6. Kim Y, Schulz R. Family caregivers' strains: comparative analysis of cancer caregiving with dementia, diabetes, and frail elderly caregiving. J of Aging and Health 2008;20(5):483–503.
7. Mitchell SL, Teno JM, Kiely DK, et al. The clinical course of advanced dementia. N Engl J Med 2009;361(16):1529–38.
8. Givens JL, Jones RN, Shaffer ML, et al. Survival and comfort after treatment of pneumonia in advanced dementia. Arch Intern Med 2010;170(13):1107–9.
9. Luchins DJ, Hanrahan P, Murphy K. Criteria for enrolling dementia patients in hospice. J Am Geriatr Soc 1997;45:1054–9.
10. Hanrahan P, Raymond M, McGowan E, et al. Criteria for enrolling dementia patients in hospice: a replication. Am J Hosp Palliat Care 1999;16(1):395 400.
11. Mitchell SL, Kiely DK, Hamel MB, et al. Estimating prognosis for nursing home residents with advanced dementia. JAMA 2004;291:2734–40.
12. Fast facts concept #150. Medical College of Wisconsin Web site. Available at: http://www.mcw.edu/fastFact/ff_150.htm. Accessed August 10, 2010.
13. Finucane T, Christmas C, Travis K. Tube feeding in patients with advanced dementia. JAMA 1999;282(14):1365–70.
14. Li I. Feeding tubes in patients with severe dementia. Am Fam Physician 2002; 65(8):1605–10.
15. Kuo S, Rhodes RL, Mitchell SL, et al. Natural history of feeding-tube use in nursing home residents with advanced dementia. J Am Med Dir Assoc 2009; 10:264–70.
16. Gillick MR, Volandes AE. The standard of caring: why do we still use feeding tubes in patients with advanced dementia? J Am Med Dir Assoc 2008;9:364–7.
17. Mitchell SL, Buchanan JL, Littlehale S, et al. Tube-feeding versus hand-feeding nursing home residents with advanced dementia: a cost comparison. J Am Med Dir Assoc 2004;5:S23–9.
18. Volandes AE, Paasche-Orlow MK, Barry MJ, et al. Video decision support tool for advance care planning in dementia: randomized controlled trial. BMJ 2009;338:b2159.
19. Volandes AE, Mitchell SL, Gillick MR, et al. Using video images to improve the accuracy of surrogate decision-making: a randomized controlled trial. J Am Med Dir Assoc 2009;10(8):575–80.
20. Improving palliative care in nursing homes. Center to Advance Palliative Care; June 2007. Available at: www.capc.org/support-from-capc/capc_publications/nursing_home_report.pdf. Accessed August 10, 2010.
21. Gillick MR. Adapting advance medical planning for the nursing home. J Palliat Med 2004;7(2):357–61.
22. Mitchell SL. A 93 year-old man with advanced dementia and eating problems. JAMA 2007;298(21):2527–36.
23. Corcoran A. Advance care planning at transitions in care: challenges, opportunities, and benefits. Ann Longterm Care 2010;18(4):26–9.
24. Miller SC, Gozalo P, Mor V. Hospice enrollment and hospitalization of dying nursing home patients. Am J Med 2001;111:38–44.

25. Mitchell SL, Teno JM, Roy J, et al. Clinical and organizational factors associated with feeding tube use among nursing home residents with advanced cognitive impairment. JAMA 2003;290:73–80.
26. Teno JM, Clarridge BR, Casey V, et al. Family perspectives on end-of-life care at the last place of care. JAMA 2004;291:88–93.
27. Reynolds KS, Hanson LC, DeVellis RF, et al. Disparities in pain management between cognitively intact and cognitively impaired nursing home residents. J Pain Symptom Manage 2008;35:388–96.
28. Miller SC, Mor V, Wu N, et al. Does receipt of hospice care in nursing homes improve the management of pain at the end of life? J Am Geriatr Soc 2002;50:507–15.
29. Miller SC, Mor V, Teno J. Hospice enrollment and pain assessment and management in nursing homes. J Pain Symptom Manage 2003;26:791–9.
30. Buchanan RJ, Choi M, Wang S, et al. End-of-life care in nursing homes: residents in hospice compared to other end-stage residents. J Palliat Med 2004;7:221–32.
31. Warden V, Hurley AC, Volicer L. Development and psychometric evaluation of the pain assessment in advanced dementia (PAINAD) scale. J Am Med Dir Assoc 2003;4:9–15.
32. Feldt KS. The checklist of nonverbal pain indicators. Pain Manag Nurs 2000;1: 13–21.
33. Hurley AC, Volicer BJ, Hanrahan PA, et al. Assessment of discomfort in advanced Alzheimer patients. Res Nurs Health 1992;15(5):369–77.
34. American Geriatrics Society Panel on the Pharmacological Management of Persistent Pain in Older Persons. Pharmacological management of persistent pain in older persons. J Am Geriatr Soc 2009;57:1331–46.
35. Douzjian M, Wilson C, Shultz M, et al. A program to use pain control medication to reduce psychotropic drug use in residents with difficult behavior. Ann Longterm Care 1998;6(5):174–9.
36. Manfredi PL, Breuer B, Wallenstein S, et al. Opioid treatment for agitation in patients with advanced dementia. Int J Geriatr Psychiatry 2003;18(8):700–5.
37. Kitwood T, Bredin K. Towards a theory of dementia care: personhood and well-being. Ageing Soc 1992;12:269–87.
38. Sabat SR. Excess disability and malignant social psychology; a case study of Alzheimer's disease. J Community Appl Soc Psychol 1994;4(3):157–66.
39. Kitwood T. Towards a theory of dementia care: the interpersonal process. Ageing Soc 1993;13(1):51.
40. Teri L, Uomoto JM. Reducing excess disability in dementia patients. Clin Gerontol 1991;10(4):49–63.
41. Reifler BV, Larson E. Excess disability in dementia of the Alzheimer's type. In: Light E, Lebowitz B, editors. Alzheimer's disease and family stress. Rockville (MD): Taylor and Francis Press; 1990. p. 363–82.
42. Sabat SR, Harre R. The construction and deconstruction of self in Alzheimer's disease. Ageing Soc 1992;12(4):443.
43. Post SG. The moral challenge of Alzheimer's disease: ethical issues from diagnosis to dying. Baltimore (MD): JHU Press; 2000.
44. Beatty WW, Brumback RA, Vonsattel JP. Autopsy-proven Alzheimer disease in a patient with dementia who retained musical skill in life. Arch Neurol 1997; 54(12):1448.
45. Venneri A, Shanks MF. Preservation of golf skills in a case of severe left lobar frontotemporal degeneration. Neurology 2001;57:521–4.
46. Bosche-Domènech A, Nagel R, Sánchez-Andrés JV. Prosocial capabilities in Alzheimer's patients. J Gerontol B Psychol Sci Soc Sci 2010;65B:119–28.

47. Beatty WW, Rogers CL, Rogers RL, et al. Piano playing in Alzheimer's disease: longitudinal study of a single case. Neurocase 1999;5(5):459–69.
48. Beatty WW, Winn P, Adams RL, et al. Preserved cognitive skills in dementia of the Alzheimer type. Arch Neurol 1994;51(10):1040–6.
49. Cuddy LL, Duffin J. Music, memory, and Alzheimer's disease: is music recognition spared in dementia, and how can it be assessed? Med Hypotheses 2005; 64(2):229–35.
50. Heyn P. The effect of a multisensory exercise program on engagement, behavior, and selected physiological indexes in persons with dementia. Am J Alzheimers Dis Other Demen 2003;18(4):247–51.
51. Baker R, Bell SL, Baker E, et al. A randomised controlled trial of the effects of multi-sensory stimulation (MSS) for people with dementia. Br J Clin Psychol 2001;40(1):81–96.
52. Roumen VM. Multisensory stimulation for elderly with dementia: a 24-week single-blind randomized controlled pilot study. Am J Alzheimers Dis Other Demen 2008; 23:372–6.
53. Graf A, Wallner C, Schubert V. The effects of light therapy on mini-mental state examination scores in demented patients. Biol Psychiatry 2001;50:725–7.
54. Lyketsos C, Veiel LL, Baker A, et al. A randomised controlled trial of bright light therapy for agitated behaviours in dementia patients residing in long-term care. Int J Geriatr Psychiatry 1999;14:520–5.
55. Burns A, Byrne J, Ballard C, et al. Sensory stimulation in dementia: an effective option for managing behavioral problems. Br Med J 2002;325(7376): 1312–3.
56. Haffmanns PM, Sival RC, Lucius SA, et al. Bright light therapy and melatonin in motor restless behaviour in dementia: a placebo-controlled study. Int J Geriatr Psychiatry 2001;16:106–10.
57. Kasl-Godley J, Gatz M. Psychosocial interventions for individuals with dementia: an integration of theory, therapy, m and a clinical understanding of dementia. Clin Psychol Rev 2000;20(6):755–82.
58. Spira AP, Edelstein B. Behavioral interventions for agitation in older adults with dementia: an evaluative review. Int Psychogeriatr 2006;18(12):195–225.
59. Volicer L, Simard J, Pupa JH, et al. Effects of continuous activity programming on behavioral symptoms of dementia. J Am Med Dir Assoc 2006;7(7):426–31.
60. Rogers JC, Holm MB, Burgio LD, et al. Excess disability during morning care in nursing home residents with dementia. Int Psychogeriatr 2000;12(2):267–82.
61. Paquet C, St-Arnaud-McKenzie D, Ma ZF, et al. More than just not being alone: the number, nature, and complementarity of meal-time social interactions influence food intake in hospitalized elderly patients. Gerontologist 2008;48(5): 603–11.
62. Powell JA. Communication interventions in dementia. Rev Clin Gerontol 2000; 10(2):161–8.
63. Sabat SR. The experience of Alzheimer's disease life through a tangled veil. Malden (MA): Wiley-Blackwell; 2001.
64. Bartol MA. Dialogue with dementia: nonverbal communication in patients with Alzheimer's disease. J Gerontol Nurs 1979;5(4):21–31.
65. Hummert ML, Wiemann JM, Nussbaum JF. Interpersonal communication in older adulthood: interdisciplinary theory and research. Sage Publications; 1994.
66. Sabat SR. Facilitating communication with an Alzheimer's disease sufferer through the use of indirect repair. In: Hamilton HE, editor. Language and communication in old age. New York (NY): Social Science Press; 1999.

67. Altus DE, Engelman KK, Mathews RM. Using family-style meals to increase participation and communication in persons with dementia. J Gerontol Nurs 2002;28(9):47–53.
68. Vorthems RC. Clinically improving communication through touch. J Gerontol Nurs 1991;17(5):6–10.
69. Bastings AD. Time slips: creative storytelling with people with dementia. UWM Center on Age and Community; 2004.
70. Holm AK, Lepp M, Ringsberg KC. Dementia: involving patients in storytelling—a caring intervention: a pilot study. J Clin Nurs 2005;14(2):256–63.
71. Palo-Bengtsson L, Ekman SL. Emotional response to social dancing and walks in persons with dementia. Am J Alzheimers Dis Other Demen 2002;17(3):149–53.
72. Van de Winckel A, Feys H, de Weerds WS, et al. Cognitive and behavioral effects of music-based exercises in patients with dementia. Clin Rehabil 2004;18(3): 253–60.
73. Lepp M, Ringsberg KC, Holm AK, et al. Dementia—involving patients and their caregivers in a drama programme: the caregivers' experiences. J Clin Nurs 2003;12(6):873–81.
74. Bastings AD. Forget memory: creating better lives for people with dementia. Baltimore (MD): Johns Hopkins U Press; 2009.

Medications in Long-Term Care: When Less is More

Thomas W. Meeks, MD[a,*], John W. Culberson, MD[b,c], Monica S. Horton, MD, MSc[d,e]

KEYWORDS

• Long-term care • Inappropriate prescribing • Polypharmacy
• Psychotropics • Opiates • Sedatives

HISTORY OF MEDICATION REDUCTION IN LONG-TERM CARE

The Nursing Home Reform Act (OBRA-87) enacted in 1987 called for sweeping changes in the standards of care in nursing homes in accordance with new, more demanding federal regulations. For example, OBRA-87 called for a new approach to the use of antipsychotics in persons with dementia. Because antipsychotics were regarded as frequently inappropriate chemical restraints in long-term care (LTC), OBRA-87 mandated dose reductions in antipsychotics in an effort to discontinue them whenever possible. OBRA-87 proposed that a safer, more supportive environment in LTC settings would facilitate such reductions in antipsychotic doses.[1]

Overall rates of potentially inappropriate prescribing in older adults have ranged from 12% to 40%, depending on the setting, criteria, and population sampled.[2] Developing from burgeoning concerns for polypharmacy and potential iatrogenic toxicity of medication in older adults, expert consensus lists of potentially inappropriate pharmacotherapy in the elderly (PIPE) began to emerge. In general, drugs with activity in the central nervous system (CNS) were commonly placed on these PIPE lists, and hence our focus on such medications in this review.

This work was supported by the following Geriatric Academic Career Awards: (1) K01 HP00047-02 (Dr. Meeks) (2) K01 HP00080-02 (Dr. Culberson) (3) K01 HP00114-02 (Dr. Horton).
The authors have no conflicts of interest to disclose.
[a] Department of Psychiatry, Division of Geriatric Psychiatry, University of California, 9500 Gilman Drive, La Jolla, San Diego, CA 92093, USA
[b] Department of Medicine, Baylor College of Medicine, One Baylor Plaza, BCM620, Houston, TX 77030, USA
[c] Extended Care Line, Michael E. DeBakey VA Medical Center, 2002 Holcombe, 110, Houston, TX 77030, USA
[d] University of Texas Health Science Center, 7703 Floyd Curl Drive, San Antonio, TX 78229, USA
[e] South Texas Veterans Health Care System, 7400 Merton Minter, San Antonio, TX 78229, USA
* Corresponding author. 9300 Campus Point Drive, MC 7602, La Jolla, CA 92037.
E-mail address: tmeeks@ucsd.edu

Clin Geriatr Med 27 (2011) 171–191
doi:10.1016/j.cger.2011.01.003 geriatric.theclinics.com

In 1991, Dr Mark Beers spearheaded a group of 12 experts in geriatrics to develop the first well-recognized PIPE list, intended specifically for older adults in LTC settings.[3] This list was subsequently referred to as the Beers list and future iterations made this probably the most well-recognized PIPE list among practitioners in geriatrics. For example, in 1997, another PIPE list, updated and expanded to include community-dwelling older adults, was published.[4] Much of the 1997 version of the Beers list was incorporated into the Centers for Medicare and Medicaid Services' Interpretive Guidelines for Long-Term Care Facilities to evaluate a nursing home's compliance with medication-related regulation. Most recently, in 2002, another iteration of the Beers list was issued, this time more explicitly explaining the process of arriving at the recommendations.[5] A 5-step modified Delphi method of expert panel consensus was implemented to generate 2 categories for medications: (1) should generally be avoided in all elderly patients and (2) should generally be avoided in elderly patients with a specific illness/symptom.

Zhan and colleagues[6] in 2001 published their own PIPE list specifically citing a criticism of previous Beers PIPE lists that they lacked the sufficient sensitivity and specificity of any explicit criteria. In an effort to overcome this limitation, they convened a 7-person panel of experts in geriatrics, pharmacoepidemiology, and pharmacy, who ultimately categorized PIPE into 3 categories: (1) always to be avoided, (2) rarely appropriate, and (3) some indications but often inappropriate. A more recent PIPE list has emerged from the Healthcare Effectiveness Data and Information Set (HEDIS) 2006.[7] This list came about as only a small part of a large national program, the National Committee on Quality Assurance. The HEDIS 2006 PIPE list and subsequent updated iterations were developed using the Delphi method to examine and categorize drugs to avoid in older adults. Comparisons among the various PIPE lists are delineated in **Table 1**.

The concerns regarding antipsychotic use in older adults with dementia have been amplified substantially since OBRA-87 because of their recent black-box warnings. In 2003, a warning was issued for risperidone (Risperdal) regarding its increased risk of cerebrovascular adverse events including stroke. Soon thereafter similar black-box warnings for cerebrovascular adverse events were issued for olanzapine (Zyprexa) and aripiprazole (Abilify). Subsequent warnings advised that, as a class, antipsychotics increased the risk of mortality from 2.6% to 4.5% (vs placebo) over the course of 10 to 12 weeks.[8] Never has the issue of the potential adverse events of CNS-acting agents among older adults been so front and center in geriatrics.

PREVALENCE OF NEUROPSYCHIATRIC ILLNESSES IN LTC

The use of psychotropic medications in LTC is common in part because neuropsychiatric illnesses are prevalent in this setting. Dementia affects 50% or more of LTC residents, with the most common causes being (in order) Alzheimer disease (AD), Lewy-body dementia, vascular dementia, and frontotemporal dementia.[9] Dementia-associated neuropsychiatric symptoms, such as psychosis, aggression, and depression, occur in 80% to 100% of patients with dementia at some point in the illness course.[10] Such neuropsychiatric symptoms remain one of the most challenging aspects of dementia to manage as they worsen patient and caregiver quality of life, often resulting in hastened placement of the patient outside the home. Furthermore, no treatments have been approved by the US Food and Drug Administration (FDA) for any dementia-related neuropsychiatric symptom. All commonly used off-label treatments carry the burden of substantial potential toxicity, lack of proven efficacy, or both. Also common in dementia, delirium was noted to have a 21.8% 1-month

Table 1
Psychotropic medications listed on some of the most prominent lists of potentially inappropriate medications for use in older adults

Drug	Beers 1991	Beers 1997	Zhan 2001	Beers 2002	HEDIS 2009
{Barbiturates}	*	⇑	1	⇑	√
{Benzodiazepines}	•				
Diazepam	•	⇑	2	⇑	√
Flurazepam	•	⇑	1	⇑	√
Chlordiazepoxide	•	⇑	2	⇑	√
Quazepam				⇑	
Halazepam				⇑	
Chlorazepate				⇑	
Meprobamate	•	⇑	1	⇑	√
Oxazepam	*	⇓*		⇑*	
Temazepam	*	⇓*		⇑*	
Triazolam	*	⇓*		⇑*	
Lorazepam		⇓*		⇑*	
Alprazolam		⇓*		⇑*	
Diphenhydramine	*	⇓/⇓*/⇑*	3	⇑	√
Hydroxyzine		⇓/⇓*/⇑*	3	⇑	√
Zolpidem		⇓*			
{Sedatives}		⇑*			
Amitriptyline	•	⇑	3	⇑	√
Doxepin		⇑	3	⇑	
Desipramine		⇓*			
Fluoxetine				⇑	
Bupropion				⇑*	
{SSRIs}		⇓*		⇓*	
{MAOIs}		⇓*		⇑*	
{TCAs}		⇑*/⇑*/⇑*		⇑*/⇑*/⇑*/⇓*	
Haloprediol	*	*			
Thiothixene				⇑*	
Thioridazine	*	⇓*		⇑	√
Mesoridazine				⇑	√
Chlorpromazine		⇓*		⇑*	
{Typical APs}				⇑*	
Clozapine		⇓*		⇑*	
Olanzapine				⇓*	
{Amphetamines}		⇑*		⇑	√
Tacrine				⇑*	

Beers lists: •, avoid in general; *, avoid in certain situations or doses; ⇑, high potential for adverse effect; ⇓, low potential for adverse effects.
HEDIS 2009: √, included among high-risk medications to avoid in elderly patients.
Zhan criteria: 1, always avoid; 2, rarely appropriate; 3, sometimes indicated.
Abbreviations: AP, antipsychotic; MAOI, monoamine oxidase inhibitor; SSRI, selective serotonin reuptake inhibitor; TCA, tricyclic antidepressant; {xxxx}, a class of medications in general.

prevalence in LTC settings in Iowa, although precise prevalence estimates are not well established.[11]

The prevalence of major depressive disorder (MDD) in LTC seems to range from 10% to 15%, whereas that of subsyndromal depression (also associated with significant morbidity) has ranged from 33% to 61% in various LTC studies.[12] There have been few large-scale studies of antidepressants in LTC and/or among persons with comorbid dementia. Anxiety disorders may also affect older adults in LTC. One report diagnosed an anxiety disorder in 2.3% of older adults on admission to LTC.[13] Data from studies in 1996 and 2005, respectively, provided similar estimates of the prevalence of anxiety disorders among older LTC residents, including, among the first sample, a 2.8% prevalence of generalized anxiety disorder (GAD) and 1.9% prevalence of panic disorder (total 4.7%),[14] and a 5.7% prevalence of all *Diagnostic and Statistical Manual of Mental Disorders (Fourth Edition)* anxiety disorders in the 2005 study.[15]

More serious and persistent mental illness is less prevalent in LTC settings. The reasons are likely multifactorial, including discriminatory exclusion of persons with such diagnoses from certain LTC facilities as well as early mortality of persons with illnesses such as bipolar disorder and schizophrenia. The data on the prevalence of bipolar disorder in LTC are scant, with only 1 article from 2005 reporting a prevalence of 0.5% on admission to LTC (lower than the 1%–2% rate reported among general adult populations).[13] Similar prevalence estimates for schizophrenia (0.5%) were reported in the same study of persons undergoing LTC admission, again lower than the 1% prevalence widely quoted in younger adult populations.[13] Few data also exist regarding the epidemiology of substance use diagnoses among older adults on admission to or during the course of stay in LTC.

MEDICATION REDUCTION: WHY, WHEN, HOW, AND WHAT?

Why?

There are several reasons why reducing medications among LTC residents should be a potential therapeutic goal for geriatricians. A typical LTC resident is on 7 or more prescription medications.[16] Older adults are more susceptible to adverse medication side effects because of various age-related changes in the pharmacokinetic and pharmacodynamic effects of drugs; adverse reactions are almost 7 times more common in adults in their 70s than among those in their 20s. An example is the commonly unrecognized cumulative anticholinergic effects of several medications, which may lead to increased cognitive decline, delirium, constipation, and urinary retention, among other effects.[17] This finding is particularly germane to older adults because, with age, the brain progressively loses cholinergic reserve, constipation commonly becomes an age-related symptom that decreases quality of life, and age-associated prostatic hypertrophy leaves older men vulnerable to iatrogenic urinary retention.

Polypharmacy (being on multiple simultaneous medications) is not de facto bad practice in the care of certain older adults, but there are high rates of older adults in LTC receiving probably inappropriate (harmful or of no clear benefit) medications.[16] The increased morbidity, hospitalization rates, mortality, and health care expenditures associated with inappropriate prescribing patterns among older adults certainly warrant increased vigilance for PIPE.[18]

One often unspoken issue that promotes polypharmacy is physician discomfort when no specific therapy (usually expected in the form of a medication in the United States) can change the patient's course of illness. Prescribing a medication may give clinicians and patients/family members a false sense of reassurance that at least something tangible was done. Geriatricians in particular should gain a comfort level permitting them to suggest no pharmacotherapy when it is not truly indicated. For instance, effects of long-term preventive medications may require more time to confer significant benefits than the patient's life expectancy (eg, statins for prevention of cardiovascular disease).

When?

It is good practice to establish a routine frequency (eg, twice yearly) for reviewing LTC residents' medication lists for inappropriate or unnecessary medications. Other important times to conduct such a review are during transitions of care (eg, admission to an LTC facility, discharge from a hospitalization). Patients with psychiatric disorders or disorders with persistent pain warrant even more vigilance. It is also important not to forget PRN (as needed) medications and to justify their ongoing use or discontinue them.

How?

Changes in medication therapy should involve discussions with patients and/or proxy decision makers regarding a medication's risk-benefit profile for that specific patient. Depending on the medication at hand, discontinuation may be achieved abruptly or may require a gradual taper (eg, with long-term use of benzodiazepines or opiates.) Successful systematic programs for reduction of certain potentially inappropriate medications are discussed in further detail later.

What?

The answer to this question is the core part of this review: describing which medications are common offenders in PIPE lists as well as potentially more appropriate alternatives. The discussion is organized according to medication classes commonly seen on PIPE lists. There are no absolutes in prohibitions against using most medications in older adults; nonetheless, avoiding or discontinuing many of the medications discussed later is more often more appropriate care for LTC residents than not doing so. Several CNS-acting medication classes are discussed in more detail.

Antipsychotics

As described in the history of medication reduction in LTC, antipsychotic medications have generally been at the forefront of medications targeted for reduction as a result of inappropriate use in LTC. The concerns have spanned from OBRA-87 to the more recent black-box warnings for antipsychotics as a class (typical and atypical) regarding about a 2% increased absolute risk of mortality in older persons with dementia (again, that includes ≥50% of LTC residents). The cause of death in most cases was infection (eg, pneumonia) or sudden cardiac death. Although direct causal pathways are unknown, excessive sedation among persons commonly already compromised in swallowing function could easily lead to aspiration pneumonia.

Antipsychotics are also known to affect cardiac conduction, often prolonging the QT_c interval (the corrected QT interval on electrocardiogram), which may lead to fatal arrhythmias such as torsades de pointes. A postulated mechanism is antipsychotic interference with cardiac potassium channels leading to prolonged QT intervals.[19] There are differences in the propensity to cause significant QT_c prolongation among various antipsychotics, prompting the inclusion of certain agents on various PIPE lists and/or withdrawal of some medications from the market (eg, thioridazine [Mellaril] and mesoridazine [Serentil]). A large study reported that persons aged 30 to 74 years with varied diagnoses taking antipsychotics (vs antipsychotic-naive persons) had a doubled incidence rate of sudden cardiac death, although it remained a rare event (absolute rates: nonusers, 0.143%; typical antipsychotic users, 0.294%; atypical antipsychotic users, 0.28%).[20] Among atypical antipsychotics, ziprasidone (Geodon) has received the most attention for potential QT_c prolongation, with reports of average prolongations of 10 ms. This finding, combined with fewer studies among older adults, twice-daily dosing, and need for concomitant food intake to ensure adequate absorption, has made ziprasidone a rare choice for older adults prescribed an atypical antipsychotic.

The discussion of potential toxicity of antipsychotics among LTC residents becomes even more germane in light of evidence questioning whether they are even effective for their most common (off-label) use in older adults: dementia-associated psychosis and agitation/aggression. The multisite CATIE-AD (Clinical Antipsychotic Trials in Intervention Effectiveness–Alzheimer Disease) trial compared risperidone, olanzapine, quetiapine (Seroquel), and placebo for psychosis and/or agitation in persons with AD.[21] There was no difference in overall effectiveness (time to treatment discontinuation) between any of the active treatments or placebo. Superior efficacy in symptom reduction with risperidone and olanzapine was offset by early treatment discontinuation because of adverse events. Other evidence supports modest efficacy of atypical antipsychotics for psychosis and/or agitation in dementia; a 2006 review of 15 randomized controlled trials (RCTs) reported that, combining data for individual drugs, psychosis scores improved significantly with risperidone treatment (average dose 0.5–1.5 mg/d), and that global neuropsychiatric symptoms improved with aripiprazole (average dose 5–15 mg/d) and risperidone.[22]

Despite the obvious limitations of antipsychotics when used for dementia-related neuropsychiatric symptoms, there is no FDA-approved medication for treating psychosis or aggression in dementia. Because these symptoms are common and produce a variety of potential adverse effects themselves, clinicians are now often left in a quandary. A proposed algorithm for the careful consideration of the off-label use of an atypical antipsychotic among older adults with dementia has been proposed (**Fig. 1**).[8] No other pharmacotherapy has shown a better evidence-based risk-benefit profile for similar symptoms.

Psychosocial/behavioral treatments are underused in part because they are time-intensive and poorly reimbursed, but they are also generally more difficult to study empirically than medications. This finding leaves unanswered questions as to the efficacy of proposed psychosocial/behavioral therapies for dementia-associated psychosis/agitation. In a recent review, the best empirical evidence for RCTs using psychosocial/behavioral therapies was for: (1) caregiver psychoeducation/support, (2) music therapy, (3) cognitive stimulation therapy, (4) Snoezelen therapy, (5) behavioral management-based techniques, and (6) staff training/education.[23] There have also been systematic studies targeting reduction/cessation of antipsychotics in LTC, with effective results.[24–26] This finding reinforces the notion that even if deemed appropriate for a given patient at a given time, trial tapers off antipsychotics should be considered every 3 to 6 months.

The clearest indications for antipsychotics in older adults are for schizophrenia or bipolar disorder. Quetiapine and aripiprazole have received recent FDA approval as adjunctive therapy for MDD, but data are limited in older adults. Extrapolating from RCTs and studies of real-world prescribing patterns, antipsychotic doses in older adults with these illnesses should be one-third to one-half those used in younger patients. A large study sponsored by the National Institutes of Health recently called into question the superiority of atypical over typical antipsychotics for schizophrenia,[27] but each class has its own potential side effect liabilities. The probable exception to this comparison is clozapine (Clozaril), which has shown superior efficacy to other antipsychotics in schizophrenia as well as protective benefits against suicide.

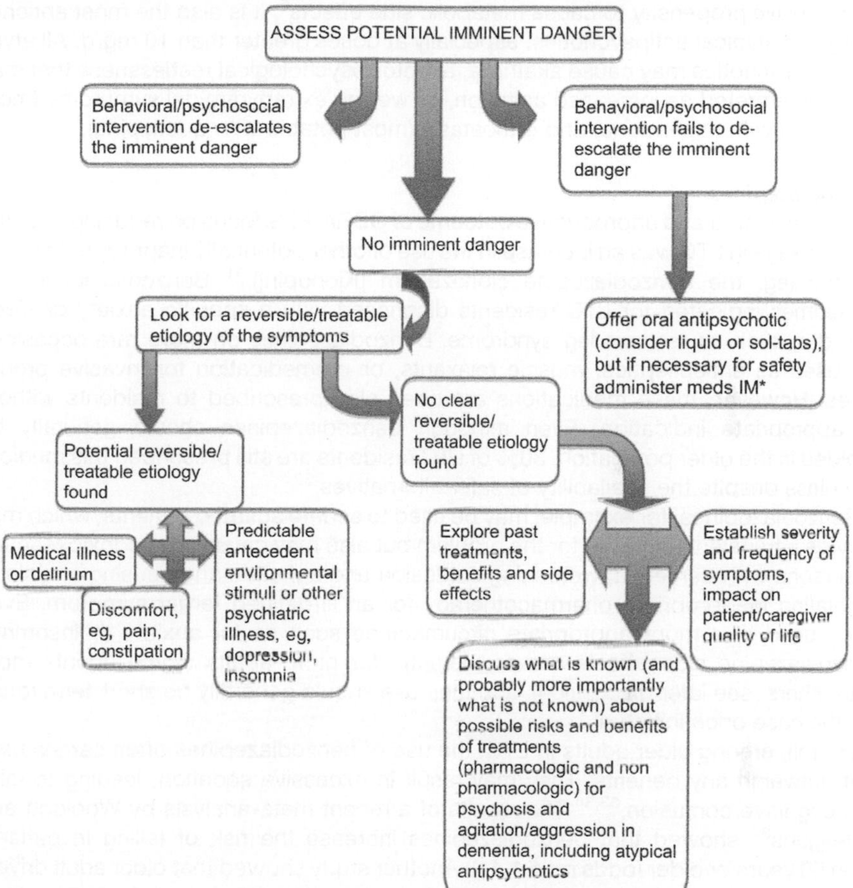

Fig. 1. A proposed algorithm for decision-making regarding the use of antipsychotics in older adults with dementia-related psychosis and/or agitation. (*) IM, intramuscularly. (*Data from* Meeks TW, Jeste DV. Beyond the black box: what is the role for antipsychotics in dementia? Curr Psychiatr 2008;7:50–65.)

However, its use in older adults is rare because of its strong anticholinergic properties, need for frequent laboratory tests (to monitor for agranulocytosis), and other unique side effects (eg, risk for seizures and cardiomyopathy).

When choosing amongst the other available antipsychotics, the side effect profile takes precedence. Typical antipsychotics appear on certain PIPE lists because of older adults' sensitivity to developing parkinsonism and tardive dyskinesia (TD). The risk of TD is 4 to 5 times higher in older versus younger patients with schizophrenia.[28] This risk is likely diminished by use of atypical versus typical antipsychotics.[29] However, atypical antipsychotics seem more likely to cause metabolic abnormalities such as hyperglycemia, dyslipidemia, and abdominal weight gain. Clinical experience along with published data such as the American Psychiatric Association/American Diabetes Association guidelines suggest that metabolic risks are highest for clozapine and olanzapine, intermediate for quetiapine and risperidone, and lowest for aripiprazole and ziprasidone.[30] Olanzapine was included in the Beers 2002 PIPE list because of its relative propensity to cause metabolic side effects[5]; it is also the most anticholinergic of atypical antipsychotics, especially at doses greater than 10 mg/d. All atypical antipsychotics may cause akathisia, a motor/psychological restlessness that may be misinterpreted as increased agitation, as well as extrapyramidal symptoms (most prominent with risperidone) and orthostasis (most notable with quetiapine).

Benzodiazepines

An unanticipated and unproductive outcome of OBRA-87's focus on reducing antipsychotic usage in LTC was an increase in the use of other potentially inappropriate medications (eg, the benzodiazepine clonazepam [Klonopin]).[31] Benzodiazepines are sometimes indicated for LTC residents diagnosed with a specific anxiety or sleep disorder, such as restless leg syndrome. Benzodiazepines on more rare occasions are used as antiepileptics, muscle relaxants, or premedication for invasive procedures. However, these medications are often also prescribed to residents without an appropriate indication. Even although benzodiazepines should generally be avoided in the older population, 30% of LTC residents are still prescribed this medication class despite the availability of safer alternatives.[32]

Benzodiazepines, for example, may be used to sedate agitated patients, which may provide a transient band-aid for the problem but also may cause a paradoxic reaction in persons with dementia, worsening confusion and agitation and causing a cycle of escalating inappropriate pharmacotherapy for an ill-defined target symptom. Even when used in a more appropriate circumstance such as for anxiety or insomnia, benzodiazepine side effects are problematic for older adults (some agents more than others, see later discussion), and their use should generally be short-term (often not the case once initiated).

Overall, among older adults in LTC, the use of benzodiazepines often carries risks that outweigh any benefits. They may result in excessive sedation, leading to falls, and cognitive confusion.[33,34] The results of a recent meta-analysis by Woolcott and colleagues[35] showed that benzodiazepines increase the risk of falling in patients aged 60 years or older (odds ratio 1.41). Another study showed that older adult drivers using benzodiazepines with a long half-life had an increased risk of motor vehicle collisions.[36] Furthermore, benzodiazepines cause physical (if not psychological) tolerance and dependence even if they are not misused, and withdrawal can be difficult. Several studies have shown effective methods of decreasing sedative and antipsychotic use through multidisciplinary teams. One Swedish study showed that regularly occurring multidisciplinary team meetings aiming to improve health care provider teamwork decreased the usage of psychotropics by 19%, and benzodiazepines by 37%.[26] Another study by Westbury and colleagues[25] used an interdisciplinary, multifaceted strategy to decrease antipsychotic and benzodiazepine use by using prescription audits, feedback, and educational sessions.

Recommendations to avoid certain benzodiazepines have been present since 1991 because there are significant inherent pharmacokinetic differences among various agents in this class as well as age-related differences in their metabolism. Meaningful pharmacokinetic differences include those related to half-lives and hepatic metabolism; for instance, temazepam (Restoril) and lorazepam (Ativan) require only hepatic glucuronidation but not cytochrome P450 activity, and are thus less susceptible to age-related alterations in metabolism or medication interactions. On the other hand, diazepam (Valium) has a problematically long half-life in older adults, especially because it stores in and is slowly released from adipose tissue, which increases relative to muscle mass with age. The Beers criteria 1991 recommended avoiding all long-acting benzodiazepines such as diazepam in older adults.[3] In 1997, the Beers criteria expanded the list of benzodiazepines one should avoid to include short-acting benzodiazepines, beyond a specified dose range.[4] In 2002, the Beers criteria were once again updated, emphasizing the need to prescribe smaller doses of benzodiazepines, if at all, particularly among persons with chronic obstructive pulmonary disease or those with a history of syncope and/or falls. The long-acting benzodiazepines are included on the HEDIS PIPE list as medications to be avoided.[37]

Benzodiazepines may be appropriate for short-term use in select psychiatric disorders (eg, panic disorder). Benzodiazepine use in palliative care is a distinct issue beyond the scope of discussion of this article, but there is generally more laxity in their use in that scenario. However, most older adults are receiving these medications without an appropriate indication. This situation is particularly concerning in a population at risk for adverse side effects with such potential risk for morbidity and mortality, such as gait impairment, respiratory suppression (eg, with comorbid obstructive sleep apnea), cognitive impairment/delirium, and falls with subsequent fractures.

Other sedatives/hypnotics

Problematic toxicity with barbiturates or related drugs such as meprobamate consistently landed them on virtually all PIPE lists, and prompted initial hope for benzodiazepines as an alternative. Given the problematic issues discussed earlier with benzodiazepines, there has been a search for a safer sedative medication. Nonbenzodiazepine sedatives have emerged as possible alternatives, such as the Z drugs zolpidem (Ambien/Ambien CR), zaleplon (Sonata), and eszopiclone (Lunesta); however, these drugs do act on benzodiazepine type 1 receptors but without the muscle relaxant or antiepileptic effects of benzodiazepines, and with some evidence for less physiologic dependence/withdrawal. However, they also significantly affect postural stability and thus risk for falling during their hours of peak onset.[38] There have also been reports of hallucinations and amnestic episodes, including sleepwalking and sleep-eating, with these Z drugs.[39,40] Although some such medications have been FDA-approved for long-term treatment of insomnia (eg, eszopiclone), their use is generally best limited in older adults in LTC settings, with particular attention to other possible causes of sleep disruption (eg, restless legs syndrome, obstructive sleep apnea, poor sleep hygiene, nocturia).

Because insomnia itself has such subjective and objective detriments for older adults, and when no primary cause of insomnia can be established, geriatricians often search for alternatives to the aforementioned treatments to alleviate this symptom. Trials of melatonin among older adults have produced mixed results,[41] but a specific melatonin receptor agonist, ramelteon (Rozerem), has produced some benefits in insomnia, primarily in reduced sleep latency. Although limited in effects on measures such as total sleep time, ramelteon use in older adults does not seem to cause the postural instability or amnesia associated with medications such as zolpidem.[42] Another commonly used drug for insomnia is trazodone (Desyrel/Oleptro). Originally developed as an antidepressant that proved too sedating at therapeutic doses, its off-label use (dosed at 50–150 mg at bedtime) for insomnia has gained popularity because of its potential to augment other antidepressants, its lack of addictive qualities, and its low cost. However, long-term data on its efficacy are lacking, and it does carry some risks such as orthostasis, residual fatigue, and priapism.[43] One option for insomnia treatment that is clearly a poor choice is a sedating antihistamine (eg, diphenhydramine [Benadryl] or hydroxyzine [Vistaril]). These medications are common on PIPE lists, because of both lack of proven efficacy for insomnia and strong anticholinergic effects among older adults. If outside medications are allowed in an LTC setting, careful scrutiny for use of over-the-counter sleep aids should be conducted. Many older adults inadvertently take such sedating antihistamines as part of PM formulations of medications such as acetaminophen.

Antidepressants

Antidepressants have not received as much attention on PIPE lists as the psychotropics discussed earlier, although MDD affects 10% to 15% of LTC residents and anxiety disorders affect about 5% of LTC residents. Many studies have documented the underdiagnosis and undertreatment of these disorders in LTC,[44] as well as, less commonly, undocumented reasons for the use of and successful discontinuation of unnecessary antidepressants.[45] The use of even newer-generation antidepressants has recently attracted attention as not being as completely benign as once believed. For instance, antidepressants as a class have a received a black-box warning for increased risk of suicidality (not usually suicide attempts or completed suicides; more often ideation or any other self-harm), but this risk was significant only up to age 24 years; antidepressants seem increasingly protective of suicidality with increasing age.[46] Other potential risks to be considered in prescribing antidepressants to older adults include reports of increased rates of hyponatremia caused by syndrome of inappropriate antidiuretic hormone (SIADH), osteoporosis, falls, and gastrointestinal (GI) bleeding (especially when on concomitant nonsteroidal antiinflammatory drugs [NSAIDs]), in particular with selective serotonin reuptake inhibitors (SSRIs).[47]

In addition to these safety concerns, there are limited and mixed data on the efficacy of antidepressants among the oldest old adults, those in institutional settings, and among older adults with comorbid dementia.[48–53] **Box 1** summarizes the suggestions for choosing antidepressants in treating MDD (or anxiety disorders) among LTC residents. Antidepressants may be used off-label in nonmajor or subthreshold depression, which may affect up to 30% to 60% of LTC residents, but their efficacy is not well established in this condition.[12] SSRIs are usually used as a first-line treatment of late-life MDD as well as most anxiety disorders, including GAD, panic disorder, social anxiety disorder, posttraumatic stress disorder, and obsessive-compulsive disorder, with GAD being the most common presentation of clinically significant anxiety in late life. It is important when assuming care of a patient admitted on an antidepressant that the indication be clearly established, that the time course of treatment and past treatment history be obtained, and that some subjective (if possible objective) measure of symptomatic and functional response to the medication be assessed over time.

Analgesics

Pain is one of the most common symptoms among LTC residents. Optimal assessment and treatment of pain is complicated by the: (1) broad variety of causes causing pain, (2) diagnostic uncertainty and frequently fluctuating course of symptoms and response to treatment, (3) availability of multiple treatment options, and (4) presence of regulatory and administrative guidelines.[55] The challenge to LTC providers is to identify the most efficacious treatments for pain and minimize medication toxicities and interactions. Most residents identified as receiving polypharmacy are receiving analgesic medications that may have significant toxicities and adverse drug interactions.[56]

Expert recommendations for treating pain in LTC have been described in detail by the American Geriatrics Society Panel on Pharmacologic Management of Persistent Pain in Older Persons (AGS Panel).[57] Although analgesic medications can reduce pain intensity/frequency and enhance older adults' quality of life, the identification and treatment of an underlying cause of the pain may permit pain management with fewer analgesics, lower doses, or medications with a lower risk of serious adverse consequences. Optimization of medication management requires an accurate assessment of the level of pain. A pain scale that combines descriptive and behavioral measurements and is valid across the range of cognitive and communicative abilities encountered in LTC ensures more accurate assessment of pain and the efficacy of interventions. In each case, the provider must consider the level of discomfort acceptable to the resident.[58]

Although the general principles of pain management apply to both acute and chronic pain, each provides its own challenge in LTC. Persistent pain is often more difficult to treat than acute pain, and requires a combination of drug and nonpharmacologic approaches to reduce the requirement for analgesic medications. Patient and staff education, frequent reassessment, and goal setting can lower expectations of the complete elimination of pain in favor of achieving tolerable pain control. The interdisciplinary team and the LTC resident collaborate to arrive at pertinent, realistic, and measurable goals for treatment, such as reducing pain sufficiently to allow the resident to ambulate comfortably to the dining room for each meal or to participate in 30 minutes of physical therapy.[59]

Often, the perception of control of pain is improved through the use of regularly scheduled dosing as opposed to as-needed orders. Patients who require frequent as-needed doses should be encouraged to consider taking their analgesic medication on a regular schedule. Pain that has become severe requires higher doses of medications to achieve satisfactory control.[59] Long-acting preparations minimize fluctuations in efficacy caused by pharmacokinetics and often result in more effective pain control at lower overall doses. The use of multiple medications is justified if the dose requirements, and therefore side effects and toxicities, are reduced. Often, several trials must be attempted before determining the optimal combination for a particular resident.[57] Careful assessment of efficacy permits the practitioner to eliminate all analgesic medications that are not contributing to dynamic pain control.

An interdisciplinary care plan that includes physical therapy modalities such as cold compresses, heat, ultrasound, and kinesiotherapy is an indispensable part of effective pain management. Increasing flexibility of muscles can improve their range of motion, and strengthening can improve support and stabilization around the joint. Treatment with heat and cold compresses increases circulation and reduces inflammation. This strategy may result in less pain with functional movement. Physical and occupational therapists may be able to suggest specific modifications of existing equipment or provide assistive devices to provide support during functional activity, which reduces the pain of movement.[60] Although evidence regarding the benefits of massage therapy, chiropractic manipulation, or acupuncture is mixed, these techniques decrease overall medication requirements for many LTC residents.[59]

Transcutaneous electrical nerve stimulation is a noninvasive method intended to reduce both intermittent and persistent pain. Although controversy exists as to its effectiveness, several systematic reviews have confirmed its effectiveness for chronic musculoskeletal pain.[61] Practitioners who are unfamiliar or uncomfortable with the use of this device can obtain consultation with pain management specialists. These practitioners can also perform a variety of temporary or permanent nerve blocks and present novel options for pain control in an older adult with particularly challenging pain management issues. Specialized surgical intervention is an effective option in some circumstances.[62] Spinal decompression, vertebroplasty, or surgical fixation of a severely damaged joint may provide a significant reduction in pain in select patients. In addition, a variety of braces and prosthetic devices may be customized for individual resident's needs by a trained prosthetist.[60]

Box 1
Guidelines for choosing antidepressants when indicated and removing potentially inappropriate antidepressants in LTC

First-line Medications

SSRIs

- Best overall risk-benefit profile and best evidence base for efficacy (typical side effects may be transient GI upset, headache, anxiety/insomnia, and more persistent sexual side effects)
- New concern for accelerating bone loss and increasing fall risk thus far has not changed their status as first-line medications (other antidepressants are not clearly absent of these risks)

  Increased vigilance for patients after recommended screening for osteoporosis

  Monitor vitamin D levels and discuss calcium/vitamin D supplements with primary care

  Gait assessments such as simple timed get-up-and-go test[54]
- Avoid SSRIs with long-term NSAID use or a history of significant GI bleeding
- For new-onset altered mental status or general lethargy, consider SSRI-induced hyponatremia caused by SIADH
- Among SSRIs, favored medications are recommended based on moderate half-lives and decreased potential for medication interactions through hepatic CYP450 (cytochrome P450, a hepatic enzyme system) inhibition:
- Citalopram (Celexa)

  Few CYP450 inhibition/medication interactions; itself metabolized primarily by CYP450 2C19 and 3A4

  A racemic mixture of s-citalopram and r-citalopram, with possibly more antihistamine (sedating) effects than pure s-citalopram; available as inexpensive generic (eg, $4/mo at major retailers)

  In older adults, typical starting dose is 10 mg/d titrated over weeks to a target dose of 20 to 40 mg/d, with a maximum dose being 60 mg/d
- Escitalopram (Lexapro)

  Virtually no CYP450 inhibition/medication interactions; itself metabolized primarily by CYP450 2C19

  Expensive (>$100/mo), no generic available

  In older adults, typical starting dose is 5 to 10 mg/d titrated over weeks to a target dose of 10 to 20 mg/d
- Sertraline (Zoloft)

  Minimal CYP450 inhibition/medication interactions (modest inhibition at 2B6, 2C19, and 2D6); itself metabolized primarily by CYP450 2B6 and 2C19

  Available as inexpensive (<$10/mo) generic

  In older adults, typical starting dose is 25 mg/d titrated over weeks to a target dose of 50 to 150 mg/d, with a maximum dose being 200 mg/d

Potential First-line or Second-line Medications

SSRIs

- Fluoxetine (Prozac)

  On the Beers 2002 list primarily because of its long half-life (and that of its metabolite norfluoxetine), which can be problematic if discontinuation because of side effects is necessary, as well as its inhibition of CYP450 1A2, 2B6, 2C19, 2D6, and 3A4

Dose of 20 to 40 mg/d, with a maximum dose being 60 mg/d; available as inexpensive generic (eg, $4/mo at major retailers)

- Paroxetine (Paxil)

  The most anticholinergic SSRI, which cumulatively with other medications may cause many negative effects; among shortest half-lives of the SSRIs, which increase risk for discontinuation symptoms; also strong inhibitor of CYP450 2B6 and 2D6

  If used, typical starting dose is 10 mg/d titrated over weeks to a target dose of 20 to 40 mg/d, with a maximum dose being 60 mg/d; available as inexpensive generic (eg, $10–15/mo)

Serotonin-Norepinephrine Reuptake Inhibitors (SNRIs)

- As a class, probably have some of the same risks as SSRIs re: osteoporosis, GI bleeding, fall risk, SIADH
- Also the noradrenergic reuptake inhibition seems to carry some potential for increasing heart rate and blood pressure
- The dual SNRI action seems to confer some analgesic effects (especially in neuropathic pain disorders) as a result of altered serotonin/norepinephrine transmission in the spinal cord
- Venlafaxine (Effexor XR)

  Serotonin reuptake inhibition primarily at initial doses; norepinephrine reuptake inhibition begins generally at doses 150 mg/d or greater

  Minimal CYP450 inhibition/drug interactions and itself metabolized primarily by CYP450 2D6; mostly renal excretion; shorter half-life increases risk for discontinuation symptoms

  If used, typical starting dose is 37.5 mg/d titrated over weeks to a target dose of 75 to 225 mg/d, with a maximum dose being 300 mg/d

- Desvenlafaxine (Pristiq)

  Active hepatic metabolite of venlafaxine with more balanced serotonin and norepinephrine reuptake inhibition at starting dose

  New medication with minimal experience in older adults

  Starting dose (50 mg/d) is also maximum dose shown to have benefit

- Duloxetine (Cymbalta)

  More balanced serotonin and norepinephrine reuptake inhibition at starting doses

  Moderate CYP450 2D6 inhibition; possible increased risk for hepatotoxicity, so best avoided in persons with compromised liver function (eg, heavy alcohol users)

  FDA-approved for treatment of fibromyalgia and diabetic neuropathy pain

  If used, typical starting dose is 30 mg/d titrated over weeks to a target dose of 60 mg/d, with a maximum dose being 120 mg/d

Other Atypical Antidepressants

- Mirtazapine (Remeron)

  Complex mechanism of action: α_2-adrenergic receptor antagonist (which disinhibits norepinephrine release at presynaptic receptors and disinhibits serotonin release at postsynaptic receptors); 5-HT_{2A}/5-HT_C serotonin receptor blockade seems to facilitate dopamine and norepinephrine release in the prefrontal cortex; 5-HT_3 blockade prevents nausea/GI upset as a side effect; increased serotonin levels are targeted toward 5-HT_{1A} receptors, believed to be the key receptors for anxiolytic/antidepressant effects

  Side effects include sedation (caused by antihistamine effects and 5-HT_A receptor blockade) and weight gain (caused by antihistamine effects and 5-HT_C receptor

Box 1
(continued)

blockade); may be useful for older adults with anorexia and insomnia as part of major depression; sedation may increase fall risk; decreased sexual side effects versus SSRIs

Minimal CYP450 inhibition; itself metabolized by CYP450 1A2, 2D6, and 3A4

If used, typical starting dose is 7.5 to 15 mg at bedtime titrated over weeks to a target dose of 15 to 45 mg at bedtime; available as generic (eg, $15–20/mo)

- Bupropion (Wellbutrin)

Described as an inhibitor of norepinephrine and dopamine reuptake, although these effects are weak, leaving its mechanism of action controversial

Often used for fatigue, amotivation, apathy (alone or as an augmentation to other antidepressants); dosed in the morning because activating and later dosing can cause insomnia; not approved to treat any anxiety disorder; may worsen anxiety in some persons; tends to be weight neutral or even decrease appetite; seems devoid of sexual side effects; slight increased risk of seizures compared with other antidepressants

Significant inhibition of CYP450 2D6; itself metabolized primarily by 2B6 and 2D6

If used, typical starting dose is 100 mg/d in the morning titrated over weeks to a target dose of 150 to 300 mg/d; maximum dose 450 mg/d (available in immediate release, sustained release, and extended release formulations)

Less Preferred, Possibly Appropriate at Times

Secondary Tricyclic Antidepressants (TCAs)

- TCAs were a class that preceded SSRIs and have largely been supplanted in modern psychiatry by newer antidepressants because newer medications have shown equivalent efficacy, a lower side effect burden, and lower toxicity in overdose
- They generally work by dual reuptake inhibition of serotonin and norepinephrine, although each agent has different degrees of relative serotonin versus norepinephrine effects; secondary TCAs tend to have more norepinephrine than serotonin reuptake inhibition; this dual reuptake effect makes them effective in certain pain disorders, similar to newer SNRIs
- TCAS are on most PIPE lists because of effects on nontherapeutic receptors (eg, anticholinergic effects such as cognitive impairment and constipation; α_1-adrenergic receptor blockade, causing orthostasis and fall risk; and sodium channel blockade in the cardiac conduction system, increasing risk for arrhythmias and sudden cardiac death); tend to prolong QT_c intervals
- Nortriptyline (Pamelor)

For TCAs, has low potential for causing orthostasis (and falls) and anticholinergic effects in older adults

Primarily metabolized by CYP450 2D6; is a metabolite of the tertiary TCA amitriptyline

If used, typical starting dose is 10 to 25 mg at bedtime titrated over weeks to a target dose of 50 to 150 mg/d; dosing guided by target blood levels of 50 to 150 ng/mL

- Desipramine (Norpramin)

For TCAs, has low potential for causing orthostasis (and falls) and anticholinergic effects in older adults

Primarily metabolized by CYP450 2D6; is a metabolite of the tertiary TCA imipramine

If used, typical starting dose is 10 to 25 mg daily (often norepinephrine effects can be activating, requiring morning dosing) titrated over weeks to a target dose of 100 to 200 mg/d; dosing guided by target blood levels of 150 to 300 ng/mL

Almost Always Inappropriate

Tertiary TCAs

- These medications are common on PIPE lists in particular (eg, amitriptyline [Elavil], doxepin [Sinequan]) because of the reasons discussed earlier. Tertiary TCAs tend to have more balanced serotonin-to-norepinephrine reuptake inhibition, but they also tend to have more potent blockade at the nontherapeutic receptor sites mentioned earlier that produce unwanted side effects

Monoamine Oxidase Inhibitors (MAOIs)

- The first antidepressant drugs discovered, MAOIs work by inhibiting the breakdown of all 3 monoamines dopamine, serotonin, and norepinephrine. Although they may prove effective in persons with treatment refractory major depression, especially atypical depression, they have several major limitations. They must be taken with a strict tyramine-free diet to avoid a potentially lethal hypertensive reaction. When taken as directed, the opposite problem is often limiting in older adults: orthostatic hypotension. They also have multiple potential drug interactions that require close vigilance by the patient to avoid reactions such as serotonin syndrome
- Older examples include phenelzine (Nardil) and tranylcypromine (Parnate). A newer patch for selegeline (Emsam), more selective for MAO type B (more responsible for dopamine metabolism), has been approved for major depression, but the only advantage seems to be lack of need for dietary restriction at the starting and lowest dose (only 6 mg/d). Doses of 9 mg and 12 mg/d also exist and carry the same restrictions as older MAOIs. The role of Emsam in geriatric depression is poorly established

Cognitive-behavioral therapy performed by a psychologist or informally by a provider or staff can also benefit the resident by providing a feeling of greater control over their pain, and provide nonpharmaceutical alternatives to increase increasing quality of life. Relaxation techniques, reminiscing, diversions, activities, music therapy, and coping techniques can be effective alternative means to achieve pain relief.[62]

Despite the frequent use of analgesic medication, there is considerable evidence that physicians fail to adequately control chronic pain in geriatric patients. Studies of Minimum Data Set information have found that 25% to 49% of nursing home residents have persistent pain, and that persons suffering daily pain were more likely to have severe impairment of activities of daily living, depressive symptoms, and less frequent involvement in activities. One-quarter received no analgesics, and the most commonly prescribed analgesic was acetaminophen, which was given as needed. Male residents, racial minorities, and cognitively impaired individuals were at increased risk.[63]

Topical Analgesics and Local Injections

Some causes of chronic pain may be treated effectively with topical agents, intra-articular injections of steroid or hyaluronic acid, and trigger-point intramuscular steroid injections. This strategy may potentially lower the systemic analgesic dose required to achieve adequate pain control. Capsaicin, topical lidocaine 5% patches, and topical NSAIDs may provide relief for patients with musculoskeletal and neuropathic pain.[59]

Acetaminophen

The low toxicity and risk of drug interactions of acetaminophen make this agent an excellent choice for mild to moderate pain; however, the short half-life provides less than optimal dosing if analgesia is required for persistent pain. The potential for hepatotoxicity at doses greater than 4 g/d can limit the optimal use of combination drugs containing acetaminophen. For these reasons, acetaminophen and acetaminophen-containing compounds are most effective for acute intermittent pain control.[62]

NSAIDs

The risk of GI bleeding, renal dysfunction, and cardiovascular complications requires careful consideration before initiating therapy with NSAIDs. These agents have a variety of half-lives, and once-daily or twice-daily dosing represents a major advantage. The AGS Panel recommends that nonselective and cyclooxygenase 2 selective inhibitor NSAIDs be considered rarely, and used with extreme caution in highly selected individuals.[57] Long-term use of full-dosage, longer half-life NSAIDs is considered potentially inappropriate in older adults according to the Beers criteria.[5] Generally, representatives of this drug class are best used sporadically for acute intermittent pain at doses on the low end of the dosage recommendations.[59]

Opiate Analgesics

Opiates are essential to providing safe, effective pain control in the LTC setting. Despite the wide variety of individual agents and delivery systems available, many practitioners limit their prescribing options, and thus miss an opportunity to discover an optimal combination for a particular resident.[63] Low potency agents such as codeine or tramadol are often combined with acetaminophen and therefore provide a reasonable progression, particularly in moderate intermittent pain. Drug interactions and the presence of baseline cognitive impairment may increase the bolus effect that occurs with the initial doses of analgesics with activity at opioid receptors. The presence of pain may also increase the likelihood of delirium. Impairment often subsides as tolerance develops after the initial few doses. Side effects such as constipation require prophylactic use of laxatives and stool softeners.[57]

Hydrocodone, hydromorphone, and oxycodone are commonly considered for severe pain. These opiates require frequent dosing and are not optimal for persistent pain management. Long-acting morphine sulfate (MS Contin) is dosed twice daily and therefore has the pharmacokinetic advantage of more stable blood levels. This treatment often provides greater efficacy and permits the development of tolerance to sedative and cognitive side effects of opiates. Transdermal delivery systems enable the opiate fentanyl to be applied as a single patch every 2 to 3 days. This strategy eliminates the need for residents, practitioners, and staff to focus on the clock in anticipation of the return of pain symptoms. With appropriate titration of dose in opiate-tolerant patients, it is not uncommon for adequate pain control to be achieved with a single agent.[62] Once stable pain control is achieved, the need for frequent dosing should be limited, although an order for a short-acting opiate is usually appropriate in the event of breakthrough pain. Education of residents, families, and staff often determines the success of this care plan.[59]

Fear of abuse or diversion is a major barrier to long-term opiate treatment in chronic nonmalignant pain. Residents, family members, and staff may confuse physical dependence, a natural consequence of appropriate chronic opiate analgesia at appropriate and effective doses, with abuse. It is common for prescribing practitioners to misinterpret drug seeking by patients with poorly managed chronic pain as a symptom of abuse.[64] Several studies have shown minimal risk of abuse or drug-seeking behavior in patients treated with long-term opiate therapy who do not have a previous history of substance abuse. Although individuals with a history of alcohol-use disorders are at increased risk to abuse opiates, even in this small group of LTC residents, opiates are essential for providing safe, effective pain control.[65] The prescription of schedule II agents is subject to specific state law and administrative regulations. The medical director of each facility can assist with the establishment of a clear protocol to review and continue the prescription of these agents based on clinical assessment.[58] The Federation of State Medical Boards provides guidelines for the prescription of opiate analgesics in the treatment of persistent nonmalignant pain.[66]

Antidepressants and Anticonvulsants

The presence of chronic pain is almost universally accompanied by symptoms of depression, and all residents with persistent pain syndromes should be routinely screened for depression. Once identified, the depression should be adequately treated with standard therapies. Successful treatment of depression permits an accurate assessment of resident pain and can reduce the need for analgesic medications.[59] TCAs have been found to reduce pain associated with postherpetic neuralgia and diabetic neuropathy; however, their adverse effect profile often prohibits the use of these medications in older residents. SSRIs are not so effective in the treatment of pain as mixed serotonin and norepinephrine reuptake inhibitors such as duloxetine and venlafaxine. Anticonvulsants such as gabapentin and pregabalin have been shown to reduce neuropathic pain from a variety of conditions and have low side effect profiles.[57] These pain-modulating medications are long-acting, and careful titration to maximal tolerated dosages with frequent monitoring is essential before determining the need for additional medications.

Other Common Adjuvant Medications

The use of systemic steroids for acute musculoskeletal pain with an inflammatory component is well established. A short course (≤2 weeks) averts significant adrenal suppression; symptoms often return after cessation of treatment. Optimal use of physical therapy modalities may decrease the likelihood that additional medication is necessary. Longer courses of steroid should be reserved for chronic inflammatory disorders such as rheumatoid arthritis or malignant bone pain. Osteoarthritis should not be treated with chronic systemic steroid therapy.[57] Serious side effects caused by long-term use (eg, insulin resistance, osteoporosis, central obesity, neuropsychiatric effects) makes it essential to use the lowest possible steroid dose and consider the use of additional agents and modalities to provide effective pain management.

Persistent pain associated with osteoporosis and vertebral compression fractures has been shown anecdotally to improve with calcitonin. Because this agent also has efficacy in increasing bone mass, it may be an attractive option for some LTC residents.[59] Bisphosphonates may reduce persistent pain for patients with bone metastases and reduce the need for other analgesics. Cyclobenzaprine, carisoprodol, and other skeletal muscle relaxants are considered to be potentially inappropriate in older adults because their efficacy is insufficient to outweigh their adverse effect profile (sedation, addictive qualities, anticholinergic effects).[5] Although these agents may relieve skeletal muscle pain, their effects are largely unrelated to muscle relaxation. Baclofen has documented skeletal muscle relaxant efficacy in patients with severe spasticity caused by CNS or neuromuscular disorders and is useful in reducing the need for other analgesic medications.[57] Benzodiazepines should not be used for pain management in older individuals unless there is a significant general anxiety component, and even then with caution and usually not indefinitely.

Factors that can be modified in pursuit of optimal pain control in LTC settings include: (1) knowledge about pain and management through direct education of patient, family, staff, and administration, (2) algorithm development and implementation of pain management pathways, (3) treatment modifications that involve the full spectrum of pharmacologic and nonpharmacologic tools, and (4) system modifications to measure and provide feedback for continuous improvement.[67]

SUMMARY

The reduction of psychotropic drugs in the LTC setting requires a process of systematic review and cultural change beyond that of federal regulation and warnings. Each member of the interdisciplinary team must consider behavioral modification and environmental change to be an essential part of the health care plan for each resident. Practitioners, nursing staff, family members, and residents must come to see medication as a complementary or secondary treatment of behavioral problems and pain. Anxiety, depression, and pain are frequent antecedents and/or consequences of chronic illness and functional decline. The LTC environment can be developed to include opportunities for positive interaction and alternative activities that may significantly decrease the necessity of medications affecting the CNS.

Some residents continue to require psychotropic medications to maximize their quality of life and/or to maintain a safe environment in the LTC community. Careful assessment of the clinical condition of each resident and their specific response to a chosen regimen of medication must be accompanied by a willingness to modify that regimen over time. A routine of periodic chart reviews for potentially unnecessary medications could greatly reduce the burden of iatrogenic illness. Although it is often difficult to predict clinical response, the consequences of excessive medication are significant; the LTC practitioner can take the lead to involve the entire interdisciplinary team in reducing these medications whenever possible.

REFERENCES

1. Haour F, Lang B. Role of hormonal receptors in the regulation of the corpus luteum (author's transl). Sem Hop 1978;54:1063–70 [in French].
2. Pugh MJ, Hanlon JT, Zeber JE, et al. Assessing potentially inappropriate prescribing in the elderly Veterans Affairs population using the HEDIS 2006 quality measure. J Manag Care Pharm 2006;12:537–45.
3. Beers MH, Ouslander JG, Rollingher I, et al. Explicit criteria for determining inappropriate medication use in nursing home residents. UCLA division of geriatric medicine. Arch Intern Med 1991;151:1825–32.
4. Beers MH. Explicit criteria for determining potentially inappropriate medication use by the elderly. An update. Arch Intern Med 1997;157:1531–6.
5. Fick DM, Cooper JW, Wade WE, et al. Updating the beers criteria for potentially inappropriate medication use in older adults: results of a US consensus panel of experts. Arch Intern Med 2003;163:2716–24.
6. Zhan C, Sangl J, Bierman AS, et al. Potentially inappropriate medication use in the community-dwelling elderly: findings from the 1996 Medical Expenditure Panel Survey. JAMA 2001;286:2823–9.
7. National Committee for Quality Assurance. HEDIS volume 2, technical specifications. Washington, DC: National Committee for Quality Assurance; 2006.
8. Meeks TW, Jeste DV. Beyond the black box: what is the role for antipsychotics in dementia? Curr Psychiatr 2008;7:50–65.
9. Cotter VT. The burden of dementia. Am J Manag Care 2007;13(Suppl 8):S193–7.

10. Jeste DV, Meeks TW, Kim DS, et al. Research agenda for DSM-V: diagnostic categories and criteria for neuropsychiatric syndromes in dementia. J Geriatr Psychiatry Neurol 2006;19:160–71.
11. Culp KR, Cacchione PZ. Nutritional status and delirium in long-term care elderly individuals. Appl Nurs Res 2008;21:66–74.
12. Meeks TW, Vahia IV, Lavretsky H, et al. A tune in "a minor" can "b major": a review of epidemiology, illness course, and public health implications of subthreshold depression in older adults. J Affect Disord 2011;129(1–3):126–42.
13. Fullerton CA, McGuire TG, Feng Z, et al. Trends in mental health admissions to nursing homes, 1999–2005. Psychiatr Serv 2009;60:965–71.
14. Cheok A, Snowdon J, Miller R, et al. The prevalence of anxiety disorders in nursing homes. Int J Geriatr Psychiatry 1996;11:405–10.
15. Smalbrugge M, Jongenelis L, Pot AM, et al. Comorbidity of depression and anxiety in nursing home patients. Int J Geriatr Psychiatry 2005;20:218–26.
16. Chutka DS, Takahashi PY, Hoel RW. Inappropriate medications for elderly patients. Mayo Clin Proc 2004;79:122–39.
17. Macdiarmid SA. Concomitant medications and possible side effects of antimuscarinic agents. Rev Urol 2008;10:92–8.
18. Gallagher PF, Barry PJ, Ryan C, et al. Inappropriate prescribing in an acutely ill population of elderly patients as determined by Beers' criteria. Age Ageing 2008;37:96–101.
19. Alvarez PA, Pahissa J. QT alterations in psychopharmacology: proven candidates and suspects. Curr Drug Saf 2010;5:97–104.
20. Ray WA, Chung CP, Murray KT, et al. Atypical antipsychotic drugs and the risk of sudden cardiac death. N Engl J Med 2009;360:225–35.
21. Schneider LS, Tariot PN, Dagerman KS, et al. Effectiveness of atypical antipsychotic drugs in patients with Alzheimer's disease. N Engl J Med 2006;355:1525–38.
22. Schneider LS, Dagerman K, Insel PS. Efficacy and adverse effects of atypical antipsychotics for dementia: meta-analysis of randomized, placebo-controlled trials. Am J Geriatr Psychiatry 2006;14:191–210.
23. Livingston G, Johnston K, Katona C, et al. Systematic review of psychological approaches to the management of neuropsychiatric symptoms of dementia. Am J Psychiatry 2005;162:1996–2021.
24. Ruths S, Straand J, Nygaard HA, et al. Stopping antipsychotic drug therapy in demented nursing home patients: a randomized, placebo-controlled study–the Bergen District Nursing Home Study (BEDNURS). Int J Geriatr Psychiatry 2008;23:889–95.
25. Westbury J, Jackson S, Gee P, et al. An effective approach to decrease antipsychotic and benzodiazepine use in nursing homes: the RedUSe project. Int Psychogeriatr 2010;22:26–36.
26. Schmidt I, Claesson CB, Westerholm B, et al. The impact of regular multidisciplinary team interventions on psychotropic prescribing in Swedish nursing homes. J Am Geriatr Soc 1998;46:77–82.
27. Lieberman JA, Stroup TS, McEvoy JP, et al. Effectiveness of antipsychotic drugs in patients with chronic schizophrenia. N Engl J Med 2005;353:1209–23.
28. Jeste DV. Tardive dyskinesia rates with atypical antipsychotics in older adults. J Clin Psychiatry 2004;65(Suppl 9):21–4.
29. Jeste DV, Lacro JP, Bailey A, et al. Lower incidence of tardive dyskinesia with risperidone compared with haloperidol in older patients. J Am Geriatr Soc 1999;47:716–9.

30. American Diabetes Association, American Psychiatric Association, American Association of Clinical Endocrinologists, et al. Consensus development conference on antipsychotic drugs and obesity and diabetes. Diabetes Care 2004; 27:596–601.
31. Borson S, Doane K. The impact of OBRA-87 on psychotropic drug prescribing in skilled nursing facilities. Psychiatr Serv 1997;48:1289–96.
32. Briesacher BA, Soumerai SB, Field TS, et al. Medicare part D's exclusion of benzodiazepines and fracture risk in nursing homes. Arch Intern Med 2010; 170:693–8.
33. Ancoli-Israel S, Cooke JR. Prevalence and comorbidity of insomnia and effect on functioning in elderly populations. J Am Geriatr Soc 2005;53:S264–71.
34. Avidan AY, Fries BE, James ML, et al. Insomnia and hypnotic use, recorded in the minimum data set, as predictors of falls and hip fractures in Michigan nursing homes. J Am Geriatr Soc 2005;53:955–62.
35. Woolcott JC, Richardson KJ, Wiens MO, et al. Meta-analysis of the impact of 9 medication classes on falls in elderly persons. Arch Intern Med 2009;169: 1952–60.
36. Hebert C, Delaney JA, Hemmelgarn B, et al. Benzodiazepines and elderly drivers: a comparison of pharmacoepidemiological study designs. Pharmacoepidemiol Drug Saf 2007;16:845–9.
37. Use of high risk medications in the elderly. Available at: http://www.ncqa.org/portals/0/hedisqm/HEDIS2008/Vol2/NDC/Table%2520DAE-A.doc. Accessed September 28, 2010.
38. Mets MA, Volkerts ER, Olivier B, et al. Effect of hypnotic drugs on body balance and standing steadiness. Sleep Med Rev 2010;14:259–67.
39. Hwang TJ, Ni HC, Chen HC, et al. Risk predictors for hypnosedative-related complex sleep behaviors: a retrospective, cross-sectional pilot study. J Clin Psychiatry 2010;71:1331–5.
40. Toner LC, Tsambiras BM, Catalano G, et al. Central nervous system side effects associated with zolpidem treatment. Clin Neuropharmacol 2000;23: 54–8.
41. Meeks TW, Wetherell JL, Irwin MR, et al. Complementary and alternative treatments for late-life depression, anxiety, and sleep disturbance: a review of randomized controlled trials. J Clin Psychiatry 2007;68:1461–71.
42. Zammit G, Wang-Weigand S, Rosenthal M, et al. Effect of ramelteon on middle-of-the-night balance in older adults with chronic insomnia. J Clin Sleep Med 2009; 5:34–40.
43. Tuya AC. The management of insomnia in the older adult. Med Health R I 2007; 90:195–6.
44. Kramer D, Allgaier AK, Fejtkova S, et al. Depression in nursing homes: prevalence, recognition, and treatment. Int J Psychiatry Med 2009;39:345–58.
45. Ulfvarson J, Adami J, Wredling R, et al. Controlled withdrawal of selective serotonin reuptake inhibitor drugs in elderly patients in nursing homes with no indication of depression. Eur J Clin Pharmacol 2003;59:735–40.
46. Stone M, Laughren T, Jones ML, et al. Risk of suicidality in clinical trials of antidepressants in adults: analysis of proprietary data submitted to US Food and Drug Administration. BMJ 2009;339:b2880.
47. Chemali Z, Chahine LM, Fricchione G. The use of selective serotonin reuptake inhibitors in elderly patients. Harv Rev Psychiatry 2009;17:242–53.
48. Kasper S, Lemming OM, de Swart H. Escitalopram in the long-term treatment of major depressive disorder in elderly patients. Neuropsychobiology 2006;54:152–9.

49. Weintraub D, Rosenberg PB, Drye LT, et al. Sertraline for the treatment of depression in Alzheimer disease: week-24 outcomes. Am J Geriatr Psychiatry 2010;18: 332–40.
50. Lyketsos CG, DelCampo L, Steinberg M, et al. Treating depression in Alzheimer disease: efficacy and safety of sertraline therapy, and the benefits of depression reduction: the DIADS. Arch Gen Psychiatry 2003;60:737–46.
51. Oslin DW, Ten Have TR, Streim JE, et al. Probing the safety of medications in the frail elderly: evidence from a randomized clinical trial of sertraline and venlafaxine in depressed nursing home residents. J Clin Psychiatry 2003;64:875–82.
52. Streim JE, Oslin DW, Katz IR, et al. Drug treatment of depression in frail elderly nursing home residents. Am J Geriatr Psychiatry 2000;8:150–9.
53. Burrows AB, Salzman C, Satlin A, et al. A randomized, placebo-controlled trial of paroxetine in nursing home residents with non-major depression. Depress Anxiety 2002;15:102–10.
54. Podsiadlo D, Richardson S. The timed "Up & Go": a test of basic functional mobility for frail elderly persons. J Am Geriatr Soc 1991;39:142–8.
55. Herman AD, Johnson TM, Ritchie CS, et al. Pain management interventions in the nursing home: a structured review of the literature. J Am Geriatr Soc 2009;57: 1258–67.
56. Dwyer LL, Han B, Woodwell DA, et al. Polypharmacy in nursing home residents in the United States: results of the 2004 National Nursing Home Survey. Am J Geriatr Pharmacother 2010;8:63–72.
57. American Geriatrics Society Panel on Pharmacological Management of Persistent Pain in Older Persons. Pharmacological management of persistent pain in older persons. J Am Geriatr Soc 2009;57:1331–46.
58. Centers for Medicare and Medicaid Services/Survey and Certification Group. Baltimore (MD): Department of Health and Human Service; 2010. Ref: S&C-09–22.
59. American Medical Directors Association. Pain management clinical practice guideline. Columbia (MD): AMDA; 2009.
60. Kisner C, Colby LA. Therapeutic exercise, foundations and techniques. 3rd edition. Philadelphia: FA Davis; 1996.
61. Johnson M, Martinson M. Efficacy of electrical nerve stimulation for chronic musculoskeletal pain: a meta-analysis of randomized controlled trials. Pain 2007;130:157–65.
62. Ferrell BA, Charette SL. Pain management. In: Halter JB, Ouslander JG, Tinetti ME, et al, editors. Hazzard's geriatric medicine and gerontology. 6th edition. New York: McGraw-Hill; 2009. p. 359–371.
63. Won AB, Lapane KL, Vallow S, et al. Persistent nonmalignant pain and analgesic prescribing patterns in elderly nursing home residents. J Am Geriatr Soc 2004; 52:867–74.
64. Trescot AM, Boswell MV, Atluri SL, et al. Opioid guidelines in the management of chronic non-cancer pain. Pain Physician 2006;9:1–39.
65. Podichetty VK, Mazanec DJ, Biscup RS. Chronic non-malignant musculoskeletal pain in older adults: clinical issues and opioid intervention. Postgrad Med J 2003; 79:627–33.
66. Federation of State Medical Boards of the United States I. Model policy for the use of controlled substances for the treatment of pain. 2004. Available at: http://www.fsmb.org/pdf/2004_grpol_Controlled_Substances.pdf. Accessed September 15, 2010.
67. Won A, Lapane K, Gambassi G, et al. Correlates and management of nonmalignant pain in the nursing home. SAGE Study Group. Systematic Assessment of Geriatric drug use via Epidemiology. J Am Geriatr Soc 1999;47:936–42.

Evidence-Based Medicine (EBM): What Long-Term Care Providers Need to Know

Huai Y. Cheng, MD, MPH

KEYWORDS

• Evidence-based medicine • Long-term care facility
• Nursing homes • EBM

Evidence-based medicine (EBM) has been exponentially disseminated to every field of medicine over past 2 decades.[1–7] EBM is now a part of postgraduate competency through practice-based learning.[8] However, its potential use in the long-term care setting was only recently appreciated in the literature.[1,9,10] EBM may play an important role in reforming nursing homes and improving quality care.[1–5,9,10]

The simple search term "EBM," limited to English and human in Medline, generated 49,304 citations, which narrowed to only 173 when "nursing homes" was added, indicating that EBP is not rare and is being implemented in long-term care. It has been a great effort that each article in this special issue presents evidence-based recommendations to long-term care providers to guide their daily practice. In contrast to the evidence-based approach to individual geriatric conditions addressed in the other articles in this issue, this article briefly introduces the basic concept of EBM; addresses some potential benefits, harms, and challenges of its practice in a long-term care setting; and promotes its appropriate use among providers of long-term care. For those who already know the EBM basics and are interested in become experts, several textbooks on EBM are recommended.[11–13] Attending an EBM workshop, such as one run by McMaster University,[14] could also be helpful. Many Internet resources are also useful, including PIER: The Physicianas' Information and Education Resource (pier.acponline.org), Clinical Evidence (www.clinicalevidence.bmj.com), UpToDate

This work was supported by Geriatric Academic Career Award funded by Health Resources & Services Administration and Bureau of Health Professions of USA (Grant Number: 1 K01HP00086-01).
Disclosure of conflict of interests: none.
Department of Palliative Care and Rehabilitation Medicine, MD Anderson Cancer Center, 1515 Holcombe Boulevard, Unit 1414/FCT5.6057, Houston, TX 77030, USA
E-mail address: wcheng@rocketmail.com

Clin Geriatr Med 27 (2011) 193–198
doi:10.1016/j.cger.2011.01.004 **geriatric.theclinics.com**
0749-0690/11/$ – see front matter

(www.uptodate.com), Evidence-Based Medicine Guidelines (http://onlinelibrary.wiley.com), The Cochrane Library (http://www.thecochranelibrary.com), Clinical Guidelines (http://www.guideline.gov/), and ACP Journal Club (www.acpjc.org). KC Clearinghouse (http://ktclearinghouse.ca/cebm/syllabi/geriatric) has a page introducing the EBM concept and framework for the geriatric population, which can be very useful for long-term care providers.

THE EBM CONCEPT

The concept of EBM was developed in 1991 by Professor Gordon Guyatt at McMaster University.[15] EBM is defined as the integration of the best available evidence with clinical expertise, patient values and preferences, and clinical circumstances (**Fig. 1**).[16] The concept is that EBM offers health care providers a framework to make the best decisions for individual patients. From this perspective, evidence-based clinical practice or evidence-based practice (EBP) is also used.[17,18] EBM and EBP are used interchangeably in this article.

The concept of EBM is particularly relevant to long-term care, in which patients often have multiple coexisting conditions, including medical diseases, mental and psychological disorders, functional decline, and multiple symptoms. Their preferences may be different from those of patients receiving non–long-term care, such as wanting care that provides more comfort rather than prolongs life.

Research findings are one part of the available evidence. Because evidence is lacking for many situations, long-term care providers may have to use their clinical

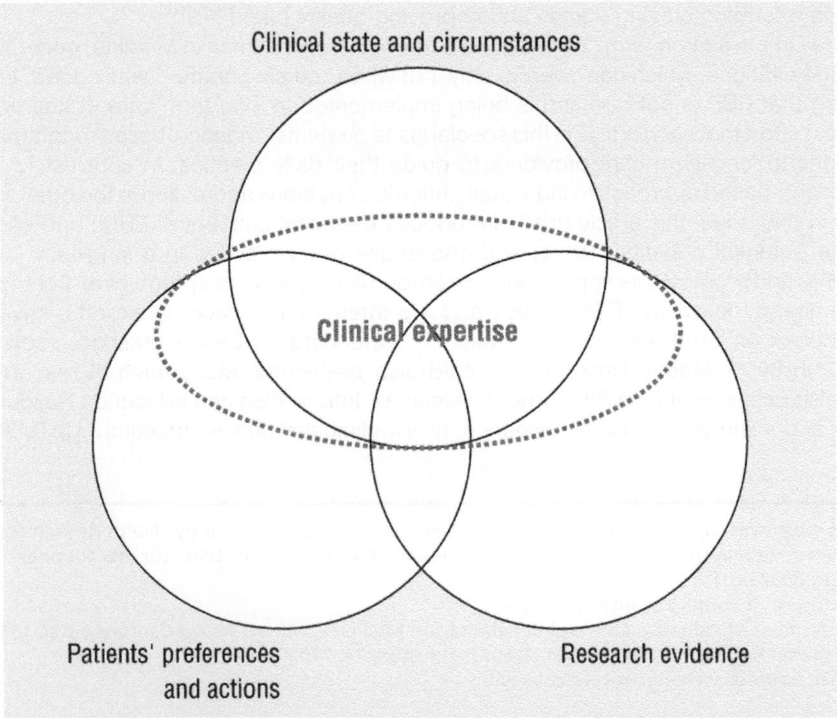

Fig. 1. Definition of EBM. (*From* Haynes RB, Devereaux PJ, Guyatt GH. Physicians' and patients' choices in evidence based practice. BMJ 2002;324:1350; with permission.)

experience and judgment to decide what is best for their frail patients. The application of EBM obviously extends beyond results of randomized controlled trials or systematic reviews, such as Cochrane reviews. EBP is important in the context of long-term care.

Although the strongest evidence on therapeutic interventions in general is provided by systematic reviews of either multiple or single, large, well-performed randomized controlled trials, few have been conducted in the long-term care setting.[9,19] A search of Medline using the simple terms "randomized controlled trials" and "nursing home," and limited to English and human from 1968 to 2009, showed that only 300 trials were conducted in nursing homes (**Table 1**).[20] More non-drug randomized controlled trials were conducted than drug trials. Some randomized controlled trials tested the efficacy of intervention for psychological disorders and vaccinations. The results from these randomized controlled trials can be integrated with clinical decision making in managing these conditions.

No single trial has tested drug efficacy in treating hypertension, congestive heart failure, hyperlipidemia, and other cardiovascular diseases in the nursing home setting, although many residents take cardiovascular drugs. Therapeutic decisions for patients with these diseases may be difficult for long-term care providers. Additionally, randomized controlled trials addressing some conditions might be impossible or inappropriate to perform in the long-term care setting. For example, whether inserting a feeding tube for a nursing home patient with advanced dementia could prolong life or improve quality of life could be difficult to evaluate in randomized controlled trials. Under these circumstances, decision making can be challenging, and the evidence must come from non–randomized controlled trials. Provider experience and patient values and preferences may contribute substantially to the decision making process for long-term care providers who wish to treat the whole patient. Evidence from non–randomized controlled trials has been used to support decision making for certain conditions.

Improvement of quality care and pay for performance have become important topics in the long-term care literature.[1–7] EBM can be used to develop clinical guidelines to standardize clinical practice and hopefully control medical expenditure (ie, *regulatory EBM*).[21] However, this is an area of controversy, and the concerns about using EBM to regulate long-term care practice and measure quality of care[6,7] should be considered.

EBM APPLICATION IN LONG-TERM CARE FACILITIES

The practice of EBM in long-term care settings, especially nursing homes, is unique in many ways. Long-term care is more tightly regulated than other settings. Patients

Table 1
Summary of selected randomized controlled trials at nursing homes (1968–2009)

Trial Types	2001–2009	1968–2000	Total
Drug trials (n)[a]	59	45	104
Vaccine trials	4	6	10
Non-drug trials (n)[b]	131	53	184
Mixed drug and non-drug trials	2	None	2
Total	196	104	300

[a] Prescribed medications, over-the-counter drugs, and nutritional supplements.
[b] Involving exercise, smoking cessation, and physical therapy.

receiving long-term care are usually old and frail, often have multiple conditions, and take many pills. Providing high-quality care for these patients is challenging.[1–7] The potential benefits, harms, and challenges in practicing EBM in long-term care facilities are discussed briefly.

A recent report by the Institute of Medicine summarized the concerns regarding quality of care in the long-term care setting.[22] Nursing home reform, improvement of care and pay for performance, and implementation of EBM in long-term care settings have been recent topics of interest.[1–7,10] The needs for high-quality and standardized care in long-term care facilities clearly should and must be met. Some clinical practice guidelines have been developed and some randomized controlled trials have been conducted in the long-term care setting. However, implementation of these guidelines requires long-term care providers to understand the evidence and comply with the recommendations. Understanding of the basic EBM concept could help long-term care providers use the evidence appropriately, offer them a new way to practice medicine, and help them make better decisions for their older patients and the families, potentially improving the quality of care in these settings.

Despite this potential benefit, practicing EBM in a long-term care setting has many challenges.[1,9,10] First, practicing EBM might require training and education for providers and perhaps other staff members. A formal EBM workshop for long-term care providers is urgently needed. Money and time are limiting factors. The good news is that the *Journal of American Medical Director Association*, a leading journal of long-term care providers, recently published some valuable review articles on EBM.[1,9,10]

Second, EBM has not been well tested to show that it improves outcomes and quality of care in general medicine and long-term care. Little evidence is available from high-quality randomized controlled trials performed in the long-term care setting.[20] Furthermore, most randomized controlled trials are efficacy trials, meaning they are conducted in ideal conditions, rather than effectiveness trials, meaning they are conducted in the real world. Also, achieving clinical outcomes depends on multiple factors.[23] The results from the research population might not be applicable to individual patients in the real world, which could make providers unwilling to use EBM. More randomized controlled trials must be performed in the long-term care setting.[9,19]

Third, old and frail patients in long-term care facilities often have multiple coexisting problems, including medical diseases, psychological and mental disorders, functional decline, and multiple symptoms. Unfortunately, most clinical practice guidelines, randomized controlled trials, and meta-analyses are disease- or organ-based. The targeted outcomes are often prevention of mortality and morbidity. This kind of evidence might not be applicable to a long-term care setting, where providers treat the whole person, and often according to the patient's individual goals of care, such as prolonging life, improving and maintaining function, or relieving symptoms.[24] These goals can sometimes present a conflict for an individual patient. For example, treating hypertension to prolong life and prevent stroke may cause some well-known side effects, such as constipation and fatigue secondary to antihypertensive drugs, leading to decreased comfort.

Furthermore, because of frequent cognitive impairment among patients in long-term care facilities, the patients are unable to express their major issues and preferences to providers, and therefore shared or patient-centered decision making can be difficult. Under these circumstance, providers must speak to the individual with power of attorney or the health proxy, such as a family member.

Finally, many important clinical questions in long-term care facilities are difficult to answer based on evidence from randomized controlled trials, which could be frustrating to long-term care providers. Therefore, evidence from non–randomized controlled trials must be used, such as from those examining the benefit or harm of tube feeding, the secondary prevention of cardiovascular diseases, outcomes of palliative care, and hospice care. The danger is if this easily obtained evidence becomes the only focus and results in the "Idries Shah effect," in which some treatments become the norm, but not because they are actually better, rather because the evidence for them was better tested.[21]

Practicing EBM in the long-term care setting could also cause some potential and unexpected harm. First, whether the evidence based on research in middle-aged or healthy old patients can be applied to old and frail patients receiving long-term care is unclear. The benefit for patients not receiving long-term care might not be reproducible for old and frail patients who are receiving this care, and harm might become more common and potentially worse. Good examples are aggressive treatment of diabetes mellitus and hypertension.

Second, providers must be careful to not simply follow disease-based guidelines when treating older persons. These may not take into consideration drug–drug and drug–disease interactions. For example, treating one problem may cause another problem in some older patients, depending on their comorbid conditions and current medications. Therefore, long-term care providers must examine the results for non–long-term care patients carefully.

Third, government, insurance, or other agencies may potentially misuse EBM in policymaking (ie, *regulatory EBM*),[21] such as when using EBM to determine pay for performance, which could cause many unexpected problems in the long-term care setting.[6,7]

SUMMARY

EBM has been widely used in medicine for 2 decades. Recently, EBM has become a central part of reforming nursing homes and quality improvement.[1–7,10] It can be very important for long-term care providers to practice EBM. This article introduces the concept of EBM; addresses some potential benefits, harms, and challenges of practicing EBM in the long-term care setting; and promotes EBM and its appropriate use among long-term care providers.

REFERENCES

1. Levenson SA. The basis for improving and reforming long-term care, part 2: clinical problem solving and evidence-based care. J Am Med Dir Assoc 2009; 10:520–9.
2. Levenson SA. The basis for improving and reforming long-term care, part 1: the foundation. J Am Med Dir Assoc 2009;10:459–65.
3. Levenson SA. The basis for improving and reforming long-term care, part 3: essential elements for quality care. J Am Med Dir Assoc 2009;10:597–606.
4. Levenson SA. The basis for improving and reforming long-term care, part 4: identifying meaningful improvement approaches (segment 1). J Am Med Dir Assoc 2010;11:84–91.
5. Levenson SA. The basis for improving and reforming long-term care, part 4: identifying meaningful improvement approaches (segment 2). J Am Med Dir Assoc 2010;11:161–70.
6. Levenson S. "Pay for performance": can it help improve long-term care? J Am Med Dir Assoc 2006;7:262–4.

7. Dolinar RO, Leininger SL. Pay for performance means compliance-based care. J Am Med Dir Assoc 2006;7:328–33.
8. Outcome project. ACGME. Available at: http://www.acgme.org/outcome/comp/compFull.asp. Accessed August 1, 2010.
9. Messinger-Rapport BJ. Evidence-based medicine: is it relevant to long-term care? J Am Med Dir Assoc 2004;5:328–32.
10. Levenson SA, Morley JE. Evidence rocks in long-term care, but does it roll? J Am Med Dir Assoc 2007;8:493–501.
11. Guyatt G, Rennie D, Meade M, et al. Users' guides to the medical literature—a manual for evidence-based clinical practice. 2nd edition. New York: McGraw Hill Medical; 2009.
12. Straus SE, Richardson WS, Glasziou P, et al. Evidence-based medicine—how to practice and teach EBM. 3rd edition. Edinburgh (UK): Elsevier Churchill Livingstone; 2005.
13. Heneghan C, Badenoch D. Evidence-based medicine toolkit. 2nd edition. Malden (MA): Blackwell Publishing; 2006.
14. How to teach evidence-based clinical practice workshop. McMaster University. Available at: http://ebm.mcmaster.ca. Accessed August 2, 2010.
15. Guyatt G. Evidence-based medicine. ACP J Club 1991;114:A16.
16. Haynes RB, Devereaux PJ, Guyatt GH. Physicians' and patients' choices in evidence based practice. BMJ 2002;324:1350.
17. Guyatt GH, Rennie D. Users' guides to the medical literature: a manual of evidence-based clinical practice. Chicago: AMA Press; 2002.
18. Atkins D, Kamerow D, Eisenberg GM. Evidence-based medicine at the Agency for Health Care Policy and Research. ACP J Club 1998;128:A14–6.
19. Cheng HY. Assessing the quality of evidence from randomized, controlled drug and nutritional supplement trials conducted among nursing home residents between 1968 and 2004: what can we learn? J Am Med Dir Assoc 2009;10:28–35.
20. PubMed. NIH. Available at: http://www.ncbi.nlm.nih.gov/pubmed/. Accessed December 18, 2009.
21. Dickenson D, Vineis P. Evidence-based medicine and quality of care. Health Care Anal 2002;10:243–59.
22. Institute of Medicine. Committee on proving quality in long-term care. Improving the quality of long-term care. Washington, DC: National Academy Press; 2001.
23. Graham RP, James PA, Cowan TM. Are clinical practice guidelines valid for primary care? J Clin Epidemiol 2000;53:949–54.
24. Gillick MR. Choosing appropriate medical care for the elderly. J Am Med Dir Assoc 2001;2:305–9.

Update on Teaching in the Long-Term Care Setting

Gwendolen T. Buhr, MD, MHS[a,*], Miguel A. Paniagua, MD[b]

KEYWORDS

• Nursing homes • Teaching • Long-term care
• Medical education

TEACHING IN THE LONG-TERM CARE SETTING

The teaching nursing home was "a new and exciting concept" in the 1980s.[1] Although some teaching nursing homes had existed previously,[2] the concept of the teaching nursing home formally began in 1982 when the Robert Wood Johnson Foundation funded a Teaching Nursing Home Program.[3] This initiative supported partnerships between 11 schools of nursing and skilled nursing facilities, which taught students long-term care for older adults. The National Institute on Aging also funded teaching nursing homes at about the same time, this time partnering medical schools and skilled nursing facilities.[3] Neither of the funding streams lasted for long enough to create enduring partnerships in many cases. However, evaluation of the teaching nursing homes indicated that they met their two main goals—to foster clinical research and to train health care professional students using interprofessional teaching strategies[4]—specifically demonstrating improvements in increased research productivity, nursing home resident outcomes, student attitudes toward older adults, and strengthened geriatric clinical experiences and curricula.[5,6] Many of the teaching nursing homes had home care components so that a broader view of long-term

Dr Paniagua was supported in part by funds from the Department of Health and Human Services (DHHS), Health Resources and Services Administration (HRSA), Bureau of Health Professions (BHPr), under Geriatric Academic Career Award number 1 K01 HP 00118-01. Dr Buhr was supported by a Geriatric Academic Career award 1 K01 HP00111-01. The information or content and conclusions are those of the authors and should not be construed as the official position or policy of, nor should any endorsements be inferred by the DHHS, HRSA, BHPR, or the US Government.

[a] Division of Geriatrics, Department of Medicine, Duke University Medical Center, DUMC Box 3003, Durham, NC 27710, USA

[b] Division of Gerontology and Geriatric, Department of Internal Medicine, Saint Louis University School of Medicine, Internal Medicine Residency Program, Fourteenth Floor, Desloge Tower, 1402 South Grand Boulevard, St Louis, MO 63104, USA

* Corresponding author.

E-mail address: buhr0001@mc.duke.edu

Clin Geriatr Med 27 (2011) 199–211
doi:10.1016/j.cger.2011.01.005 **geriatric.theclinics.com**
0749-0690/11/$ – see front matter

care as services provided in a wide range of settings was considered.[3,4] Since the 1980s, there have been fewer reports of the teaching nursing home, although the model is sustained at many schools of medicine, nursing, and academic medical centers.[6]

Long-term care has become a critically important area of geriatrics for the nation, as many of the frailest and most vulnerable elders are cared for in nursing homes. In 2004 there were 1.5 million older adults living in 16,000 nursing homes across the United States.[7] Unfortunately, there are far too few physicians, nurses, and other health care professionals with appropriate training in long-term care to care for that population, let alone educate learners in these venues. With respect to residency training, a 1998 survey of resident physicians completing their final year of training found that 31% of internal medicine (IM) residents and 20% of family medicine (FM) residents considered themselves unprepared to care for nursing home patients, compared with 0% and 4%, respectively, who felt unprepared to care for hospital inpatients.[8] Furthermore, these graduates felt unprepared for several long-term care associated tasks such as participation in quality improvement (40%/29%) and collaboration with nonphysician caregivers (18%/11%).[8]

Although the geriatric content has increased in medical schools in the United States, students are still receiving insufficient long-term care content. A survey of medical schools in 1999 and 2000 showed that 69% of medical schools had a teaching nursing home and 65% had curricular content in interdisciplinary teams.[9] In the 2007 American Association of Medical Colleges' (AAMC), Medical School Graduation Questionnaire, 38.4% of students felt unprepared to care for older adults in long-term care.[10] The 2010 AAMC Medical School Graduation Questionnaire indicates that most graduating students believed that their instruction in the care of geriatric patients (83.5%), and long-term health care (80.2%) was adequate, yet only about one-third of students had any experience with home care or nursing home care during medical school.[11] In addition, a significant portion of these medical school graduates believed that their instruction in quality improvement (29.1%), teamwork with other health professionals (9.9%), and health care systems (39.8%) was inadequate. A recent study found by using focus groups of third and fourth year medical students and IM residents that the trainees felt a need to know more about the different sites of care, specifically home care, nursing homes, assisted living, and hospice, as well as the level of care required for each patient in these settings.[12] The purpose of this qualitative study was to compare trainee perceptions of geriatric medicine experiences in relation to established core competencies in geriatrics, specifically those of the American Geriatrics Society.[13] In this study one student was quoted as saying, "I was very grateful for the opportunity in Medical School to go into a nursing care facility or hospice care or go into patients' homes...and see what happens at many different sites and therefore feel comfortable with the decision making process."[12] Although neither quantifiable nor generalizable, this study makes the case for using a needs analysis for a negotiated set of goals with trainees in a geriatric training program, and underscores the unique potential of site-specific experiences in long-term care education.

CURRENT REQUIREMENTS AND STRUCTURE OF LONG-TERM CARE CONTENT FOR PHYSICIAN TRAINEES

Postgraduate physician trainees get variable exposure to long-term care overall. Even if geriatrics is included in the curriculum, the long-term care perspective and a complete range of long-term care setting experiences is often missing. The Accreditation Council for Graduate Medical Education (ACGME) requires that FM residents "learn about, and practically apply, a multidisciplinary approach to the care of older patients in the hospital, the family medicine center (FMC), the long-term care facility, and the home."[14] Furthermore, they are required to care for at least 2 patients in a nursing home over a minimum of 24 consecutive months. In addition, each FM resident must perform 2 home visits.[14] By contrast, the ACGME only requires that IM training programs contain clinical experience that includes "an assignment in geriatric medicine."[15] There is no mention of the nursing home or long-term care in these requirements. As a result of the difference in requirements, FM programs universally have a required longitudinal experience, whereas the IM programs most commonly have a 1-month block rotation in geriatrics with a reported range of zero to 100% nursing home content in curricula, although some programs include long-term care specific topics in didactic instruction alone.

In 2002, a survey of IM residency programs indicated that 67% had a required nursing home component in their geriatrics rotation, which was offered in the block format 83% of the time.[16] Training also occurred at other long-term care sites including home care (44%), assisted living (23%), hospital-based skilled nursing facilities (38%), and senior centers (20%).[16] Comparable results were obtained from another survey in 2005.[17]

A similar survey was sent to FM program directors in 2001 and 2004,[18,19] with the latter revealing FM programs used nursing home (97%), home care (88%), assisted living (46%), hospital-based skilled nursing facilities (44%), and senior centers (28%) as teaching venues.[18] In 90% of the experiences, the nursing home rotation was longitudinal.[18]

There is no consensus on whether longitudinal experiences or block rotations are more effective at teaching desired content. The two are differentiated by both the timing and content of exposures. Longitudinal rotations are characterized by intermittent exposures (weekly to monthly) over an extended time period (1–3 years), whereas block rotations usually have repeated exposures over a 1-month time period. The block rotation often contains assigned readings and didactic instruction that are matched with the clinical content, whereas in longitudinal rotations, didactic instruction is often unrelated to the particular clinical experiences. In support of block rotations, one study showed that a geriatrics block rotation was more effective at increasing geriatric knowledge, as evidenced on in-training examinations. Further, the increased knowledge obtained in the block rotation was found to be retained at the time of graduation.[20] These data suggest that an organized, intensive geriatric block rotation, in which key concepts are repeated through multiple clinical exposures, relevant didactic instruction, and assigned readings, may lead to better learning and retention of geriatrics, This approach contrasts sharply with the usual longitudinal experiences, in which FM residents see a wide variety of patients with the geriatric cases mixed in, and geriatric didactic material scattered throughout the training period. In one study of third-year medical students in a 4-week geriatrics clerkship, multimodal curricula and assessments were used to positively affect knowledge, skills, and attitudes toward geriatrics. Pre-post knowledge improvement was significant ($P<.001$). Skills outcomes based on faculty observations and student self-assessment were positive overall, although only 50% of students rated themselves as improved in physical examination skills. Although attitudes were measured as students' satisfaction with the clerkship rather than their attitudes toward older adults or geriatrics, two-thirds of the students felt that the rotation was important for their education, indicating a positive attitude toward geriatrics. This study was an example of a block rotation leading to improvement in geriatric knowledge, skills, and attitudes.[21]

Regarding longitudinal rotations, the *Future of General Internal Medicine Report and Recommendations* called for longitudinal experiences across the spectrum of care.[17] In support of this recommendation, one study found that a longitudinal long-term care rotation for IM residents was effective in increasing geriatric knowledge (from 46.3% to 59%).[22] This curriculum consisted of a preassigned article, and a half-day a month of a 30-minute interactive case-based lecture, followed by nursing home rounds during which the resident was expected to conduct an assessment for one of the two assigned longitudinal patients to apply the information from the lecture.[22] Other studies have reached similar conclusions in favor of longitudinal rotation formats.[23] It is notable that the breadth of longitudinal geriatrics experiences described in the literature is vast, and these experiences are not standardized to one particular methodology (ie, mentor programs or didactics for preclinical students, patient encounters in graduate medical education, or a geriatric scholar program).

EDUCATIONAL DOMAINS EASILY TAUGHT IN LONG-TERM CARE

The ACGME sets standards that should be met by physicians seeking postgraduate medical specialization. Predictably, these standards historically focused on patient care, medical knowledge, and professionalism. In addition, many groups have recently published geriatric competencies for health professionals.[24–26] Many of these competencies can be fulfilled in the long-term care setting. **Table 1** lists the pertinent competencies compared side by side. For example, the long-term care patient population has a high prevalence of dementia, delirium, and depression, necessitating diagnosis and treatment in addition to the determination of decision-making capacity.[27] Most nursing home residents take between 5 and 9 medications, with one-quarter taking 9 or more,[28] facilitating the teaching of medication management competencies. As many as 3 out of 4 nursing home residents fall each year,[29] making the nursing home the ideal environment to learn about the risks and differential diagnosis for falls. In addition, the frail nursing home population requires a considered approach to treatment given their limited life expectancy, multiple comorbidities, and limited functional status.

In addition to the clinical competencies, the ACGME, in response to increasing pressure to ensure that physicians will be prepared to practice in the rapidly changing health care environment, has approved competencies in several key areas including (1) practice-based learning and improvement, (2) interpersonal and communication skills, and (3) systems-based practice.[30] These competencies are also effectively taught in the long-term care environment. Several examples are detailed in the following sections on quality improvement, interprofessional teamwork and group dynamics, health systems, and transitions of care.

Quality Improvement

"Practice-based learning and improvement" includes self-assessment of knowledge and expertise, and using quality improvement (QI) methods to make practice improvements. The completion of QI projects is one method of addressing these competencies. It is difficult for learners to understand the QI process through didactic instruction alone; rather, learners should experience the process to grasp the concepts and adopt the practices of QI. Therefore, successful teaching strategies have employed didactic instruction in combination with experiential learning.[31] In one curriculum, geriatric fellows were given a 1-hour interactive lecture, followed by monthly mentoring to complete an assignment to lead a brief QI project involving their long-term care practice using the Plan-Do-Study-Act cycle. This strategy resulted in improved self-efficacy in QI knowledge.[32] In a systematic review of QI curricula, 7 studies involving residents were reviewed. Each study combined didactic instruction with participation in QI activities.[31] Five curricula were integrated into a 4-week ambulatory or elective rotation, while 2 held weekly or biweekly meetings for a year. All 5 reported improvement in either perceived knowledge or scores on a QI knowledge test. The investigators recommended that future curricula teach collaborative skills, provide opportunities for trainees to work with an interprofessional team, and facilitate experiential learning.[31] These recommendations are all easily accomplished in the long-term care setting.

Interprofessional Teamwork and Group Dynamics

Appropriate care of frail older adults requires an interprofessional team of clinicians. Interprofessional training includes the principles of teamwork (establishing the team's mission, values, and goals), understanding group dynamics, and developing key interpersonal and communication skills that facilitate working effectively as member of an interprofessional health care team (eg, role negotiation, conflict management, problem solving, and decision making).[23] For education in teamwork to be effective, it must be grounded in clinical practice.[33] The nursing home has been an ideal place to integrate trainees into the interprofessional team and teach the concepts.[23] One unique study attempted to characterize the baseline attitudes of 591 multisite physician, social work, and nurse practitioner trainees toward interdisciplinary geriatric team work prior to their exposure to interdisciplinary team training. Validated attitudinal scales that measure attitudes toward team value, efficiency, and the physician role were used. All groups had a generally positive attitude toward the interdisciplinary teams' usefulness and benefit to patient care, though the physician trainees were at least twice as likely to consider the team as a means to assist physician care planning than either the nursing or social work trainees. The study has limitations in that trainees from other disciplines commonly found on interdisciplinary teams were not included. However, the study does make a case for early involvement of interdisciplinary team members in the education of physicians in training, so as to ensure the reinforcement of the concept of shared team decision making as fundamental in the team process of care.[34]

Health Systems

"Systems-based practice" entails working effectively in various health care settings (including nursing homes), advocating for optimal patient care quality, and identifying system errors and potential solutions. Long-term care is less technological and is often an unknown entity for medical trainees. The focus groups of medical students and IM trainees discussed by Drickamer and colleagues[12] illustrate that the trainees perceived a need to know more about the different sites of care. The investigators concluded that there should be education in the process of care, which includes knowledge of a variety of care settings including home care, assisted living, and nursing home.[12] First-hand experiences with long-term care settings and the requirements for each level of care are one way to deliver this important objective.

Transitions of Care

Long-term care is an ideal arena to teach transitions of care, as patients in long-term care commonly experience transitions to and from the hospital, clinic, and emergency department. Drickamer and colleagues[12] found that trainees expressed a need to know more about the discharge process and the data needed to determine the next site of care. A systematic review of the literature, which focused on best practices

Table 1
Examples of geriatric competencies easily taught in long-term care

Partnership for Health in Aging Multidisciplinary Competencies	AAMC Geriatric Competencies for Medical Students	Minimum Geriatric Competencies for IM-FM Residents
Health promotion and safety	Medication management	Medication management
1. Recognize the principles and practices of safe, appropriate, and effective medication use in older adults 2. Assess specific risks and barriers to older adult safety, including falls, elder mistreatment, and other risks in care environments 3. Apply knowledge of the indications and contraindications for, risks of, and alternatives to the use of physical and pharmacologic restraints with older adults	1. Explain impact of age-related changes on drug selection and dose based on knowledge of age-related changes in renal and hepatic function, body composition, and central nervous system sensitivity **Falls, balance, gait disorders** 2. In a patient who has fallen, construct a differential diagnosis and evaluation plan that addresses the multiple etiologies identified by history, physical examination, and functional assessment **Hospital care for elders** 3. Explain the risks, indications, alternatives, and contraindications for physical and pharmacologic restraint use 4. Explain the risks, indications, alternatives, and contraindications for indwelling (Foley) catheter use in the older adult patient 5. Conduct a surveillance examination of areas of the skin at high risk for pressure ulcers and describe existing ulcers	1. Prescribe appropriate drugs and dosages considering: age-related changes in renal and hepatic function, body composition, and central nervous system sensitivity; common side effects in light of patient's comorbidities, functional status, and other medications; and drug-drug interactions **Hospital patient safety** 2. Before using or renewing physical or chemical restraints on geriatric patients, assess for and treat reversible causes of agitation. Consider alternatives to restraints such as additional staffing, environmental modifications, and presence of family members
Evaluation and assessment	Cognitive and behavioral disorders	Cognitive, affective, and behavioral health
4. Choose, administer, and interpret a validated and reliable tool/instrument appropriate for use with a given older adult to assess: (a) cognition, (b) mood, (c) physical function, (d) nutrition, and (e) pain 5. Demonstrate knowledge of the signs and symptoms of delirium and whom to notify if an older adult exhibits these signs and symptoms	6. Compare and contrast among the clinical presentations of delirium, dementia, and depression 7. Formulate a differential diagnosis and implement initial evaluation in a patient who exhibits delirium, dementia, or depression 8. In an older patient with delirium, urgently initiate a diagnostic workup to determine the root cause (etiology)	3. Appropriately administer and interpret the results of at least one validated screening tool for each of the following: delirium, dementia, and depression 4. In patients with dementia and/or depression, initiate treatment and/or refer as appropriate

6. Develop verbal and nonverbal communication strategies to overcome potential sensory, language, and cognitive limitations in older adults	9. Perform and interpret a cognitive assessment in older patients for whom there are concerns regarding memory or function 10. Develop an evaluation and nonpharmacologic management plan for agitated demented or delirious patients	5. Evaluate and formulate a differential diagnosis and workup for patients with changes in affect, cognition, and behavior (agitation, psychosis, anxiety, apathy)
Care planning and coordination across the care spectrum (including end-of-life care)	Health care planning and promotion	Complex or chronic illness(es) in older adults
7. Develop treatment plans based on best evidence and on person-centered and person-directed care goals 8. Evaluate clinical situations where standard treatment recommendations, based on best evidence, should be modified with regard to older adults' preferences and treatment/care goals, life expectancy, comorbid conditions, and/or functional status 9. Develop advanced care plans based on older adults' preferences and treatment/care goals, and their physical, psychological, social, and spiritual needs 10. Recognize the need for continuity of treatment and communication across the spectrum of services and during transitions between care settings, using information technology where appropriate and available	11. Define and differentiate among types of code status, health care proxies, and advance directives in the state where one is training 12. Accurately identify clinical situations where life expectancy, functional status, patient preference or goals of care should override standard recommendations for screening tests in older adults 13. Accurately identify clinical situations where life expectancy, functional status, patient preference or goals of care should override standard recommendations for treatment in older adults **Atypical presentation of disease** 14. Generate a differential diagnosis based on recognition of the unique presentations of common conditions in older adults, including acute coronary syndrome, dehydration, urinary tract infection, acute abdomen, and pneumonia **Palliative care** 15. Assess and provide initial management of pain and key nonpain symptoms based on patient's goals of care 16. Identify the psychological, social, and spiritual needs of patients with advanced illness and their family members, and link these identified needs with the appropriate interdisciplinary team members	6. Identify and assess barriers to communication such as hearing and/or sight impairments, speech difficulties, aphasia, limited health literacy, and cognitive disorders. When present, demonstrate ability to use adaptive equipment and alternative methods to communicate (eg, with the aid of family/friend, caregiver) 7. Discuss and document advance care planning and goals of care with all patients with chronic or complex illness, and/or their surrogates 8. Determine whether an older patient has sufficient capacity to give an accurate history, make decisions, and participate in developing the plan of care **Transitions of care** 9. In transfers to the hospital from the skilled nursing or extended care facilities, ensure that the caretaking team has correct information on the acute events necessitating transfer, goals of transfer, medical history, medications, allergies, baseline cognitive and functional status, advance care plan and responsible primary care provider

(*continued on next page*)

Table 1
(continued)

Partnership for Health in Aging Multidisciplinary Competencies	AAMC Geriatric Competencies for Medical Students	Minimum Geriatric Competencies for IM-FM Residents
		Palliative and end of life care
	17. Present palliative care (including hospice) as a positive, active treatment option for a patient with advanced disease	10. In patients with life-limiting or severe chronic illness, assess pain and distressing nonpain symptoms (dyspnea, nausea, vomiting, fatigue) at regular intervals, and institute appropriate treatment based on their goals of care
		11. In patients with life-limiting or severe chronic illness, identify with the patient, family and care team when goals of care and management should transition to primarily comfort care
Interdisciplinary and team care	Self-care capacity	Ambulatory care
11. Communicate and collaborate with older adults, their caregivers, health care professionals, and direct-care workers to incorporate discipline-specific information into overall team care planning and implementation	18. Develop a preliminary management plan for patients presenting with functional deficits, including adaptive interventions and involvement of interdisciplinary team members from appropriate disciplines, such as social work, nursing, rehabilitation, nutrition, and pharmacy	12. Identify older persons at high safety risk, including unsafe driving or elder abuse/neglect, and develop a plan for assessment or referral
Health care systems and benefits	**Hospital care for elders**	
12. Provide information to older adults and their caregivers about the continuum of long-term care services and supports such as community resources, home care, assisted living facilities, hospitals, nursing facilities, subacute care facilities, and hospice care	19. Compare and contrast potential sites for discharge	

in training residents in geriatrics, identified that longitudinal care of patients from the hospital or ambulatory care setting to the nursing home, assisted living, home, or subacute facility is a good way for residents to develop a greater understanding of the care provided at each site and the issues involved with transition from one site to another.[23]

EDUCATIONAL METHODS IN LONG-TERM CARE

Most programs of long-term care education integrate didactic and experiential learning. A survey of directors of IM and FM residency programs in 1992 revealed that the most commonly employed instructional strategies in required nursing home experiences were direct patient care (91%), bedside rounds (86%), and lectures (86%).[35] Role models, individual instruction, group discussion, site visits, case presentations, case conferences, and assigned readings were also used more than half of the time.[35] This survey is almost 20 years old; however, the same methods are still being used with the addition of online learning.

Learning through direct patient care is common in medical education, especially postgraduate medical education. Such learning can be structured and guided, or informal and unstructured. The goal is for trainees to learn the knowledge and skills necessary to care for frail older adults in long-term care, which is accomplished by engaging in the actual hands-on work that maintains standards of high-quality patient care. By participating in patient care at the long-term care site, the trainees have the opportunity to learn from other professionals and from patients in context. However, simply placing trainees into the clinical arena without a formal curriculum or support is not sufficient. The old aphorism in clinical teaching, "see one, do one, teach one," is no longer acceptable. Brandt, Farmer, and Buckmaster created a 5-phase model for cognitive apprenticeships, a form of which is a structured direct patient care experience (as cited in Merriam and colleagues[36]). In the first phase the instructor demonstrates the activity ("see one"). Phase 2 involves the trainee doing the activity ("do one"), but with support or scaffolding from the instructor. The support is gradually removed in phase 3, so that in phase 4, the instructor assists only when asked by the trainee. The final phase involves generalizing the new skill to a different situation ("teach one").

Bedside teaching is a teaching strategy that can accompany direct patient care. It is defined as clinical teaching in the presence of a patient. Trainees believe that bedside teaching is an essential component of medical education to teach physician-patient communication, physical examination skills, clinical reasoning, and professionalism.[37] Janicik and Fletcher[38] have developed a model for best bedside teaching practices. The model includes 3 domains: (1) attending to the patient comfort, (2) focused teaching, and (3) group dynamics. The session begins by asking the patient's permission ahead of time; it remains patient centered, avoiding technical language while offering direct explanations to the patient; and it ends outside the room with a debriefing.[38]

Both direct patient care and bedside teaching are forms of experiential learning. The rationale that underscores the impetus for experiential learning is that experiences are critical for learning. Kolb's learning cycle for experiential learning is a widely known model; it has the following 4 steps in sequence: (1) concrete experience, (2) observation and reflection on the experience, (3) integration of ideas and concepts from the reflective observations, and (4) incorporation of the new ideas and concepts into actual practice, a process called active experimentation.[36] This model emphasizes reflecting on the experience as key to learning.

Didactics are also commonly employed to teach long-term care, examples of which include lecture, group discussion, and case conferences. Lecture is an efficient way to transmit information to a group of people in a relatively short amount of time that is familiar to most adults. Lecture has been shown to affect knowledge retention, but not physician behavior.[39] The technique is more effective when it was made more interactive with case discussion, role play, or if time was included for hands-on practice.[40] One way to teach trainees about the interprofessional team in long-term care is to have them interview members of the team individually, or in groups, and then teach their peers about the discipline that they interviewed.

BARRIERS TO LONG-TERM CARE EDUCATIONAL PROGRAMS

Several barriers are often cited that prevent improvements in geriatric and long-term care training; these include lack of adequately trained teachers and mentors, the belief that geriatrics is not important, and a lack of funding.[17] The first of these is underscored by a report from the Institute of Medicine (IOM) that outlined recommendations to improve the care of the aging population in the future.[41] This report highlighted the shortage of health care workers with appropriate training in geriatrics. Consequently, one of the recommendations was that hospitals should encourage the training of residents in all settings where older adults receive care, including nursing homes, assisted living facilities, and patients' homes.[41] There is, nevertheless, a financial disincentive for using the nursing home, assisted living facility, or home as training sites, because Medicare rules state that a faculty preceptor must accompany a resident to the setting in order for the clinician to receive reimbursement for the visit. This level of one-on-one supervision off site is difficult to provide for many programs.[41] In fact, 15% of IM program directors rated reimbursement constraints as a significant barrier to implementing a geriatric medicine curriculum in 2005.[17]

The most significant barrier reported by IM program directors in the 2005 survey was conflicting time demands with other curricula: 34% reported this barrier in 2005 compared with 46% in 2002.[17] While it is encouraging that most program directors are successfully integrating geriatrics into the residency curricula, there remains a significant number who encounter barriers, perhaps reflecting the belief that geriatrics is not important. Program planning is a social activity influenced by local politics and power.[42] Long-term care and geriatrics traditionally have suffered from negative attitudes, lack of interest, and little power within the medical establishment. It is encouraging that attitudes have improved over the years,[17] but planners of long-term care curricula should continue to work to gain representation and power in the planning process. There has been some increase in power, thanks to the recent report from the IOM highlighting the dire need for geriatric trained health care providers, thus establishing a needs assessment. Program planners can also gain buy-in from those who decide on the curricula by highlighting the areas easily taught in long-term care already discussed: QI, interprofessional teamwork and group dynamics, health systems, and transitions of care.

SUMMARY

As the American population ages, it becomes more essential that health professionals be trained in long-term care. Long-term care education began in earnest in the 1980s with the Teaching Nursing Home Programs. Although many of the original partnerships formed in these programs have not been continued, many of the effects of strengthened geriatric clinical experience and curricula for trainees are sustained today.

Long-term care is currently taught via block rotations, longitudinal rotations, and didactics. Educational leaders favor longitudinal experiences, because medical residents will be expected to provide longitudinal care to older adults in long-term care on graduation. However, to have more impact on physician behavior, the longitudinal experiences should combine interactive didactic techniques matched with hands-on practice that contains faculty scaffolding.

"Practice-based learning and improvement," "interpersonal and communication skills," and "systems-based practice" are 3 ACGME competencies that program directors may be struggling to teach and that are effectively taught in the long-term care setting. This fact should be leveraged by program planners negotiating for curricular time for long-term care education. Even if the ideal long-term care educational program is not possible immediately, it is important for planners to provide some long-term care education so that a minimal standard of competence can be achieved. This approach will also allow long-term care educators a place at the curriculum planning table, where they will have the opportunity to shape the future through learning interventions and innovations in long-term care education.

REFERENCES

1. Schneider EL. The teaching nursing home: a new approach to geriatric research, education, and clinical care. New York: Raven Press; 1985.
2. Duthie EH, Priefer B, Gambert SR. The teaching nursing home. One approach. JAMA 1982;247(20):2787–8.
3. Klein SM. A national agenda for geriatric education: white papers. New York: Springer Pub. Co; 1997.
4. Butler RN. The teaching nursing home. JAMA 1981;245(14):1435–7.
5. Mezey MD, Mitty EL, Bottrell M. The teaching nursing home program: enduring educational outcomes. Nurs Outlook 1997;45(3):133–40.
6. Mezey MD, Mitty EL, Burger SG. Rethinking teaching nursing homes: potential for improving long-term care. Gerontologist 2008;48(1):8–15.
7. Jones AL, Dwyer LL, Bercovitz AR, et al. The national nursing home survey: 2004 overview. National Center for Health Statistics. Vital Health Stat 2009;13(167):1–155.
8. Blumenthal D, Gokhale M, Campbell EG, et al. Preparedness for clinical practice: reports of graduating residents at academic health centers. JAMA 2001;286(9): 1027–34.
9. Eleazer G, Doshi R, Wieland D, et al. Geriatric content in medical school curricula: results of a national survey. J Am Geriatr Soc 2005;53:136–40.
10. Geriatrics Workforce Policy Studies Center. Table 5.4 Students responses regarding preparedness to care for older adults, 2001–2007. Available at: http://129.137.5.214/GWPS/files/Table%25205_4.pdf. Accessed October 26, 2010.
11. Association of American Medical Colleges. 2010 GQ Medical school graduation questionnaire all schools summary report. Available at: http://www.aamc.org/data/gq/allschoolsreports/gq_alllschools_2010.pdf. Accessed October 19, 2010.
12. Drickamer MA, Levy B, Irwin KS, et al. Perceived needs for geriatric education by medical students, internal medicine residents and faculty. J Gen Intern Med 2006;21(12):1230–4.
13. The Education Committee Writing Group of the American Geriatrics Society. Core competencies for the care of older patients: recommendations of the American Geriatrics Society. Acad Med 2000;75(3):252–5.

14. Acgme. ACGME program requirements for graduate medical education in family medicine. 2007. Available at: http://www.acgme.org/acWebsite/downloads/RRC_progReq/120pr07012007.pdf. Accessed April 29, 2010.
15. Acgme. ACGME program requirements for graduate medical education in internal medicine. 2009. Available at: http://www.acgme.org/acWebsite/downloads/RRC_progReq/140_internal_medicine_07012009.pdf. Accessed April 29, 2010.
16. Warshaw G, Murphy J, Buehler J, et al. Geriatric medicine training for family practice residents in the 21st century: a report from the Residency Assistance Program/Harfford Geriatrics Initiative. Fam Med 2003;35(1):24–9.
17. Warshaw GA, Bragg EJ, Thomas DC, et al. Are internal medicine residency programs adequately preparing physicians to care for the baby boomers? A national survey from the Association of Directors of Geriatric Academic Programs Status of Geriatrics Workforce Study. J Am Geriatr Soc 2006;54(10):1603–9.
18. Bragg EJ, Warshaw GA, Arenson C, et al. A national survey of family medicine residency education in geriatric medicine: comparing findings in 2004 to 2001. Fam Med 2006;38(4):258–64.
19. Li I, Arenson C, Warshaw G, et al. A national survey on the current status of family practice residency education in geriatric medicine. Fam Med 2003;35(1):35–41.
20. Steinweg KK, Cummings DM, Kelly SK. Are some subjects better taught in block rotation? A geriatric experience. Fam Med 2001;33(10):756–61.
21. Struck BD, Bernard MA, Teasdale TA. Effect of a mandatory geriatric medicine clerkship on third-year students. J Am Geriatr Soc 2005;53(11):2007–11.
22. Baum EE, Nelson KM. The effect of a 12-month longitudinal long-term care rotation on knowledge and attitudes of internal medicine residents about geriatrics. J Am Med Dir Assoc 2007;8(2):105–9.
23. Thomas DC, Leipzig RM, Smith LG, et al. Improving geriatrics training in internal medicine residency programs: best practices and sustainable solutions. Ann Intern Med 2003;139(7):628–34.
24. Leipzig RM, Granville L, Simpson DE, et al. AAMC Geriatric competencies for medical students 2009. Available at: http://www.pogoe.org/Minimum_Geriatric_Competencies. Accessed October 30, 2010.
25. Semla TP, Barr JO, Beizer JL, et al. Partnership for Health in Aging: multidisciplinary competencies in the care of older adults at the completion of the entry-level health professional degree. Available at: http://www.americangeriatrics.org/files/documents/health_care_pros/PHA_Multidisc_Competencies.pdf. Accessed October 29, 2010.
26. Williams B, Warshaw G, Medina-Walpole A, et al. Minimum geriatric competencies for IM-FM residents 2009. Available at: http://www.pogoe.org/IMFM_Competencies. Accessed October 30, 2010.
27. Evans JM, Chutka DS, Fleming KC, et al. Medical care of nursing home residents. Mayo Clin Proc 1995;70(7):694–702.
28. Lau DT, Kasper JD, Potter DE, et al. Potentially inappropriate medication prescriptions among elderly nursing home residents: their scope and associated resident and facility characteristics. Health Serv Res 2004;39(5):1257–76.
29. Rubenstein LZ, Josephson KR, Robbins AS. Falls in the nursing home. Ann Intern Med 1994;121(6):442–51.
30. ACGME Board. Common program requirements: general competencies 2007. Available at: http://www.acgme.org/outcome/comp/GeneralCompetenciesStandards21307.pdf. Accessed May 1, 2010.
31. Boonyasai RT, Windish DM, Chakraborti C, et al. Effectiveness of teaching quality improvement to clinicians: a systematic review. JAMA 2007;298(9):1023–37.

32. Yanamadala M, Buhr G. Can geriatric fellows learn continuous quality improvement (CQI) principles within a structured curriculum? [abstract]. J Am Geriatr Soc 2010;58(Suppl 1):s156.
33. Tsukuda RA. A perspective on health care teams and team training. In: Siegler EL, Hyer K, Fulmer T, et al, editors. Geriatric interdisciplinary team training. New York: Springer Pub. Co; 1998. p. 21–37.
34. Leipzig RM, Hyer K, Ek K, et al. Attitudes toward working on interdisciplinary healthcare teams: a comparison by discipline. J Am Geriatr Soc 2002;50(6): 1141–8.
35. Counsell SR, Katz PR, Karuza J, et al. Resident training in nursing home care: survey of successful educational strategies. J Am Geriatr Soc 1994;42(11): 1193–9.
36. Merriam SB, Caffarella RS, Baumgartner LM. Learning in adulthood: a comprehensive guide. 3rd edition. San Francisco (CA): Jossey-Bass; 2007.
37. Williams KN, Ramani S, Fraser B, et al. Improving bedside teaching: findings from a focus group study of learners. Acad Med 2008;83(3):257–64.
38. Janicik RW, Fletcher KE. Teaching at the bedside: a new model. Med Teach 2003; 25(2):127–30.
39. Casebeer L, Centor RM, Kristofco RE. Learning in large and small groups. In: Davis D, Barnes BE, Fox RD, editors. The continuing professional development of physicians: from research to practice. Chicago: American Medical Association Press; 2003. p. 169–90.
40. Davis D, O'Brien MAT, Freemantle N, et al. Impact of formal continuing medical education: do conferences, workshops, rounds, and other traditional continuing education activities change physician behavior or health Care Outcomes? JAMA 1999;282(9):867–74.
41. Institute of Medicine. Retooling for an aging America: building the health care workforce. Washington, DC: National Academies Press; 2008.
42. Cervero RM, Wilson AL. Working the planning table: negotiating democratically for adult, continuing, and workplace education. 1st edition. San Francisco (CA): Jossey-Bass; 2006.

Nausea and Other Nonpain Symptoms in Long-Term Care

Matthew J. Gonzales, MD[a,*], Eric Widera, MD[b,c]

KEYWORDS

- Geriatric • Long-term care • Palliative care • Management
- Nursing home

Long-term care facilities are becoming increasingly important as sites to improve the quality of end-of-life care. Nearly 1 of every 4 deaths in the United States occurs in a long-term care facility.[1] This number is expected to increase in the near future. The experiences of patients who die in long-term care facilities are notable for the patients' brief lengths of stay,[2] poor control of symptoms,[3,4] high rates of hospitalization and burdensome treatments,[3] and low use of hospice and palliative care services.[3,5] There has been a great deal of attention to improve the quality of end-of-life care in nursing homes by improving the timely assessment and management of various sources of suffering. Most of this literature has traditionally focused on one key symptom: pain. However, pain is only one of the many distressing symptoms long-term care residents experience at the end of their lives. It is important that all providers caring for residents in nursing homes understand the burden of nonpain symptoms and their management to improve the care of these individuals.

This article (1) summarizes the current literature on the frequency of nonpain symptoms in long-term care settings, particularly the data concerning residents at the end of their lives; (2) reviews the challenges to effectively assess and treat nonpain symptoms in nursing homes; (3) discusses an approach to address these challenges; and (4) reviews 3 common types of symptoms in nursing home residents at the end of

Dr Widera is supported by a Geriatrics Academic Career Award from the Health Resources and Services Administration, and by the Hartford Foundation as a Center of Excellence Faculty Scholar.

Commercial Financial Disclosure: None.

[a] Division of Hospital Medicine, Department of Medicine, University of California San Francisco, 521 Parnassus Avenue, Suite C-126, UCSF, Box 0903, San Francisco, CA 94941, USA

[b] Geriatrics and Extended Care, Department of Veterans Affairs Medical Center, VA Medical Center 181G, 4150 Clement Street, San Francisco, CA 94121, USA

[c] Division of Geriatrics, University of California San Francisco, 4150 Clement Street, San Francisco, CA 94121, USA

* Corresponding author.

E-mail address: matthew.gonzales@ucsf.edu

Clin Geriatr Med 27 (2011) 213–228
doi:10.1016/j.cger.2011.01.006 geriatric.theclinics.com

life within the context of this approach. Although this article focuses on residents at the end of life, many of these principles can be applied throughout the long-term care population.

SYMPTOM PREVALENCE

Symptoms at the end of life are common. The long-term care setting is no exception to this rule.[3,4,6–12] **Table 1** summarizes the data on the prevalence of symptoms at the end of life in the long-term care setting derived from 3 methods: (1) retrospective interviews of either facility staff or family members; (2) chart audits; and (3) minimum data set (MDS) analyses.[13] Caution is warranted in the interpretation of reported symptom prevalence data, because any of these methods can be problematic. For instance, MDS long-stay assessments are performed infrequently and assess only the presence or absence of a symptom within the designated look back period, which is 7 days for most symptoms. Thus if a resident suffered from daily nausea and intermittent vomiting for 2 months, but no vomiting in the week before the MDS assessment, nausea would not be included as an experienced symptom in the assessment. MDS data likely define the lowest prevalence of end-of-life symptoms in the long-term care setting. In general, data from chart audits or after-death interviews of care providers and family members indicate a higher prevalence of symptoms.

The presence of a symptom may not give a clear picture of the effect the symptom has on a resident's quality of life, and thus may not be the best indicator of the amount of suffering conferred by the symptom. A study by Brandt and colleagues[14] explored the degree of symptom burden within the last 2 days of life in nursing home residents as assessed by the resident's medical provider shortly after death. Symptoms were defined as burdensome when the symptom was rated greater than or equal to 60 on a 100-point visual analogue scale. The prevalence of burdensome symptoms was reported to be 51.3% and 28.4% at 48 and 24 hours before death, respectively. The most common burdensome symptoms at 48 to 24 hours before death were pain (30%), depression (30%), anxiety (25%), dyspnea (21%), and nausea (17%). The most common burdensome symptoms within 24 hours of death were dyspnea (23%), pain (22%), anxiety (21%), and nausea (17%).

Taken as a whole, symptom prevalence data show a clear need for improving nonpain symptom control in the long-term care setting at the end of life. Even though pain is frequently cited as the most common symptom experienced at the end of life, dyspnea is almost as common. In addition, nausea, constipation, depression, and anxiety significantly contribute to resident suffering.

CHALLENGES

Reducing the burden of symptoms in the long-term setting is important, yet it can be especially difficult to effectively recognize, evaluate, and treat nonpain symptoms in the long-term care setting. Several studies have reported underuse of proven therapies to treat nonpain symptoms in nursing home residents at the end of life.[4,10] These facilities are distinctly different from either the acute hospital or home setting. Approaches that may work in other settings may be more challenging to implement in the long-term care setting.

One of the main challenges in the effective management of nonpain symptoms is a high rate of serious comorbid conditions in nursing home residents. Almost 1 in 10 nursing home residents in the United States have cancer.[5] Progressive neurodegenerative conditions such as Alzheimer dementia are common, as are other diseases that impair functional status. These comorbidities affect every aspect of symptom

Table 1
Symptom prevalence at the end of life in long-term care facilities

Study	Population	Method of Assessment	Period of Assessment	Pain (%)	Nausea (%)	Dyspnea (%)	Constipation (%)
Mitchell et al, 2004[3]	2730 NH residents 65 years and older with advanced dementia who died within 1 year of admission	Last MDS assessment completed within 120 days before death	7 days before their last MDS assessment	16.9	n/a	12.7	n/a
Mitchell et al, 2004[6]	NH residents 65 years and older who died within 1 year of admission	Last MDS assessment completed within 120 days before death	7 days before their last MDS assessment				
	1609 with advanced dementia			11.5[a]	n/a	8.2	13.7
	883 with terminal cancer			56.6[a]	n/a	27.6	32.7
Caprio et al, 2008[7]	325 recently deceased NH, RC/AL residents	After-death interview with facility staff	Last month of life	45	n/a	44	n/a
Cartwright et al, 2006[8]	25 recently deceased AL residents	After-death interview with a family member	Last week of life	75	n/a	46	54
Duncan et al, 2009[9]	1022 NH residents with cancer	First MDS assessment recorded within 90 days after admission	7 days before the MDS assessment	50.6	3.4	13.2	n/a
	9910 NH residents without cancer			44.2	1.3[b]	10.1	n/a
Hall et al, 2002[10]	185 residents who died within an NH	Chart audit	Last 48 hours of life	44	n/a	62	n/a
Hanson et al, 2008[11]	674 recently deceased NH, RC/AL residents	After-death interview with facility staff and family	Last month of life	59	8	51	n/a
Rodriguez et al, 2010[4]	303 NH residents 65 years and older receiving hospice and palliative care	Facility staff reviewing medical records and MDS assessments	Unknown	n/a	7.2	n/a	8.8
Reynolds et al, 2002[12]	80 recently deceased NH residents	After-death interview with facility staff and family	Last 3 months of life	86	n/a	75	n/a

Abbreviations: AL, assisted-living facility; n/a, not assessed in the study; NH, nursing home; RC, residential care.
[a] Evaluated daily or almost daily pain, not just the presence of pain.
[b] Evaluated only vomiting and not nausea.

management, from assessment to treatment, and must be taken into account. For instance, in a study of nursing home residents, documentation of pain and analgesic use decreased as the degree of cognitive impairment increased. This discrepancy was not explained by differences in diagnoses that commonly result in pain.[15]

The recognition of nonpain symptoms in the long-term care setting presents a unique challenge. In particular, the problem of high staff turnover complicates both the screening and assessment of symptom burden. In general the higher the staff turnover rate within a nursing home, the lower the quality of care.[16] In addition, there is an overall lack of palliative care training among nursing home staff. Attention to nonpain symptoms is not the main focus of the daily routines in the long-term care setting. This situation is made worse by a regulatory environment that focuses most of its efforts on maintaining or improving function with little attention paid to improving the symptom-related quality of life.[17,18]

Once bothersome symptoms are recognized, the ability to perform a diagnostic workup in the long-term care setting is limited. Particularly, the lack of physician or midlevel provider presence limits what evaluations can be undertaken. In addition, long-term care facilities are not set up to provide rapid results from diagnostic evaluations. Given the lack of both provider and diagnostic resources, the perception is that it is often easier to refer the resident to an acute care facility.

Other issues are faced if the decision is made to provide treatment of the individual symptom within the long-term care facility. This situation is a particular challenge when considering pharmacologic intervention in this population, who in general have decreased renal function and increased sensitivity to side effects and polypharmacy issues. In addition, biases exist in health care providers around the prescription of opioids, including fear of exacerbating comorbid conditions or precipitating adverse effects.[19] Even nonpharmacologic therapies, such as environmental modifications, can present problems, because long-term care facilities are traditionally highly structured environments resistant to change.

SYMPTOM MANAGEMENT STRATEGY

Although the long-term setting presents some unique challenges, successful symptom management at the end of life is possible. We suggest an approach for the assessment and management of symptoms common at the end of life. In general, the necessary steps include early recognition and assessment of symptoms, tailored evaluation of the resident, initiation of therapy (both pharmacologic and nonpharmacologic), and frequent reassessment.

It is valuable to use a combination of resident reports, caregiver reports, and direct observation when assessing symptoms, because long-term care residents often have difficulty communicating their needs due to functional problems like cognitive impairment and hearing loss. However, even people with moderate to severe dementia may be able to communicate the severity of symptoms such as pain that they are currently experiencing.[20] In addition, behavioral cues are often helpful to assess for symptom burden when residents are unable to adequately verbally communicate discomfort. This observation can be particularly important in the assessment of terminal dyspnea.[21]

After an initial assessment documents the presence of symptoms, a more comprehensive assessment and diagnostic evaluation are indicated, because the treatment of these symptoms is most successful when the underlying cause is identified and addressed. The evaluation requires obtaining a history from both the resident and caregivers that includes details of comorbid health conditions, concurrent medications, and previous response to therapies. A detailed description of the rate of onset, frequency of occurrence, severity, associated symptoms, exacerbating or alleviating factors, and effect of the nonpain symptom is helpful both diagnostically and therapeutically. A focused physical examination is necessary to evaluate for common causes of nonpain symptoms in nursing home residents. Diagnostic evaluation with laboratory or radiology studies may be helpful, but a thorough history and physical examination alone leads to an understanding of the underlying process. If diagnostic interventions are necessary, it is critically important that they are tailored to the individual resident's preferences and goals for their care.

As with many therapeutic plans in palliative care, there is not a single unified approach that fits all patients. Rather, thoughtfully considering the goals of the patient and family along with the practicality of therapy in the nursing home setting is critical to ensuring high-quality care. Optimal symptom control requires evidence-based pharmacologic and nonpharmacologic interventions that focus on the whole person, as well as the needs and concerns of the resident's loved ones. Once a treatment plan has been initiated, it is important to ensure adequate, frequent reassessment.

This article applies the approach outlined earlier to 3 common symptoms seen at the end of life in the long-term care setting. Where possible the relevant articles from the literature pertaining to symptoms at the end of life in the long-term care setting are included. Where these data do not exist we have included best practices from the palliative medicine literature and our clinical experience. Even although it is not specifically addressed in this article, the addition of a multidisciplinary hospice team that coordinates care with the nursing home staff is an underused, yet valuable, way of improving the quality of end-of-life care for terminally ill residents.[22–25]

NAUSEA

Nausea is a subjective sensation that usually occurs before vomiting. Nausea is triggered by at least 1 of 4 pathways and then relayed to a final common pathway that produces emesis. This final common pathway is known as the vomiting center, which is located in the midbrain. The vomiting center helps to coordinate the parasympathetic and motor efferent activity necessary to produce a vomiting reflex. It is believed that nausea in the absence of vomiting likely arises from stimulation of this center at a low level that is not sufficient to cause triggering of the vomiting reflex.[26]

Four inputs relay information to the vomiting center: the chemoreceptor trigger zone, cortex, peripheral pathways, and vestibular system. Each of the 4 inputs detects a different stimulus and relays that information by way of neurotransmitters to the vomiting center. There is much overlap between the neurotransmitters. This overlap helps to explain why different antiemetic agents can be effective for treating multiple causes of nausea. A recent comprehensive review by Wood and colleagues[27] provides insight into the interrelationships between the neural pathways that mediate nausea and vomiting.

Screening for nausea is important to the successful treatment of this condition. Whereas vomiting is a clear symptom that can be recognized objectively by long-term care staff, nausea is a subjective symptom and must be enquired about. No formalized scales exist to help in the assessment of nausea in residents with cognitive impairment. It is important to consider other symptoms that may be markers for nausea. For example, chronic anorexia may represent constant low-grade nausea.

Evaluation of nausea should include a focused history and physical examination. It is critically important to pay attention to the pattern of nausea and other associated symptoms, such as concurrent constipation, because these may lend diagnostic clues to the underlying cause. If they are within a patient's goals of care, prudent laboratory testing and radiology evaluation may be helpful. Identification of infectious causes for nausea should also prompt staff to consider infection control measures to prevent viral or bacterial outbreaks commonly seen in the long-term care setting, such as *Clostridium difficile* or *norovirus*.[28]

Although the pathophysiology of nausea is well understood, the implementation of this understanding is often lacking at the bedside. Determining the most likely cause of nausea is critically important because the various pharmacologic antiemetic agents affect different neurotransmitters and are thus more effective in combating certain causes. Standardized approaches to the identification and treatment of nausea based on etiology have been successful.[29,30] Although some data suggest empiric therapy with a dopamine antagonist,[31] we suggest a mechanism-based approach, particularly for residents in the long-term care setting, where minimization of polypharmacy and side effects is important. The most common causes of nausea and their first-line antiemetics are listed in **Table 2**.

There are limited data to suggest that combination therapy to block multiple receptors is superior to changing agents when faced with nausea unresponsive to the first selected agent.[32,33] This is our experience as well. Although no clinical trial data support the use of continuous or around-the-clock administration of antiemetics, in our clinical practice this is often more effective than intermittent or as-needed administration.

Corticosteroids are also used in the management of nausea and vomiting.[34] Their mechanism of action in affecting these symptoms is unclear. Corticosteroids have been used successfully in the treatment of chemotherapy-induced nausea[35] and in the end-of-life setting.[36] Although not well understood, the addition of corticosteroids to an antiemetic regimen is often helpful in palliation of nausea.

Although medication and constipation-induced nausea are common in all settings, medication is likely to play a significant role in those residents who are in the long-term setting. One of the more common medications used in the long-term care setting is oral zinc supplementation, which has been associated with nausea. One recent small study reported that residents who received 440 mg/d of zinc sulfate for the treatment of pressure ulcers were 12.5 times more likely to experience nausea/vomiting than those residents who did not receive the zinc sulfate.[37] Another commonly used class of medications associated with significant nausea is the acetylcholinesterase inhibitors, such as donepezil. Clinical trials that evaluated the use of this drug noted a high incidence of nausea, ranging from 10% to 22%, particularly around the time of dose escalation.[38–40]

Environment modification is considered important in the management of nausea. Often simple, practical approaches are recommended by various authorities in the field.[26,27,41,42] These include avoidance of strong odors, presentation of small, attractive meals, and cool, carbonated drinks. Although independent data on the efficacy of these interventions are lacking, there is little harm in advising these environmental changes before initiation of pharmacologic therapy.

Acupuncture and acupressure have been shown to reduce postoperative nausea and vomiting[43] and chemotherapy-induced nausea,[44] but there is only minimal literature to support their use in the end-of-life setting.[45,46] Trials are being designed to better assess this question given the low side effect profile of this intervention.

After any intervention has occurred it is critically important that reassessment of symptom burden be undertaken. It may not be possible for this reassessment to be

Table 2
Common causes of nausea and their pharmacologic treatments

Cause	Mechanism	First-line Therapy: Class	First-line Therapy: Examples
Toxic/metabolic (including opioid-induced)	CTZ	Dopamine antagonist	Metoclopramide 5–10 mg by mouth/intravenously/subcutaneously every 6 h Haloperidol 0.5–2 mg by mouth/intravenously/ subcutaneously every 6 h Prochlorperazine 5–10 mg by mouth/intravenously/rectally every 8 h
Malignant bowel obstruction	CTZ	Dopamine antagonist	Metoclopramide 5–10 mg by mouth/intravenously/subcutaneously every 6 h[a] Haloperidol 0.5–2 mg by mouth/intravenously/subcutaneously every 6 h Dexamethasone 8 mg by mouth/intravenously daily Consider octreotide, nasogastric tube, venting gastrostomy
Chemotherapy	CTZ	Serotonin receptor antagonist	Ondansetron 4–8 mg by mouth/intravenously every 6 h
Constipation	—	—	Bowel agent (see **Table 3**)
Anticipatory	Cortex	Benzodiazepine	Lorazepam 0.5–1 mg by mouth/intravenously every 6 h[b]
Gut inflammation	Peripheral pathways	Serotonin receptor antagonist Dopamine antagonist	Ondansetron 4–8 mg by mouth/intravenously every 6 h Prochlorperazine 5–10 mg by mouth/intravenously/rectally every 8 h
Motion-induced labyrinthitis	Vestibular	Anticholinergic	Promethazine 12.5–25 mg by mouth every 4 h Scopolamine 1.5-mg patch every 72 h
Increased intracranial pressure (brain tumor)	Stimulation of vomiting center	Glucocorticoids	Dexamethasone 8–16 mg by mouth/intravenously divided every day every 6 h
Gastric stasis	Gastroparesis	Dopamine antagonist	Metoclopramide 5–10 mg by mouth/intravenously/subcutaneously before meals and at bedtime

Abbreviations: CTZ, chemoreceptor trigger zone; NK1, neurokinin.
[a] Avoid in complete bowel obstruction.
[b] Weak antiemetic, avoid as a single agent.

performed by a physician, but the physician should leave specific orders to ensure response to therapy is adequate.

DYSPNEA

Dyspnea is the subjective sense of difficulty breathing.[47] It likely results from a mismatch between afferent information from receptors and respiratory motor activity.[48] It can be affected by interactions with multiple physiologic, psychological, social, and environmental factors.[47,49,50] Dyspnea is often experienced at the end of life, independent of the terminal diagnosis[51] and is seen frequently in the long-term care setting.[12] In one study, nearly one-fourth of family members of deceased nursing home residents reported that the resident did not receive any or enough help with dyspnea.[52]

Dyspnea, like pain, is a symptom for which the only reliable indicator is resident self-report. This observation is particularly important because objective measures (ie, tachypnea or oxygen saturation) may not reflect the degree of discomfort experienced by residents. Residents may be found to be hypoxemic but not dyspneic, or dyspneic but not hypoxemic. Dyspnea is most often assessed as either present or absent; however, there are several scales, such as the Borg 0 to 10 scale or the visual analogue scale, which gives an indication of the severity or intensity of breathlessness. There is no evidence to support the use of any one of these instruments over another.[53] Although resident self-report is the gold standard, the assessment of dyspnea in patients in whom self-report is not possible should include assessment for dyspnea-associated behaviors such as nasal flaring, accessory muscle use, or tachypnea.[21] In clinical practice, most nursing homes do not regularly assess and document dyspnea in any manner; however, considering the prevalence of these symptoms in nursing home residents, frequent and routine assessment is warranted.

Evaluation should begin with a history that includes the resident's perspective of their dyspnea. This history should include what dyspnea means to the resident in relationship to their underlying illness, its effect on activities of daily living, and concerns regarding possible treatment modalities, such as opioids or oxygen. Psychological and spiritual distress should also be explored because they may exacerbate feelings of breathlessness and may indicate the need for greater interdisciplinary support.[54] A physical examination, pulse oximetry, and the possible addition of a complete blood count and chest radiograph can often clarify underlying causes. Further diagnostic testing may or may not be warranted depending on the preferences and goals of the resident and their family, and whether results may change the course of treatment.

Treating the underlying cause of dyspnea is always preferred if it is consistent with the resident's goals of care. This treatment may include antibiotics for pneumonia; corticosteroids and bronchodilators for a chronic obstructive pulmonary disease (COPD) exacerbation; or furosemide for a heart failure exacerbation. The addition of symptom-targeted treatments is often necessary, the cornerstone of which includes the administration of opioids.[53,55] The exact mechanism by which opioids relieve dyspnea is unclear. A recent systematic review of 9 crossover trials of oral or parental opioids showed a significant positive effect on the sensation of breathlessness.[56] Although the evidence from these trials is strong, the number of patients included in these studies was small. In addition, most of these patients had COPD as their study diagnosis, although 1 included study was completed on patients with cancer.

More recent studies have been completed and are increasing the body of evidence in support of opioid use for the relief of dyspnea. One of the best-designed studies was a randomized, double-blind, placebo-controlled crossover trial of sustained-release morphine for the management of dyspnea. Patients had a significant improvement in dyspnea scores when treated with morphine.[57] This improvement is seen not only in normoxic individuals but also in hypoxic individuals.[58]

Clinical experience suggests that lower doses of opioids are useful for controlling dyspnea, but few data exist on what doses are optimal.[59] A reasonable starting dose for an opioid-naive nursing home resident would be 2 mg of oral morphine, titrated to achieve symptom relief. Although it is believed that all opioids are effective in the treatment of dyspnea, most trials have studied morphine or dihydrocodeine.

One of the largest reported concerns with the use of opioids for the treatment of dyspnea is the fear of respiratory depression. Although respiratory depression is theoretically concerning, the literature reports that when appropriately administered, opioids do not seem to cause clinically significant respiratory depression.[58,60] In addition, multiple studies show that survival time is unrelated to opioid administration.[61,62] Of the 9 studies included in a recent systematic review that measured oxygen saturation, none found a significant change in oxygen saturation.[63] Of the 4 studies included in the systematic review that included arterial blood gas tensions, only 1 study showed a statistically significant increase in the amount of blood carbon dioxide while on treatment. Although statistically significant, this finding is unlikely to represent a clinical significance, because the $Paco_2$ never rose more than 40 mm Hg.

Interest in alternative delivery methods for opioids has been raised for the management of dyspnea. Particular interest has focused on providing opioids by nebulizer in an effort to avoid or reduce systemic side effects and access the intrapulmonary opioid receptors. Although data from current meta-analyses are insufficient to rule out future study on the issue, nebulized opioids have not been shown to be of any benefit in the treatment of dyspnea.[56,63] The studies included in this Cochrane review all looked at the use of nebulized morphine. A recent pilot study on nebulized hydromorphone found a benefit when this opioid was administered.[64] Thus additional data on other opioids may still be necessary to clarify whether the lack of benefit is generalizable to the entire class of opioids or specific to morphine.

Benzodiazepines have been suggested for the management of dyspnea, but a recent Cochrane review encompassing 200 individuals showed no beneficial effect on the relief of dyspnea in patients with advanced cancer or COPD.[65] However, the authors did note a slight, nonsignificant trend toward benefit. One recently published prospective nonrandomized trial suggests some benefit to midazolam in ambulatory residents with cancer. Although this outpatient data is not generalizable to the long-term care population. The cumulative body of evidence suggests that clinicians could consider benzodiazepines as a second-line or third-line treatment when other therapies are ineffective. If however residents have the symptom cluster of dyspnea and anxiety, benzodiazepines should be judiciously considered by the clinician. Additional therapies such as nebulized furosemide[66] or antidepressants[67,68] for the treatment of dyspnea have been explored but there is not enough evidence to support their use.

Several studies have attempted to look at the use of oxygen to treat dyspnea. Supplemental oxygen can provide relief of dyspnea in patients who are hypoxemic[53] but the data on the efficacy of oxygen supplementation on the nonhypoxic residents have been less convincing. A recent Cochrane database review completed on residents with cancer was inconclusive.[69] Most recently a randomized, double-blind, multicenter trial was completed in which oxygen delivery compared with room air provided no additional symptomatic benefit for relief of refractory dyspnea in nonhypoxic residents with life-limiting illness.[70] Although oxygen does not seem to independently improve dyspnea, forced air (eg, a fan) does seem to have some benefit in the relief of dyspnea and may eliminate the need to be connected to a nasal cannula.[71,72]

CONSTIPATION

Constipation is a common symptom encountered in the long-term setting, particularly at the end of life when opioids are used for palliation of pain and dyspnea. The early recognition and assessment of constipation is critical in nursing home residents to avoid serious negative outcomes. This situation is complicated by the various definitions used throughout the literature to characterize constipation. Usually it is defined as difficulty with defecation characterized by straining or hard stools or fewer than 3 defecations per week. Straining has been suggested to be the symptom most sensitive for constipation.[73] In practice, it is helpful to note any changes to the usual pattern of bowel movements, whether in stool frequency or consistency. Other signs and symptoms that raise concern for constipation include fecal incontinence, new urinary incontinence, new or worsening abdominal or hemorrhoidal pain, or changes in mental status.

The evaluation of constipation is often divided into consideration of primary and secondary causes by history and physical examination. Primary causes of constipation are important, but often treated with the addition of laxatives irrespective of the underlying cause. In the long-term care setting, consideration of secondary causes of constipation is critical. In particular, the identification of medications associated with constipation is important. Medications commonly used in the long-term care setting associated with constipation include calcium supplementation, antacids, iron, calcium channel blockers, nonsteroidal antiinflammatory agents, and opioids. Cessation of offending medications, if possible, can be beneficial in treating constipation.

Common agents used for the treatment of constipation are listed in **Table 3**. A recent Cochrane review of 4 trials including 280 residents founds there was insufficient evidence to support the use of 1 laxative over another.[74] Although docusate is commonly used for the treatment of constipation, a recent pilot study of hospitalized patients with cancer suggests docusate may provide no additional benefit over a sennoside-based bowel protocol.[75] Docusate is also poorly tolerated if given orally, either by crushing the capsule or by giving it as a solution, as is frequently attempted at the end of life when residents begin to have difficulty swallowing pills. For this reason, we no longer recommend prescribing this agent.

At the end of life, opioid-induced constipation is common. A proactive approach is a necessity in managing opioid-induced constipation to minimize the associated negative outcomes that may include nausea, anorexia, and bowel obstruction. This approach includes anticipating constipation to be a common adverse side effect of opioids. There is often rapid development of tolerance to most of the side effects of opioids. Unfortunately, the decrease in gastrointestinal motility and thus increase in gastrointestinal transit time does not abate with continued opioid therapy. It is therefore recommended that, at a minimum, a stimulant laxative such as senna be prescribed with the use of any opioid. Although the current standard of care is the prescription of prophylactic laxative regimens in residents who are at the end of life, a recent analysis of long-term care residents suggests adherence to these standards is low.[76]

Laxative administration is common for the treatment of opioid-induced constipation, yet it does not address the underlying pathophysiology, namely the activation of the gastrointestinal μ-opioid receptors. Activation of the gastrointestinal μ-opioid receptors slows gastrointestinal transit time and induces constipation.[77,78] Recent interest has been generated in locally antagonizing this receptor to treat opioid-induced constipation. The challenge has been to find a compound that antagonizes the gastrointestinal receptor and not the central nervous system receptors. Naloxone

Table 3
Common medications to treat constipation

Medication	Dosage	Onset	Adverse Effects
Bulk Forming			
Psyllium	1–2 tablespoons dissolved in 236.5 mL (8 oz) of fluid 1–3 times/d	Days	Abdominal cramps and bloating, bowel impaction if unable to maintain recommended fluid intake
Methylcellulose	1 tablespoon dissolved in 236.5 mL (8 oz) of fluid 1–3 times/d	Days	Abdominal cramps and bloating, bowel impaction if unable to maintain recommended fluid intake
Emollients (Softeners)			
Mineral oil	15–45 mL/d	Hours	Risk of lipid pneumonia if aspirated; decreased absorption of fat-soluble vitamins and Coumadin
Osmolar Agents			
Polyethylene glycol (PEG 3350)	17 g dissolved in 236.5 mL (8 oz) of fluid 1–2 times/d	Days	Nausea, bloating, cramping, urticaria
Lactulose	15–30 mL 1–2 times/d	Days	Abdominal cramps and bloating
Sorbitol	30–150 mL of 70% solution 1 time/d	Hours	Abdominal cramps and bloating
Glycerine	1 suppository 1 time/d	Minutes	Rectal irritation, headache
Magnesium hydroxide (milk of magnesia)	30–60 mL 1 time/d (maximum 60 mL/24 h)	Hours	Magnesium toxicity (with renal insufficiency)
Magnesium citrate	150–300 mL/d (maximum 300 mL/d)	Hours	Magnesium toxicity (with renal insufficiency)
Stimulant Laxatives			
Bisacodyl	10–30 mg by mouth 1 time/d	Hours	Abdominal cramps and bloating; avoid use within 1 h of antacids or milk
	10 mg suppository 1 time/d	Hours	—
Senna[a]	2–4 tablets 1–2 times/d	Hours	Abdominal cramps and bloating, urine discoloration
Peripheral Opioid Antagonist			
Methylnaltrexone	Weight-based subcutaneous injection	Hours	Abdominal pain, nausea, hyperhidrosis

[a] Not effective in patients with ileostomies.

when administered orally in low doses undergoes extensive first-pass metabolism and has been shown to have low systemic bioavailability. Using this knowledge, 1 study found benefit in coadministration of sustained-release oxycodone with oral naloxone.[79] Subcutaneous methylnaltrexone, a quaternary amine that does not cross the blood-brain barrier, is effective in inducing laxation for 48% of patients with opioid-induced constipation.[80] The benefit of methylnaltrexone is that there is no effect on analgesic efficacy, although cost may limit its widespread adoption.

Although increased physical activity and fluid intake are commonly recommended, data for their use are limited. For many residents these interventions may be appropriate, but both of these interventions may lead to increased discomfort in a resident at the end of life. The addition of increased amounts of dietary fiber may help many in the long-term setting, but only if resident's are able to tolerate adequate amounts of fluids.

SUMMARY

Although almost one-quarter of the population of the United States dies in the long-term care setting, few specific nonpain symptom management guidelines are available. Certainly there are few randomized control trials. It is encouraging that data on this population seem to be increasing, but additional studies are needed to better characterize the symptom prevalence and best management guidelines for this population. Despite this lack of evidence in the long-term care setting, best evidence from the palliative care literature can help to guide practice.

It is critical that providers in the long-term care setting work with their staff to increase the awareness of nonpain symptoms. These symptoms present a significant burden to patients and their families. Yet through early assessment and recognition, tailored evaluation, prompt intervention, and consistent reassessment, providers can make significant progress in improving the quality of life for their long-term facility residents.

REFERENCES

1. Gruneir A, Mor V, Weitzen S, et al. Where people die: a multilevel approach to understanding influences on site of death in America. Med Care Res Rev 2007; 64(4):351–78.
2. Kelly A, Conell-Price J, Covinsky K, et al. Length of stay for older adults residing in nursing homes at the end of life. J Am Geriatr Soc 2010;58(9):1701–6.
3. Mitchell SL, Morris JN, Park PS, et al. Terminal care for persons with advanced dementia in the nursing home and home care settings. J Palliat Med 2004;7(6): 808–16.
4. Rodriguez KL, Hanlon JT, Perera S, et al. A cross-sectional analysis of the prevalence of undertreatment of nonpain symptoms and factors associated with undertreatment in older nursing home hospice/palliative care patients. Am J Geriatr Pharmacother 2010;8(3):225–32.
5. Johnson VM, Teno JM, Bourbonniere M, et al. Palliative care needs of cancer patients in U.S. nursing homes. J Palliat Med 2005;8(2):273–9.
6. Mitchell SL, Kiely DK, Hamel MB. Dying with advanced dementia in the nursing home. Arch Intern Med 2004;164(3):321–6.
7. Caprio AJ, Hanson LC, Munn JC, et al. Pain, dyspnea, and the quality of dying in long-term care. J Am Geriatr Soc 2008;56(4):683–8.
8. Cartwright JC, Hickman S, Perrin N, et al. Symptom experiences of residents dying in assisted living. J Am Med Dir Assoc 2006;7(4):219–23.

9. Duncan JG, Bott MJ, Thompson SA, et al. Symptom occurrence and associated clinical factors in nursing home residents with cancer. Res Nurs Health 2009; 32(4):453–64.
10. Hall P, Schroder C, Weaver L. The last 48 hours of life in long-term care: a focused chart audit. J Am Geriatr Soc 2002;50(3):501–6.
11. Hanson LC, Eckert JK, Dobbs D, et al. Symptom experience of dying long-term care residents. J Am Geriatr Soc 2008;56(1):91–8.
12. Reynolds K, Henderson M, Schulman A, et al. Needs of the dying in nursing homes. J Palliat Med 2002;5(6):895–901.
13. Mor V. A comprehensive clinical assessment tool to inform policy and practice: applications of the minimum data set. Med Care 2004;42(Suppl 4):III50–9.
14. Brandt HE, Ooms ME, Deliens L, et al. The last two days of life of nursing home patients–a nationwide study on causes of death and burdensome symptoms in The Netherlands. Palliat Med 2006;20(5):533–40.
15. Reynolds KS, Hanson LC, DeVellis RF, et al. Disparities in pain management between cognitively intact and cognitively impaired nursing home residents. J Pain Symptom Manage 2008;35(4):388–96.
16. Castle NG, Engberg J, Men A. Nursing home staff turnover: impact on nursing home compare quality measures. Gerontologist 2007;47(5):650–61.
17. Huskamp HA, Stevenson DG, Chernew ME, et al. A new Medicare end-of-life benefit for nursing home residents. Health Aff (Millwood) 2010;29(1):130–5.
18. Zerzan J, Stearns S, Hanson L. Access to palliative care and hospice in nursing homes. JAMA 2000;284(19):2489–94.
19. Pargeon KL, Hailey BJ. Barriers to effective cancer pain management: a review of the literature. J Pain Symptom Manage 1999;18(5):358–68.
20. Kapo J, Morrison LJ, Liao S. Palliative care for the older adult. J Palliat Med 2007; 10(1):185–209.
21. Campbell ML. Terminal dyspnea and respiratory distress. Crit Care Clin 2004; 20(3):403–17, viii–ix.
22. Miller SC, Mor V, Wu N, et al. Does receipt of hospice care in nursing homes improve the management of pain at the end of life? J Am Geriatr Soc 2002; 50(3):507–15.
23. Miller SC, Mor V, Teno J. Hospice enrollment and pain assessment and management in nursing homes. J Pain Symptom Manage 2003;26(3):791–9.
24. Baer WM, Hanson LC. Families' perception of the added value of hospice in the nursing home. J Am Geriatr Soc 2000;48(8):879–82.
25. Casarett D, Karlawish J, Morales K, et al. Improving the use of hospice services in nursing homes: a randomized controlled trial. JAMA 2005;294(2):211–7.
26. Mannix KA. Palliation of nausea and vomiting. In: Hanks G, Fallon M, Cherny NI, et al, editors. Oxford Textbook of Palliative Medicine. 4th edition. Oxford: Oxford University Press; 2010.
27. Wood GJ, Shega JW, Lynch B, et al. Management of intractable nausea and vomiting in patients at the end of life: "I was feeling nauseous all of the time. nothing was working". JAMA 2007;298(10):1196–207.
28. Widera E, Chang A, Chen HL. Presenteeism: a public health hazard. J Gen Intern Med 2010;25(11):1244–7.
29. Bentley A, Boyd K. Use of clinical pictures in the management of nausea and vomiting: a prospective audit. Palliat Med 2001;15(3):247–53.
30. Stephenson J, Davies A. An assessment of aetiology-based guidelines for the management of nausea and vomiting in patients with advanced cancer. Support Care Cancer 2006;14(4):348–53.

31. Bruera E, Seifert L, Watanabe S, et al. Chronic nausea in advanced cancer patients: a retrospective assessment of a metoclopramide-based antiemetic regimen. J Pain Symptom Manage 1996;11(3):147–53.
32. Cole RM, Robinson F, Harvey L, et al. Successful control of intractable nausea and vomiting requiring combined ondansetron and haloperidol in a patient with advanced cancer. J Pain Symptom Manage 1994;9(1):48–50.
33. Mystakidou K, Befon S, Liossi C, et al. Comparison of tropisetron and chlorpromazine combinations in the control of nausea and vomiting of patients with advanced cancer. J Pain Symptom Manage 1998;15(3):176–84.
34. Shih A, Jackson KC. Role of corticosteroids in palliative care. J Pain Palliat Care Pharmacother 2007;21(4):69–76.
35. Grunberg SM. Antiemetic activity of corticosteroids in patients receiving cancer chemotherapy: dosing, efficacy, and tolerability analysis. Ann Oncol 2007; 18(2):233–40.
36. Popiela T, Lucchi R, Giongo F. Methylprednisolone as palliative therapy for female terminal cancer patients. The Methylprednisolone Female Preterminal Cancer Study Group. Eur J Cancer Clin Oncol 1989;25(12):1823–9.
37. Houston S, Haggard J, Williford J, et al. Adverse effects of large-dose zinc supplementation in an institutionalized older population with pressure ulcers. J Am Geriatr Soc 2001;49(8):1130–2.
38. Rogers SL, Farlow MR, Doody RS, et al. A 24-week, double-blind, placebo-controlled trial of donepezil in patients with Alzheimer's disease. Donepezil Study Group. Neurology 1998;50(1):136–45.
39. Greenberg SM, Tennis MK, Brown LB, et al. Donepezil therapy in clinical practice: a randomized crossover study. Arch Neurol 2000;57(1):94–9.
40. Rogers SL, Doody RS, Mohs RC, et al. Donepezil improves cognition and global function in Alzheimer disease: a 15-week, double-blind, placebo-controlled study. Donepezil Study Group. Arch Intern Med 1998;158(9):1021–31.
41. Rhodes VA, McDaniel RW. Nausea, vomiting, and retching: complex problems in palliative care. CA Cancer J Clin 2001;51(4):232–48 [quiz: 249–52].
42. Pantilat SZ, Isaac M. End-of-life care for the hospitalized patient. Med Clin North Am 2008;92(2):349–70, viii–ix.
43. Lee A, Fan LT. Stimulation of the wrist acupuncture point P6 for preventing postoperative nausea and vomiting. Cochrane Database Syst Rev 2009;2:CD003281.
44. Ezzo JM, Richardson MA, Vickers A, et al. Acupuncture-point stimulation for chemotherapy-induced nausea or vomiting. Cochrane Database Syst Rev 2006;2:CD002285.
45. Wright LD. The use of motion sickness bands to control nausea and vomiting in a group of hospice patients. Am J Hosp Palliat Care 2005;22(1):49–53.
46. Perkins P, Vowler SL. Does acupressure help reduce nausea and vomiting in palliative care patients? Pilot study. Palliat Med 2008;22(2):193–4.
47. Dyspnea. Mechanisms, assessment, and management: a consensus statement. American Thoracic Society. Am J Respir Crit Care Med 1999;159(1): 321–40.
48. Luce JM, Luce JA. Perspectives on care at the close of life. Management of dyspnea in patients with far-advanced lung disease: "once I lose it, it's kind of hard to catch it." JAMA 2001;285(10):1331–7.
49. von Leupoldt A, Sommer T, Kegat S, et al. Dyspnea and pain share emotion-related brain network. Neuroimage 2009;48(1):200–6.
50. Gilman SA, Banzett RB. Physiologic changes and clinical correlates of advanced dyspnea. Curr Opin Support Palliat Care 2009;3(2):93–7.

51. Solano JP, Gomes B, Higginson IJ. A comparison of symptom prevalence in far advanced cancer, AIDS, heart disease, chronic obstructive pulmonary disease and renal disease. J Pain Symptom Manage 2006;31(1):58–69.
52. Teno JM, Clarridge BR, Casey V, et al. Family perspectives on end-of-life care at the last place of care. JAMA 2004;291(1):88–93.
53. Mahler DA, Selecky PA, Harrod CG, et al. American College of Chest Physicians consensus statement on the management of dyspnea in patients with advanced lung or heart disease. Chest 2010;137(3):674–91.
54. Thomas JR, von Gunten CF. Management of dyspnea. J Support Oncol 2003; 1(1):23–32 [discussion: 32–4].
55. Ben-Aharon I, Gafter-Gvili A, Paul M, et al. Interventions for alleviating cancer-related dyspnea: a systematic review. J Clin Oncol 2008;26(14):2396–404.
56. Jennings AL, Davies AN, Higgins JPT, et al. A systematic review of the use of opioids in the management of dyspnoea. Thorax 2002;57(11):939–44.
57. Abernethy AP, Currow DC, Frith P, et al. Randomised, double blind, placebo controlled crossover trial of sustained release morphine for the management of refractory dyspnoea. BMJ 2003;327(7414):523–8.
58. Clemens KE, Quednau I, Klaschik E. Use of oxygen and opioids in the palliation of dyspnoea in hypoxic and non-hypoxic palliative care patients: a prospective study. Support Care Cancer 2009;17(4):367–77.
59. Allard P, Lamontagne C, Bernard P, et al. How effective are supplementary doses of opioids for dyspnea in terminally ill cancer patients? A randomized continuous sequential clinical trial. J Pain Symptom Manage 1999;17(4):256–65.
60. Rocker G, Horton R, Currow D, et al. Palliation of dyspnoea in advanced COPD: revisiting a role for opioids. Thorax 2009;64(10):910–5.
61. Sykes N, Thorns A. The use of opioids and sedatives at the end of life. Lancet Oncol 2003;4(5):312–8.
62. Thorns A, Sykes N. Opioid use in last week of life and implications for end-of-life decision-making. Lancet 2000;356(9227):398–9.
63. Jennings AL, Davies AN, Higgins JP, et al. Opioids for the palliation of breathlessness in terminal illness. Cochrane Database Syst Rev 2001;4:CD002066.
64. Charles MA, Reymond L, Israel F. Relief of incident dyspnea in palliative cancer patients: a pilot, randomized, controlled trial comparing nebulized hydromorphone, systemic hydromorphone, and nebulized saline. J Pain Symptom Manage 2008;36(1):29–38.
65. Simon ST, Higginson IJ, Booth S, et al. Benzodiazepines for the relief of breathlessness in advanced malignant and non-malignant diseases in adults. Cochrane Database Syst Rev 2010;1:CD007354.
66. Newton PJ, Davidson PM, Macdonald P, et al. Nebulized furosemide for the management of dyspnea: does the evidence support its use? J Pain Symptom Manage 2008;36(4):424–41.
67. Smoller JW, Pollack MH, Systrom D, et al. Sertraline effects on dyspnea in patients with obstructive airways disease. Psychosomatics 1998;39(1):24–9.
68. Borson S, McDonald GJ, Gayle T, et al. Improvement in mood, physical symptoms, and function with nortriptyline for depression in patients with chronic obstructive pulmonary disease. Psychosomatics 1992;33(2):190–201.
69. Cranston JM, Crockett A, Currow D. Oxygen therapy for dyspnoea in adults. Cochrane Database Syst Rev 2008;3:CD004769.
70. Abernethy AP, Mcdonald CF, Frith PA, et al. Effect of palliative oxygen versus room air in relief of breathlessness in patients with refractory dyspnoea: a double-blind, randomised controlled trial. Lancet 2010;376(9743):784–93.

71. Bausewein C, Booth S, Gysels M, et al. Non-pharmacological interventions for breathlessness in advanced stages of malignant and non-malignant diseases. Cochrane Database Syst Rev 2008;2:CD005623.
72. Galbraith S, Fagan P, Perkins P, et al. Does the use of a handheld fan improve chronic dyspnea? A randomized, controlled, crossover trial. J Pain Symptom Manage 2010;39(5):831–8.
73. Koch A, Voderholzer WA, Klauser AG, et al. Symptoms in chronic constipation. Dis Colon Rectum 1997;40(8):902–6.
74. Miles CL, Fellowes D, Goodman ML, et al. Laxatives for the management of constipation in palliative care patients. Cochrane Database Syst Rev 2006;4:CD003448.
75. Hawley PH, Byeon JJ. A comparison of sennosides-based bowel protocols with and without docusate in hospitalized patients with cancer. J Palliat Med 2008; 11(4):575–81.
76. Max EK, Hernandez JJ, Sturpe DA, et al. Prophylaxis for opioid-induced constipation in elderly long-term care residents: a cross-sectional study of Medicare beneficiaries. Am J Geriatr Pharmacother 2007;5(2):129–36.
77. Tavani A, Bianchi G, Ferretti P, et al. Morphine is most effective on gastrointestinal propulsion in rats by intraperitoneal route: evidence for local action. Life Sci 1980; 27(23):2211–7.
78. Manara L, Bianchi G, Ferretti P, et al. Inhibition of gastrointestinal transit by morphine in rats results primarily from direct drug action on gut opioid sites. J Pharmacol Exp Ther 1986;237(3):945–9.
79. Meissner W, Leyendecker P, Mueller-Lissner S, et al. A randomised controlled trial with prolonged-release oral oxycodone and naloxone to prevent and reverse opioid-induced constipation. Eur J Pain 2009;13(1):56–64.
80. Thomas J, Karver S, Cooney GA, et al. Methylnaltrexone for opioid-induced constipation in advanced illness. N Engl J Med 2008;358(22):2332–43.

Urinary Tract Infections in Long-Term Care Residents

Gwendolen T. Buhr, MD, MHS[a,*], Liza Genao, MD[b], Heidi K. White, MD, MHS, MEd[a]

KEYWORDS

- Urinary Tract Infections • Asymptomatic bacteriuria
- Bacteriuria • Nursing homes

DEFINITIONS

A bacterial urinary tract infection (UTI) is defined as the presence of bacteria in the urine in appropriate quantitative counts. A symptomatic UTI is diagnosed when the level of bacteria in the urine is equal to or greater than 10^5 CFU/mL in a clean catch specimen, or equal to or greater than 10^2 CFU/mL in a catheterized specimen with symptoms attributable to the genitourinary tract.[1] Asymptomatic UTI is defined as the presence of bacteriuria in the same quantitative counts on 2 consecutive urine specimens without symptoms attributable to the genitourinary tract.[1] Pyuria is the presence of more than 10 white blood cells per high field of spun urine, and indicates an inflammatory response in the genitourinary tract.[1,2] Because pyuria is virtually synonymous with bacteriuria in long-term care (LTC) residents, the terms asymptomatic UTI and asymptomatic bacteriuria can be used interchangeably.

EPIDEMIOLOGY

Asymptomatic UTI is common in LTC residents, occurring in 15% to 37% of men, and 25% to 53% of women.[3] In the 5% to 15% of LTC residents with chronic indwelling urinary catheters,[4,5] asymptomatic UTI is almost universal.[6] In contrast, the rate of symptomatic UTI has been measured as 5.5% in LTC residents with an indwelling urinary catheter.[7] This is higher than the rate of symptomatic UTI measured in residents without an indwelling urinary catheter; in studies performed in community nursing homes, intermediate care wards, and Veterans Affairs (VA) nursing home

Gwendolen T. Buhr was supported by a Geriatric Academic Career award 1 K01 HP00111-01.
[a] Division of Geriatrics, Department of Medicine, Duke University Medical Center, DUMC Box 3003, Durham, NC 27710, USA
[b] Division of Geriatrics, Department of Medicine, Duke University Medical Center, Durham VA Medical Center, 508 Fulton Street, Box 182, Durham, NC 27705, USA
* Corresponding author.
E-mail address: buhr0001@mc.duke.edu

Clin Geriatr Med 27 (2011) 229–239
doi:10.1016/j.cger.2011.01.007 geriatric.theclinics.com

care units in Canada and the United States, these rates have ranged from 0.1 to 2.4 cases/1000 resident days,[8,9] or have had a point-prevalence rate of 1.1%.[7]

MICROBIOLOGY

As in younger and community-dwelling populations, *Escherichia coli* remains the most common organism isolated in noncatheterized LTC residents.[10,11] For instance, a cohort of nursing home residents from 5 nursing homes in Connecticut followed for 1 year showed that *E coli* was the most commonly isolated organism (54%). However, in the same study, other bacteria occurred with some frequency, including *Proteus mirabilis* (15%), *Klebsiella* species (14%), *Enterococcus* (4.5%), *Staphylococcus* (4.1%), *Providencia* (3.7%), and *Pseudomonas* (2.6%).[10] A similar distribution of pathogens was found in a distinct study that analyzed nursing home residents with chronic urinary incontinence.[11] Appropriate concentrations of multiple pathogens should not be dismissed as contamination. In this second study, 14% of the samples grew more than 1 pathogen.[11]

For LTC residents with chronic indwelling urinary catheters, a wider spectrum of bacteria is isolated, with the infections typically being polymicrobial.[6] To illustrate this, urease-producing Enterobacteriaceae comprised most of the isolates in one study (*P mirabilis* [60%], *Morganella morganii* [10%], and *Providencia* [50%]),[12] whereas *Enterococcus* spp (24%), *E coli* (18%), and *P mirabilis* (10%) were the most common in a second study.[13]

RISK FACTORS

A variety of factors predispose LTC residents to develop UTI, whether asymptomatic or symptomatic. Awareness of these risk factors may help to risk stratify members of the LTC population for surveillance purposes (**Box 1**). For women, the risk increases with age. Several risk factors have been found in postmenopausal, community-dwelling women that likely translate to the LTC population. Postmenopausal women have a decrease in the normal vaginal colonization by lactobacilli, which is believed to result from the lack of estrogen and is associated with an increased risk of vaginal colonization by *E coli*.[14] The strongest risk factor for UTI in postmenopausal women has been a history of UTI throughout life. In one study, the hazard ratio was 6.9 (95% confidence interval [CI] 3.5–13.6) for a lifetime history of 6 or more UTIs,[15] and another study found that a history of UTI before menopause was associated with recurrent UTI (odds ratio 4.85, 95% CI 1.7–13.84).[16] Based on these data, it has been suggested that genetic factors may predispose women to UTI, with 1 such

Box 1
Risk factors for asymptomatic and symptomatic UTI in LTC residents

Age

Postmenopausal status

Prostatic hypertrophy

History of UTI earlier in adult life (women)

Dementia

Mobility limitations

Comorbidities that result in bladder dysfunction (eg, diabetes mellitus, Parkinson disease, stroke)

genetic factor having been verified as being a nonsecretor of ABO blood antigens (odds ratio 2.9, 95% CI 1.28–6.25).[16]

Less is known about the risk factors for UTI in men. As with women, the incidence of UTI also increases with age, and, in the case of men, is associated with prostatic enlargement and bladder dysfunction.[17] Prostatic hypertrophy results in urethral obstruction and turbulent urine flow. Although increased postvoid residual volume has historically been believed to be associated with increased risk for UTI, 2 recent studies have not confirmed this association in LTC residents.[18,19]

Various risk factors have been identified that specifically predispose LTC residents to UTI. In one study, urinary incontinence was the strongest risk factor in female LTC residents (odds ratio 6.3),[20] although this has also been linked to UTI in women in the community (odds ratio 2.9).[16] Other risk factors in female LTC residents included mobility limitation (odds ratio 3.2) and dementia (odds ratio 2.4).[20] In the same study, cancer was the only risk factor in men (odds ratio 6.3).[20] In a retrospective analysis of 4 years of LTC residents in one teaching nursing home, the risk factors for UTI were stroke (relative risk 2.2, 95% CI 1.4–3.2), decreased activities of daily living (relative risk 2.6–3.2, 95% CI 1.4–4.7), and decreased mental status (relative risk 2.2, 95% CI 1.2–3.1).[21] Similarly, in a prospective surveillance study of male VA nursing home residents, bacteriuria was associated with being confused or demented and urinary or fecal incontinence.[22] In a retrospective cohort study of short-stay skilled nursing facility residents in 5 of the largest US states, the patient characteristics associated with hospitalization for UTI were older age, Parkinson disease, diabetes mellitus, dementia, renal failure, stroke, transient ischemic attack, or hemiplegia.[23]

DIAGNOSIS

In the community-dwelling population, elders present with classic signs or symptoms including urinary frequency, urgency, dysuria, and suprapubic discomfort. Some LTC residents complain of these classic symptoms, but more present with nonspecific signs or symptoms and the clinician is tasked with deciding whether a symptomatic UTI could be the explanation. Furthermore, because of the higher baseline rate of asymptomatic bacteriuria, a positive urine culture alone is insufficient for the diagnosis of UTI even when it is accompanied by pyuria on urinalysis. LTC residents often have communication barriers and multiple comorbid diseases, (including a high prevalence of chronic genitourinary symptoms such as chronic urinary incontinence, frequency, urgency, or nocturia) that can confound the diagnosis. A recent prospective cohort study that followed 551 residents from 5 nursing homes in New Haven (CT) for 1 year illustrates this difficulty.[24] The researchers recorded episodes of clinically suspected UTI and asked the staff members to list up to 3 clinical reasons for their suspicion. The most common reasons were change in mental status (39%), change in behavior (19%), change in character of the urine (15.5%), fever or chills (12.8%), change in gait or fall (8.8%), dysuria (7.8%), and change in voiding pattern (7%).[24] Only dysuria and change in character of the urine were associated with bacteriuria and pyuria on a urinalysis and culture.[24] In a multivariate model, dysuria, change in character of the urine, and change in mental status were most predictive of bacteriuria and pyuria.[24] When present, symptoms and signs specific to the genitourinary tract are strong predictors of symptomatic UTI.

As noted in the study discussed earlier, changes in the character of the urine, such as odor or increased turbidity, are associated with symptomatic UTI.[24] However, these signs alone do not always indicate symptomatic UTI because asymptomatic UTI may also be associated with the same changes.[25,26] In addition, a substantial number of incontinent LTC residents with negative urine cultures have malodorous urine.[27] Concomitant dehydration may cause the change in the character of the urine; therefore, efforts at improved hydration and continence management should be the first intervention rather than investigation of symptomatic UTI or treatment of a UTI.

Gross hematuria is often associated with a UTI; however, hematuria in itself is not sufficient to diagnose UTI. For instance, the incidence of gross hematuria in one LTC population was 31/100,000 resident days; of those, 3.3 to 5.8/100,000 resident days were diagnosed with an invasive UTI, depending on the definition used.[28] Gross hematuria was more likely to occur in men, patients with known structural abnormalities of the urinary tract, and catheterized patients.[28]

Fever without localizing genitourinary symptoms should also not be immediately attributed to a UTI. In one study, only 7% of episodes of fever were caused by UTI in LTC residents without a chronic indwelling urinary catheter.[29]

Pyuria is present in more than 90% of LTC residents with asymptomatic bacteriuria. In addition, in one study, 34% of patients without bacteriuria had pyuria; therefore, pyuria does not indicate a symptomatic UTI.[2] However, pyuria may be useful to rule out symptomatic UTI, because it is present in virtually all cases of symptomatic UTI.[26]

Because of the lack of certainty regarding the diagnosis of UTI in LTC and a presumption that LTC residents are currently overtreated for UTI, expert consensus committees have put forward recommendations, summarized in **Table 1**. Surveillance criteria for UTI were developed at a consensus conference in 1989 and published in 1991, often called the McGeer criteria.[30] The definition requires 3 of the following 5 signs or symptoms for a resident without an indwelling urinary catheter and 2 of the 5 for a resident with an indwelling urinary catheter: (1) fever or chills; (2) new or increased dysuria, frequency, or urgency; (3) new flank or suprapubic pain; (4) change in character of the urine; and (5) worsening mental or functional status.[30] The committee also advised that LTC residents with a urinary catheter should not have symptoms or signs of another infection and still receive a diagnosis of UTI. Another consensus conference convened in 2000 published guidelines for the minimum criteria for the initiation of antibiotics in LTC residents, often referred to as the Loeb[31] criteria. For LTC residents without an indwelling urinary catheter, the committee recommended the following criteria: acute dysuria alone or fever with at least 1 of 6 specified genitourinary signs or symptoms (new or worsening urgency, frequency, suprapubic pain, gross hematuria, costovertebral angle tenderness, or urinary incontinence).[31] For LTC residents with an indwelling urinary catheter, the proposed criteria included just 1 of the following signs or symptoms: fever, new costovertebral tenderness, rigors with or without identified cause, or new onset of delirium.[31] These criteria were modified slightly and applied to 24 nursing homes in

Table 1
Comparison of the expert consensus criteria for the diagnosis of acute symptomatic UTI for noncatheterized residents in the nursing home

McGeer	Loeb
3 of the following signs or symptoms:	Acute dysuria OR fever with 1 of the following:
Fever or chills	New or worsening urgency
New or increased dysuria, frequency, or urgency	Frequency
New flank or suprapubic pain	Suprapubic pain
Change in character of the urine	Gross hematuria
Worsening of mental or functional status	Costovertebral angle tenderness
	Urinary incontinence

Boise (ID) and Ontario, Canada, in a cluster randomized controlled trial using diagnostic and treatment algorithms.[32] The researchers were able to show a lower rate of antimicrobial use for suspected UTI in the intervention nursing homes compared with the usual care homes.[32]

Juthani-Mehta and colleagues[33] compared the expert consensus definitions in a cohort of nursing home residents in New Haven (CT) to determine the sensitivity and specificity. They compared the clinical criteria with residents suspected of UTI by their clinician who subsequently had greater than 100,000 CFU on urine culture plus greater than 10 white blood cells on urinalysis. In this study, only 43 of 100 participants with suspected UTI had laboratory confirmation. Because the symptoms and signs by which clinicians identified potential symptomatic UTI were not specified in this study, it is possible that some of these laboratory-confirmed cases include cases that could be asymptomatic UTI. All but 2 of the participants with confirmed UTI were treated with an antibiotic. However, an additional 37 participants without laboratory confirmation also received antibiotic therapy. The 1989 consensus conference surveillance criteria resulted in a sensitivity of 30%, a specificity of 82%, a positive predictive value of 57%, and a negative predictive value of 61%. The 2000 consensus conference minimum criteria before initiation of antibiotics resulted in a sensitivity of 19%, a specificity of 89%, a positive predictive value of 57%, and a negative predictive value of 59%. The criteria used in the cluster randomized controlled trial had a sensitivity of 30%, a specificity of 79%, a positive predictive value of 52%, and a negative predictive value of 60%.[33] Based on these analyses, all of the expert consensus recommendations have similar characteristics, and the diagnostic accuracy of UTI criteria in LTC residents could be substantially improved.

In an effort to develop a more accurate diagnostic tool, we initiated a quality improvement program in our nursing home, where the prevalence of suspected UTI was 14% and the prevalence of treated UTI was 4.4%, a rate higher than the national average of 1.1%.[7] We implemented a diagnostic algorithm targeted to the nurses, similar to the one by Loeb and colleagues[31] in the randomized controlled trial described earlier. The algorithm was derived from a fusion of the signs and symptoms most associated with UTI in the literature. The algorithm divides the symptoms into major and minor criteria, based on the probability that they are associated with UTI. The major criteria include the following: (1) fever (>37.9°C or 100°F/increase >1.5°C or 2.4°F from baseline), (2) dysuria, (3) altered mental status, (4) gross hematuria, and (5) flank pain. The minor criteria consist of the following: (1) urgency; (2) frequency; (3) incontinence; (4) behavioral changes; (5) suprapubic pain; and (6) changes in urine odor, color, or consistency. If 1 or more major criteria are present, the nurse is instructed to obtain a urinalysis and culture and to call the care provider. For the minor criteria, the algorithm recommends frequent monitoring for the emergence of major symptoms, hydration, and treatment of constipation if present. If the minor criteria persist for 24 hours then the algorithm directs the nurse to obtain a urinalysis and urine culture and to call the care provider. In the first 3 months of using the algorithm, the rate of suspected UTI decreased to 9% (30% decreased from previous months) and the rate of treated UTI was 3.85% (a 20% decrease). We hope that there will continue to be a decrease because we only had partial use of the algorithm and are working on strategies to spread its use with one-on-one teaching and reminders. We are also testing the efficacy of the algorithm in a second nursing home. This algorithm, unlike previously described consensus criteria, incorporates a process of observation and intervention over time that may enhance diagnostic accuracy. The reality of LTC, unlike ambulatory care, is that patients can be more easily observed and evaluated over time by health care personnel.

MANAGEMENT

Several well-designed randomized controlled trials have shown no benefit to treating asymptomatic bacteriuria in older LTC residents; this can be illustrated by detailing 3 studies. In the first, there was no difference in mortality in a 12-month trial in which female LTC residents were randomized to treatment versus no treatment of asymptomatic bacteriuria that had been identified on monthly cultures.[34] Furthermore, the antimicrobial therapy group experienced more adverse drug events and more cultures positive for drug-resistant organisms.[34] Second, there was no difference in mortality in a 9-year trial in which female residents of a large geriatric center (congregate housing in apartments or nursing home) or 21 continuing care retirement communities were randomized to treatment or no treatment of asymptomatic bacteriuria that had been identified on biannual urine cultures.[35] Third, there was no effect on the incidence or prevalence of symptomatic infection, and no difference in mortality, among elderly male veterans receiving treatment of asymptomatic bacteriuria in a 2-year period.[36] In addition, researchers have found no short-term improvement in chronic urinary incontinence with treatment of asymptomatic bacteriuria.[11] The Infectious Disease Society of America therefore recommends against screening for and treatment of asymptomatic bacteriuria in elderly institutionalized subjects.[1] A urine culture should not be obtained after treatment of a symptomatic UTI to document cure; the patient should be assessed clinically to determine whether the UTI is cured. The Infectious Disease Society of America also recommends against screening for asymptomatic bacteriuria in catheterized patients, and against systemic antimicrobial prophylaxis, a practice that has been shown to select for antibiotic-resistant strains.

The treatment of symptomatic UTI should be based on antimicrobial susceptibility testing. The selection of antimicrobial agent is similar to that in the younger community-dwelling population, and should take into consideration the local antimicrobial resistance patterns. In one study of antimicrobial susceptibility of urinary pathogens from residents not using an indwelling urinary catheter in 5 nursing homes in New Haven (CT), the bacteria were often resistant to the frequently prescribed oral antibiotics[10]: 60% of the *E coli* isolates were resistant to fluoroquinolones, 27% were resistant to trimethoprim-sulfamethoxazole (Bactrim; Septra), and only 7% were resistant to nitrofurantoin (Macrobid). In this study, the antibiotics that maintained the best overall susceptibility pattern were the first-generation cephalosporins and trimethoprim-sulfamethoxazole (Bactrim; Septra), although nitrofurantoin (Macrobid) should be considered if *E coli* is identified.[10] A caveat is that renal function is often impaired in LTC residents, necessitating antimicrobial dosage adjustments. In particular, nitrofurantoin (Macrobid) is contraindicated for residents with a creatinine clearance of less than 60 mL/min.

The treatment of catheter-associated UTI in residents with chronic indwelling catheters should be based initially on the individual's microbial resistance pattern established from prior cultures, with the treatment possibly altered later based on the results of the urine culture taken before the initiation of therapy. It is recommended that the catheter be exchanged before specimen collection, because this will produce a specimen that more accurately reflects bladder colonization, as well as shortening the symptomatic phase of UTI and decreasing recurrence rate.[6,37]

The duration of treatments for UTI in the LTC population are arbitrarily chosen, because they have not been defined in rigorous clinical studies. Some guidance has been gleaned from trials performed in community, but not LTC, populations. For instance, a randomized controlled noninferiority trial conducted in mostly ambulatory women with good functional and cognitive status showed that 3 days was not inferior to 7 days of treatment with ciprofloxacin (Cipro) 250 mg twice daily.[38] Most experts recommend that symptomatic UTI receive 3 to 7 days of antibiotics,[39,40] whereas, for more severe presentation, 10 to 14 days is probably appropriate.[39,40] In men with recurrent UTI, chronic bacterial prostatitis should be excluded, because this could require 6 to 12 weeks of therapy.[17] For catheter-associated UTI, based on expert recommendations, the *Infectious Diseases Society of America* (IDSA) suggests 7 days of treatment in patients who have a prompt response, and 10 to 14 days in those who have a delayed response.[6] In all cases, as with any antimicrobial therapy, it is desirable to limit exposure to the drugs as much as possible to guard against the emergence of drug-resistant organisms.

PREVENTION

Several evidence-based prevention strategies have been defined that could decrease the incidence of UTI in LTC. These strategies and the evidence supporting them are summarized in **Table 2**. Therapy to improve functional status, particularly ambulation, may be of value. A retrospective cohort study was performed in short-stay skilled nursing facilities in 5 of the largest US states to ascertain positive and negative risk factors for hospitalization for UTI.[23] Independent walking was associated with a 69% decreased risk of hospitalization for UTI; maintaining or improving walking was associated with a 39% to 76% risk reduction; and, for patients who were nonambulatory at baseline, improvement in their ability to move in bed or transfer was associated with a 38% risk reduction.[23]

Many studies have shown an increased risk of UTI with the use of chronic indwelling urinary catheters.[7,23] Therefore, eliminating the use of chronic indwelling urinary catheters whenever possible prevents UTI. If the catheter cannot be discontinued, consideration should be given to the use of condom catheterization for men without dementia.[6] This recommendation was based on a single randomized controlled trial of men in VA acute hospitals or nursing home care units in which only 75 patients were enrolled in 3.5 years (1.8% of those screened).[41] The trial had a median follow-up of 3 days and found a hazard ratio for bacteriuria, symptomatic UTI, or death of 4.84 (95% CI 1.46–16.02) for patients without dementia who had an indwelling urinary

Table 2
UTI prevention strategies in LTC

Strategy	Evidence
Improvement in walking, transfers, and bed mobility	Retrospective cohort study of short-stay LTC residents
Elimination of chronic indwelling urinary catheter	Multiple RCT showing increased risk of UTI with catheters
Replace indwelling catheter with condom catheter in men without dementia	Single RCT in VA acute hospital or nursing home
Replace chronic indwelling catheter with clean intermittent catheterization	Prospective observational studies, expert opinion/clinical practice guidelines
Vaginal estrogen preparations	2 RCTs in community-dwelling older women
Cranberry juice or tablets	Quasi-RCT in LTC with asymptomatic UTI as the outcome measure; RCT data strongest for women with recurrent UTI
Prophylactic antibiotics	RCT in younger community-dwelling women

Abbreviation: RCT, randomized controlled trial.

catheter compared with a condom catheter.[41] Clean intermittent catheterization is recommended by the IDSA rather than chronic indwelling urinary catheterization to reduce the incidence of UTI.[6] For those patients in whom a chronic indwelling urinary catheter is deemed necessary, a closed drainage system is recommended, the drainage bag should always be below the level of the bladder, and the catheter should be properly secured after insertion to prevent urethral trauma.[6,42]

Several researchers have investigated whether estrogen decreases the incidence of UTI in postmenopausal women, based on the rationale that there is a link between decreased estrogen and increased incidence of UTI (vaginal lactobacillus decrease allowing *E coli* to grow) and typical decrease in estrogen in women with advancing age. In 4 randomized controlled trials having a total of 2798 subjects, oral estrogen did not affect the incidence of UTI.[43] However, vaginal estrogen preparations, topically applied cream,[44] and an estrogen-releasing vaginal ring[45] have been successful at decreasing the number of symptomatic UTIs in postmenopausal women with a history of recurrent UTI living in the community. The relative risk reductions were 0.25 (95% CI 0.13–0.50)[44] and 0.64 (95% CI 0.47–0.86).[45] Based on these data, it is likely that vaginal estrogen decreases the occurrence of symptomatic UTI in women with recurrent UTI, although it has not been specifically studied in the LTC population.

Cranberries have long been a home remedy for UTI, and there is evidence that cranberry juice is effective for the prevention of recurrent UTI in women.[46] One study that was performed in the LTC population using a quasirandomized method showed a reduction in asymptomatic UTI with 300 mL/d of cranberry juice cocktail. However, there was no difference in this study in the number of symptomatic UTI, the clinically significant outcome. In a trial of community-dwelling women with recurrent UTI (mean age 63 years, range 45–93 years), cranberry (500 mg cranberry extract tablet) was compared with trimethoprim (100 mg). The 2 groups, cranberry tablet and trimethoprim, had an equal number of symptomatic UTI during the study.[47] This study did not include a placebo group, so the effectiveness of either intervention is unclear.

Long-term prophylactic antibiotics for the prevention of recurrent UTI in women have been shown to be effective.[48] However, most of the participants in these trials were younger than 65 years and all were community-dwelling. There are no trials of prophylactic antibiotics in the LTC population. In addition, the participants in the antibiotic groups reported frequent adverse events.

FUTURE AREAS OF RESEARCH

There are many challenges in the diagnosis, treatment, and prevention of UTI in the nursing home. Foremost is the need to better define symptomatic UTI in the nursing home and improve diagnostic accuracy. Although there has been some investigation of biomarkers (C-reactive protein, interleukin 1,6,8, and procalcitonin) and antibodies to uropathogens in urine to aid in diagnosis, these methods have yet to be found useful in the elderly LTC population. In addition, further prospective clinical trials are needed that evaluate modifiable risk factors and interventions such as mobility, cranberries, and vaginal estrogen to determine whether the incidence of UTI can be decreased in the LTC population. Other studies are needed to determine the appropriate duration for antimicrobial therapy in the LTC population.

SUMMARY

UTI is common in LTC residents. A large proportion of UTIs in the LTC population are asymptomatic. Many well-designed clinical trials have shown that there is no benefit to treating asymptomatic UTI/bacteriuria in this population, and there are compelling reasons to avoid unnecessary antimicrobial use. However, differentiating asymptomatic from symptomatic UTI is difficult, because LTC residents have chronic genitourinary complaints, multiple comorbidities, and communication barriers. Two consensus guidelines have been put forward that help to differentiate symptomatic from asymptomatic UTI, but improvement in diagnosis is still needed. Treatment of symptomatic UTI in LTC residents is similar to the community-dwelling and younger populations. There is some evidence for the efficacy of cranberry products and vaginal estrogen to prevent recurrent UTI in women, but much less is known about the risk factors and prevention strategies for men.

REFERENCES

1. Nicolle LE, Bradley S, Colgan R, et al. Infectious Diseases Society of America guidelines for the diagnosis and treatment of asymptomatic bacteriuria in adults. Clin Infect Dis 2005;40(5):643–54.
2. Ouslander JG, Schapira M, Schnelle JF, et al. Pyuria among chronically incontinent but otherwise asymptomatic nursing home residents. J Am Geriatr Soc 1996;44(4):420–3.
3. Nicolle LE. Asymptomatic bacteriuria in the elderly. Infect Dis Clin North Am 1997;11(3):647–62.
4. Hebel JR, Warren JW. The use of urethral, condom, and suprapubic catheters in aged nursing home patients. J Am Geriatr Soc 1990;38(7):777–84.
5. Warren JW, Steinberg L, Hebel JR, et al. The prevalence of urethral catheterization in Maryland nursing homes. Arch Intern Med 1989;149(7):1535–7.
6. Hooton TM, Bradley SF, Cardenas DD, et al. Diagnosis, prevention, and treatment of catheter-associated urinary tract infection in adults: 2009 International Clinical Practice Guidelines from the Infectious Diseases Society of America. Clin Infect Dis 2010;50(5):625–63.
7. Tsan L, Davis C, Langberg R, et al. Prevalence of nursing home-associated infections in the Department of Veterans Affairs nursing home care units. Am J Infect Control 2008;36(3):173–9.
8. Nicolle LE, Strausbaugh LJ, Garibaldi RA. Infections and antibiotic resistance in nursing homes. Clin Microbiol Rev 1996;9(1):1–17.
9. Stevenson KB, Moore J, Colwell H, et al. Standardized infection surveillance in long-term care: interfacility comparisons from a regional cohort of facilities. Infect Control Hosp Epidemiol 2005;26(3):231–8.
10. Das R, Perrelli E, Towle V, et al. Antimicrobial susceptibility of bacteria isolated from urine samples obtained from nursing home residents. Infect Control Hosp Epidemiol 2009;30(11):1116–9.
11. Ouslander JG, Schapira M, Schnelle JF, et al. Does eradicating bacteriuria affect the severity of chronic urinary incontinence in nursing home residents? Ann Intern Med 1995;122(10):749–54.
12. Warren JW, Tenney JH, Hoopes JM, et al. A prospective microbiologic study of bacteriuria in patients with chronic indwelling urethral catheters. J Infect Dis 1982;146(6):719–23.
13. Bregenzer T, Frei R, Widmer AF, et al. Low risk of bacteremia during catheter replacement in patients with long-term urinary catheters. Arch Intern Med 1997;157(5):521–5.
14. Pabich WL, Fihn SD, Stamm WE, et al. Prevalence and determinants of vaginal flora alterations in postmenopausal women. J Infect Dis 2003;188(7):1054–8.

15. Jackson SL, Boyko EJ, Scholes D, et al. Predictors of urinary tract infection after menopause: a prospective study. Am J Med 2004;117(12):903–11.
16. Raz R, Gennesin Y, Wasser J, et al. Recurrent urinary tract infections in postmenopausal women. Clin Infect Dis 2000;30(1):152–6.
17. Lipsky BA. Prostatitis and urinary tract infection in men: what's new; what's true? Am J Med 1999;106(3):327–34.
18. Omli R, Skotnes LH, Mykletun A, et al. Residual urine as a risk factor for lower urinary tract infection: a 1-year follow-up study in nursing homes. J Am Geriatr Soc 2008;56(5):871–4.
19. Barabas G, Molstad S. No association between elevated post-void residual volume and bacteriuria in residents of nursing homes. Scand J Prim Health Care 2005;23(1):52–6.
20. Eberle CM, Winsemius D, Garibaldi RA. Risk factors and consequences of bacteriuria in non-catheterized nursing home residents. J Gerontol 1993;48(6): M266–71.
21. Powers JS, Billings FT, Behrendt D, et al. Antecedent factors in urinary tract infections among nursing home patients. South Med J 1988;81(6):734–5.
22. Nicolle LE, Henderson E, Bjornson J, et al. The association of bacteriuria with resident characteristics and survival in elderly institutionalized men. Ann Intern Med 1987;106(5):682–6.
23. Rogers MA, Fries BE, Kaufman SR, et al. Mobility and other predictors of hospitalization for urinary tract infection: a retrospective cohort study. BMC Geriatr 2008;8:31.
24. Juthani-Mehta M, Quagliarello V, Perrelli E, et al. Clinical features to identify urinary tract infection in nursing home residents: a cohort study. J Am Geriatr Soc 2009;57(6):963–70.
25. Nicolle LE. Symptomatic urinary tract infection in nursing home residents. J Am Geriatr Soc 2009;57(6):1113–4.
26. Nicolle LE, Long-Term-Care-Committee S. Urinary tract infections in long-term-care facilities. Infect Control Hosp Epidemiol 2001;22(3):167–75.
27. Midthun SJ, Paur R, Lindseth G, et al. Urinary tract infections. Does the smell really tell? J Gerontol Nurs 2004;30(6):4–9.
28. Nicolle LE, Orr P, Duckworth H, et al. Gross hematuria in residents of long-term-care facilities. Am J Med 1993;94(6):611–8.
29. Orr PH, Nicolle LE, Duckworth H, et al. Febrile urinary infection in the institutionalized elderly. Am J Med 1996;100(1):71–7.
30. McGeer A, Campbell B, Emori TG, et al. Definitions of infection for surveillance in long-term care facilities. Am J Infect Control 1991;19(1):1–7.
31. Loeb M, Bentley DW, Bradley S, et al. Development of minimum criteria for the initiation of antibiotics in residents of long-term-care facilities: results of a consensus conference. Infect Control Hosp Epidemiol 2001;22(2):120–4.
32. Loeb M, Brazil K, Lohfeld L, et al. Effect of a multifaceted intervention on number of antimicrobial prescriptions for suspected urinary tract infections in residents of nursing homes: cluster randomised controlled trial. BMJ 2005;331(7518):669.
33. Juthani-Mehta M, Tinetti M, Perrelli E, et al. Diagnostic accuracy of criteria for urinary tract infection in a cohort of nursing home residents. J Am Geriatr Soc 2007;55(7):1072–7.
34. Nicolle LE, Mayhew WJ, Bryan L. Prospective randomized comparison of therapy and no therapy for asymptomatic bacteriuria in institutionalized elderly women. Am J Med 1987;83(1):27–33.

35. Abrutyn E, Mossey J, Berlin JA, et al. Does asymptomatic bacteriuria predict mortality and does antimicrobial treatment reduce mortality in elderly ambulatory women? Ann Intern Med 1994;120(10):827–33.
36. Nicolle LE, Bjornson J, Harding GK, et al. Bacteriuria in elderly institutionalized men. N Engl J Med 1983;309(23):1420–5.
37. Raz R, Schiller D, Nicolle LE. Chronic indwelling catheter replacement before antimicrobial therapy for symptomatic urinary tract infection. J Urol 2000; 164(4):1254–8.
38. Vogel T, Verreault R, Gourdeau M, et al. Optimal duration of antibiotic therapy for uncomplicated urinary tract infection in older women: a double-blind randomized controlled trial. CMAJ 2004;170(4):469–73.
39. Nicolle LE, Bentley D, Garibaldi R, et al. Antimicrobial use in long-term-care facilities. Infect Control Hosp Epidemiol 1996;17(2):119–28.
40. Nicolle LE. Urinary tract infections in the elderly. Clin Geriatr Med 2009;25(3): 423–36.
41. Saint S, Kaufman SR, Rogers MA, et al. Condom versus indwelling urinary catheters: a randomized trial. J Am Geriatr Soc 2006;54(7):1055–61.
42. Gould CV, Umscheid CA, Agarwal RK, et al. Guideline for prevention of catheter-associated urinary tract infections 2009. Infect Control Hosp Epidemiol 2010; 31(4):319–26.
43. Perrotta C, Aznar M, Mejia R, et al. Oestrogens for preventing recurrent urinary tract infection in postmenopausal women. Cochrane Database Syst Rev 2008; 2:CD005131.
44. Raz R, Stamm WE. A controlled trial of intravaginal estriol in postmenopausal women with recurrent urinary tract infections. N Engl J Med 1993;329(11):753–6.
45. Eriksen B. A randomized, open, parallel-group study on the preventive effect of an estradiol-releasing vaginal ring (Estring) on recurrent urinary tract infections in postmenopausal women. Am J Obstet Gynecol 1999;180(5):1072–9.
46. Jepson RG, Craig JC. Cranberries for preventing urinary tract infections. Cochrane Database Syst Rev 2008;1:CD001321.
47. McMurdo ME, Argo I, Phillips G, et al. Cranberry or trimethoprim for the prevention of recurrent urinary tract infections? A randomized controlled trial in older women. J Antimicrob Chemother 2009;63(2):389–95.
48. Albert X, Huertas I, Pereiro II, et al. Antibiotics for preventing recurrent urinary tract infection in non-pregnant women. Cochrane Database Syst Rev 2004;3:CD001209.

Pressure Ulcers in Long-Term Care

E. Foy White-Chu, MD[a,b], Petra Flock, MD[c,d], Bryan Struck, MD[e,f], Louise Aronson, MD[g,*]

KEYWORDS

- Pressure ulcers • Decubitus ulcers • Elderly • Geriatric
- Management

Pressure ulcers are common, costly, and debilitating chronic wounds, which occur preferentially in people with advanced age, physical or cognitive impairments, and multiple comorbidities.[1] Because these characteristics describe the majority of long-term care residents, pressure ulcers present a significant and frequent challenge to long-term care providers.[2] Residents with pressure ulcers have decreased quality of life and increased morbidity and mortality, and facilities with high rates of pressure ulcers have higher costs and risks of litigation.[3] For these reasons, health professionals who practice in this setting should be well versed in pressure ulcer management.

This article reviews the significance, risk factors, pathophysiology, prevention, diagnosis, and management of pressure ulcers in long-term care. The discussion includes tools used to assess pressure ulcers, the wound bed preparation paradigm, tailoring care plans to the individual patient goals of care, and legal considerations.

This project was supported by funds from the Bureau of Health Professions (BHPr); Health Resources and Services Administration (HRSA); Department of Health and Human Services (DHHS), under grant numbers K01HP00009-03 (Drs Flock, Struck, and Aronson) and KO1HP20512 (Dr White-Chu); and Geriatric Academic Career Award. The information or content and conclusions are those of the authors and should not be construed as the official position or policy of, nor should any endorsements be inferred by, the BHPr, HRSA, DHHS or the U.S. Government.

[a] Department of Medicine, Hebrew Senior Life, 1200 Centre Street, Roslindale, MA 02131, USA
[b] Division of Gerontology, Beth Israel Deaconess Medical Center, 330 Brookline Avenue, Harvard Medical School, Boston, MA 02215, USA
[c] Division of Geriatrics, University of Massachusetts Medical School, 119 Belmont Street, Worcester, MA 01605, USA
[d] Summit ElderCare, 88 Masonic Home Road, Charlton, MA 01507, USA
[e] Reynolds Department of Geriatric Medicine, University of Oklahoma Health Sciences Center, 1100 N Lindsay, Oklahoma City, OK 73104, USA
[f] Geriatrics and Extended Care, Oklahoma City VA Medical Center, 921 NE 13th VAMC 11g, Oklahoma City, OK, 73104, USA
[g] Division of Geriatrics, University of California at San Francisco, 3333 California Street, Suite 380, San Francisco, CA 94118, USA
* Corresponding author.
E-mail address: louise.aronson@ucsf.edu

Clin Geriatr Med 27 (2011) 241–258
doi:10.1016/j.cger.2011.02.001
geriatric.theclinics.com

INCIDENCE, PREVALENCE, AND COSTS

The pressure ulcer has plagued mankind for millennia. Anthropologists have found evidence of pressure ulcers on Egyptian mummies, and in the mid-1500s French physician Ambroise Paré described one of the earliest pressure ulcers in the medical literature.[4] Despite the advances of modern medicine, pressure ulcers persist. Incidence rates vary widely within and between sites of care, with reported rates of 0.4% to 38% in acute care, 0 to 17% in home care, and 2.2% to 23.9% in long-term care in 2001.[5] Data from the 2004 National Nursing Home Survey estimated that 159,000 (11%) of US nursing home residents had a pressure ulcer, with stage II the most common type.[6] Given that persons over age 85 are the fastest-growing segment of the population in the developed world, and 70% of pressure ulcers occur in adults over age 70, both the long-term care population and the number of people at risk for pressure ulcers are likely to dramatically increase in coming decades.[7]

Pressure ulcers incur substantial costs to the health care system. The National Nursing Home Survey estimated that 35% of the patients with pressure ulcers received some type of specialized care. The estimated cost per stay for hospitalized Medicare beneficiaries with a secondary diagnosis of pressure ulcer is $40,381.[8] A recent study suggested that costs for treatment of stage IV pressures were much higher than this, ranging from $124,327 to $129,248.[9] Based on this information, the total cost of pressure ulcer treatment in the United States exceeds $11 billion annually. This is consistent with a study from the Netherlands in the 1990s, which found that after cancer and cardiovascular disease, pressure ulcers were that nation's most costly condition.[10] A 2004 study estimated the cost in the United Kingdom was £2.4 billion, representing 4% of the National Health Service expenditure.[11]

Today, when a family arrives to photograph a pressure ulcer, the long-term care facility must be prepared for future litigation. When it seems that a family is contemplating legal action, the entire health care team should work with the patient and family.

As a result of these costs, the Centers for Medicare & Medicaid Services stopped payment for stage III and stage IV hospital-acquired pressure ulcers in October 2008.[8] Although similar regulations do not yet exist in long-term care, this change in payment emphasizes the importance of pressure ulcer prevention and management.

RISK FACTORS

Pressure ulcers in long-term care residents occur as a result of two types of risk factors, intrinsic and extrinsic.[12] Intrinsic factors include patient age, mobility limitations, comorbidities, nutritional status, and other contributors to skin architecture and integrity. Extrinsic factors are destructive forces affecting the skin, including moisture, pressure, shear forces, or friction.

Predisposing intrinsic factors include thinning and other structural changes of the aging skin or prolonged use of steroid medication.[13] Immobility from conditions, such as cerebrovascular accidents, spinal cord injury, multiple sclerosis, prolonged surgery, trauma, and inactivity due to advanced musculoskeletal diseases or end-stage medical diseases, increases the pressure ulcer risk. The latter also often are associated with malnutrition. Malnutrition, in particular protein malnutrition, has been identified as a contributing factor, as have medical conditions associated with poor circulation, such as diabetes mellitus and peripheral vascular disease.[14] Although diseases affecting a patient's mental status, such as advanced dementia, do not cause pressure ulcers, they often contribute, because such patients may be unable to voice discomfort from being in the same position too long.[15] A history of a previous pressure ulcer increases the risk of future pressure ulcers.[2]

There are four extrinsic risk factors for pressure ulcers. Both excessive dryness and excessive moisture, which may be caused by sweat or incontinence of urine or feces, can contribute to the development of pressure ulcers. Pressure causes damage when compression of capillaries leads to tissue ischemia. Duration and intensity of pressure, particularly over bony prominences, correlates inversely with time to infarction and tissue death. Shear forces occur when gravity pulls a patient downward while the skin remains in place—as a patient slides in bed or wheelchair, for example—causing stretching of dermal vessels and impaired perfusion. When there is friction between the skin and another surface, the stratum corneum is abraded and ulceration risk increases. This can occur in agitated patients or when immobile patients are dragged during repositioning.[16]

Several tools have been developed and validated in the risk assessment of pressure sores. Among the most commonly used tools are the Norton and Braden scales in the United States and the Waterlow score in the United Kingdom.[17–19] The oldest of those three scales, the Norton scale, assesses physical and mental conditions of a patient, activity level, mobility, and incontinence. The two newer scales, Braden and Waterlow, include assessments of nutrition, risk for friction and shear, skin condition, and, in the Waterlow score, specific medical conditions that have been associated with higher risk of developing pressure ulcers.

PHASES OF WOUND HEALING

Like all wounds, pressure sores go through three phases of healing.[20] The initial inflammatory phase includes hemostasis with vasoconstriction, platelet aggregation, and clot formation, followed by vasodilatation and phagocytosis. During the second or proliferative phase, granulation, connective tissue proliferation, contraction of the wound edges, and epithelialization take place. In the final or remodeling and maturation phase, new collagen forms, although in full-thickness wounds even after 2 years, the tensile strength of this scar tissue is less than 80% that of the original tissue. In surgical and other acute wounds, wounds move through these phases in days to weeks depending on the severity of the tissue injury. In pressure ulcers and other chronic wounds, the wound is often arrested in the inflammatory phase because they produce wound fluid that is composed of matrix metalloproteinases, which break down matrix proteins, growth factors, and cytokines.[21,22] This results in defective granulation, phenotypically altered keratinocytes, and delayed wound healing. Consequently, pressure ulcers can be present for weeks to months or years.

PREVENTION

Strategies to prevent pressure ulcers overlap with those to treat already existing ulcers. The Norton scale, Braden scale, and Waterlow score are all used to assess risk for pressure ulcers and often help identify those factors that can be corrected in order to minimize the risk of developing an ulcer. It has been shown that frequent repositioning is helpful: for patients who are bed bound the recommendation is to reposition every 2 hours; for patients who are wheelchair bound, the recommendation is to reposition every hour; and for those patients who are prone to inactivity but are cognitively intact, the recommendation is to teach them to shift weight and self-reposition every 15 minutes.[23]

Preventing excessive moisture due to incontinence may warrant a toileting schedule, frequent changing of the patient, the use of barrier creams after toileting and bathing, and use of incontinence products that keep the skin dry.[24] The use of disposable briefs has been shown advantageous in incontinent long-term care residents.[2] In rare cases of recurrent or severe ulcers and/or uncontrollable diarrhea or incontinence, placement of a rectal tube or a Foley catheter may be indicated. The opposite, too dry skin, should also be avoided and can be helped by use of moisturizing lotion after toileting or bathing.[1]

If malnutrition/protein malnutrition can be corrected, attempts to do so may reduce the risk of pressure sores.[1] In long-term care patients, the use of nutritional supplement or tube feeding for patients with pre-exisiting feeding tubes for a period longer than 21 days was associated with a lower risk of developing a pressure ulcer.[2] Improved control of underlying medical problems, such as diabetes mellitus, peripheral vascular disease, and, if feasible and medically possible, reduction or elimination of medication that affect circulation or skin texture (eg, prednisone) can help reduce the risk of pressure ulcers.

For patients who are at high risk of developing ulcers, the use of pressure-relieving cushions or mattresses can be beneficial.[25,26] Two systematic reviews found that various pressure-reducing devices, such as foam overlays, pressure-relieving foam mattresses, and alternating pressure mattress and air-fluid mattress, all reduce the likelihood of developing pressure ulcers, but no one device was superior to the others.[1,27] Therefore, the decision about which type of mattress/cushion is used should be based on a patient's individual needs, patient comfort, and the cost of the device. For example, a low air-loss mattress may be so slippery that a patient who is still be able to self-transfer on a pressure-relieving foam mattress may not be able to do so anymore, thus causing the patient further functional impairment and reliance on caregivers for transfers. All pressure-relieving/reducing devices lose their benefit if the head of bed is consistently elevated above 30°.

It has also been shown that adequate staffing levels can help reduce the incidence of pressure ulcers in long-term care facilities. In the National Pressure Ulcer Long-Term Care Study,[2] more than 0.25 hours per resident per day of registered nurse time and more than 2 hours per resident per day of nurse's aide time were associated with a lower risk of developing pressure ulcers. The same study showed that a lower than 25% licensed practice nurse turnover in a given facility was associated with better outcomes.

As is often the case in geriatric medicine, the key to prevention is a multipronged approach that requires individualized care plans addressing patients' specific medical and functional problems that can be corrected plus attention to detail in implementing strategies to minimize risk for those factors that cannot be corrected.

PRESSURE ULCER DIAGNOSIS

Pressure ulcers mainly occur over bony prominences, but not all wounds on bony prominences are pressure ulcers. For residents of long-term care facilities, who are often sedentary and live with several medical comorbidities, such as diabetes mellitus, atherosclerosis, lower-extremity edema, or heart failure, wounds have multiple causes. Differential diagnosis, especially for wounds on the lower extremities, includes venous stasis ulcers, arterial ulcers, and diabetic foot ulcers. Malignant wounds may appear anywhere. When differentiating between a pressure ulcer and other causes, it is important to try to determine the causal and complicating factors. Prevention and treatment are vastly different for pressure ulcers than for these other wound types.

Venous hypertension ulcers tend to be reddish-brown and are frequently associated with stasis dermatitis and chronic edema.[28] The hyperpigmentation is due to hemosiderin deposition, and drainage is more pronounced in the setting of edema. The venous ulcer is commonly located medially but can occur above either malleolus.[29] In contrast, arterial wounds have a punched-out appearance, may be dry, and the overall skin on the leg is shiny with sparse hair growth. The foot and legs are cool, and there may be dependent rubor. Pain is often relieved with leg dependency, because this improves the blood flow to the leg and foot.[30] Diabetic foot wounds, by their nature, occur in areas of pressure. Ill-fitting shoes are often the culprit. Similar to arterial wounds, diabetic foot wounds may be seen on the tips of the toes, in-between toes, or on the lateral foot when the shoe is too narrow. Wounds beneath the metatarsal heads, especially the first and fifth, are often due to the claw deformity that occurs with neuropathy. If patients have Charcot foot deformity, their midfoot is especially susceptible to wounds. Diabetic foot wounds are complicated by neuropathy and underlying arterial disease.[31] Finally, malignancy should be suspected whenever a cutaneous nodule is present in isolation or a lesion does not heal within an expected amount of time despite treatment of infection and underlying causes.[32]

None of these wounds should be staged, because none is pressure ulcer. This detail is important in long-term care, because pressure ulcers are a quality measure. Their rates are tracked on databases, such as Nursing Home Compare.[33] Both families and government regulators evaluate a facility's performance based on these quality measures.

PRESSURE ULCER ASSESSMENT

Although pressure ulcers tend to form over bony prominences, they may occur anywhere skin is damaged by excessive pressure, friction, shear, and/or moisture. Examples of unusual pressure ulcer locations include the scrotum or midthigh from Foley catheters and earlobes from oxygen tubing.

In the United States, the Centers for Medicare & Medicaid Services no longer reimburses for stage III or stage IV pressure ulcers that develop during hospitalization. There is speculation in the long-term care community that this payment policy may eventually extend to long-term care. Regardless, accurate staging and assessment are critical to best practices treatment. The European Pressure Ulcer Advisory Panel and the National Pressure Ulcer Advisory Panel have established a pressure ulcer classification system that is recognized by all long-term care facilities.[34] **Table 1** outlines this system. Although the Centers for Medicare & Medicaid Services Minimum Data Set (MDS) Version 2.0 required documentation out of line with this staging schema and other best practices, MDS 3.0 includes deep tissue injury and unstageable categories and prohibits reverse staging.[35]

There are many assessment frameworks available for wounds in general and pressure ulcers in particular. Keast and colleagues[36] introduced the MEASURE framework—this outlines a systematic approach for nonhealing wounds.

M = Measurement

There are a variety of measurement techniques available, including rulers, acetate tracings, and more sophisticated technologies that are computer assisted. At long-term care facilities, budgetary requirements determine the type of measurement. Regardless of the technique chosen, a uniform method of measurement should be established between providers and nurses to prevent confusion in charts as the healing process is tracked.

Table 1
Pressure ulcer staging

Stage	Description
Suspected Deep Tissue Injury	Purplish discoloration or blood-filled blister that indicates more severe underlying tissue damage; can be difficult to differentiate from stage I or in patients with dark skin tones; depth unknown.
I	Nonblanchable erythema with skin intact
II	Partial-thickness/tissue loss with red/pink wound bed; no slough
III	Full-thickness/tissue loss; slough may be present
IV	Full-thickness/tissue loss with exposed bone, tendon, or muscle or probe to bone
Unstageable	Full-thickness/tissue loss where base is covered by slough and/or eschar

National Pressure Ulcer Advisory Panel and European Pressure Ulcer Advisory Panel pressure ulcer classification system, 2007.

E = Exudate

The provider should describe the volume: none, small, moderate, or large. This can be subjective. Specific descriptions of how quickly exudate appeared on the bandage—for instance, if the bandage soaks through in less than 24 hours—can provide some objectivity to the description. The nursing team can clarify when a bandage was last changed and how quickly it is saturated. The type of exudate—serous, serosanguinous (clear mixed with bloody drainage), sanguinous, seropurulent (watery white drainage), or purulent—should also be documented. Pseudomonas often presents with green drainage and can be treated topically with dilute acetic acid (9 parts sterile water to 1 part acetic acid) cleansing prior to each dressing change until the drainage disappears.[37]

A = Appearance

The provider must specify anatomic location and educate nursing staff and other members of the team about correct anatomic terms. "Buttock" is vague, whereas "iliac crest" and "ischium" are specific terms. By documenting anatomic location, the provider and team can determine which positions may have increased the risk of the pressure ulcer as well as impact of the treatment plan to offload the pressure ulcer.

When addressing the appearance of the pressure ulcer, the provider should document the color of the wound bed and texture of the tissue. Eschar often refers to dry yellow, gray, or black tissue, whereas slough most often refers to loose stringy wet yellow, gray, or black tissue. Fibrin can often be confused for necrotic tissue, because it is yellow and strongly adherent to the wound bed. This tissue corresponds to collagen deposition, however, and can be seen in the final phases of wound healing. Often, buds of epithelial tissue are seen within the fibrin deposition. Granulation tissue is pink to red appearing. A beefy red appearance is one where the granulation tissue is red and friable or bleeds easily. Formerly believed to be healthy, this is now considered indicative of critical colonization and possible infection.

S = Suffering

The provider and team must address patient-centered concerns. Wound pain, including pain with dressing changes, must be addressed. The team should also ask the patient what impact the pressure ulcer has on everyday life. Does the ulcer, because of embarrassing odor or bandages, prevent the patient from visiting with family? Is the drainage such that clothes are getting damaged? In cases where pressure ulcers occur at the end of life, goals of care should be clarified so that family knows to expect that the pressure ulcer may progress. Despite this progression, family should be reassured that quality of life will be preserved by effectively managing pain, drainage, and odor.

U = Undermining

Undermining occurs when the wound edge no longer is firmly attached to the wound bed. Necrotic tissue is closely correlated with undermining. Shear forces also worsen undermining, and reversal of the shear force aids in reversal of undermining. Healing cannot occur until reattachment of the edge to the wound bed is established. The provider can measure undermining by gently running a probe under the wound edge. By using an anatomic clock, where the 12:00 position is cephalad, and designating where the undermining is deepest, the provider can establish a consistent description of undermining.

R = Re-evaluate

After the initial evaluation, frequent follow-up may be necessary to determine if treatment plans have been put into effect, clarify any misunderstandings, and assess plan effectiveness. Because long-term care facilities have multiple staff members on different shifts, communication may be lost if treatment plans are not continuously clarified. If a palliative care approach is selected, the provider may space out the re-evaluation of the ulcer and only make adjustments in the treatment plan if the ulcer should change.

E = Edge

Pressure ulcers on the sacrum, coccyx, and ischium are exposed to constant moisture from sweat, urine, and feces. The edges often become macerated and the wound bed may rapidly extend. Pressure ulcers on other areas of the body also may have a macerated wound edge if there is large exudate. By detailing the appearance of the wound edge, the provider and team can outline a strategy to curtail the extension and aide healing.

Although the MEASURE strategy offers a comprehensive framework to approach pressure ulcers, the Pressure Ulcer Scale for Healing is another validated tool for evaluating pressure ulcer healing.[38] It is brief, easily reproducible, and commonly used for tracking in long-term care and many of its components have been included in the MDS 3.0. It incorporates measurements, exudate amount, and tissue type. Successful pressure ulcer treatment plans in the long-term care setting must incorporate a tool to assess healing over time and address comorbidites that complicate healing as well as patient-centered concerns and goals of care.

PRESSURE ULCER INTERDISCIPLINARY MANAGEMENT

Pressure ulcer management in long-term care highlights the importance of the interdisciplinary team. Providers, nursing staff, rehabilitative therapists, and nutritionists come together to evaluate contributing factors and their potential reversibility. Personal care attendants care for patients on a daily basis to where they potentially have the most insight into patient-centered concerns.

A recent systematic review of pressure ulcer treatment found that little attention is paid to reversing underlying conditions.[39] This is unfortunate given that local wound care is ineffective if the underlying cause cannot be reversed and if patients do not adhere to their treatment regimens.[40] Reversal of underlying conditions includes excellent incontinence care, nutritional optimization, and pressure relief.

Urinary incontinence is a common problem for those living in long-term care. Urinary and fecal incontinence leads to more frequent cleaning of patients. Skin easily becomes dried and excoriated from use of cleansers. When a pressure ulcer is present, healing can be even more problematic in the setting of incontinence. Attention must be paid to the wound edge to protect from urinary and fecal soilage. For stage III and stage IV pressure ulcers, collection devices for either urinary or fecal (diarrheal) incontinence may be necessary for a short period time.[41] Nurses and providers should collaborate to trial various wound care products to see which best fits patients' needs.

No evidence exists to support supplementation of specific nutrients, but good general nutrition is essential to wound care.[39,42] A long-term care facility's nutritionist and speech therapist can collaborate to ensure that patients are able to consume enough calories and protein for wound healing. Vitamin or mineral supplements should be offered only when deficiencies are suspected or confirmed.[34,39] Zinc supplementation, if used, should not be given for more than 2 weeks because longer intake leads to copper deficiency and impaired wound healing.[43,44]

Pressure reduction and shear and friction minimization are instrumental to pressure ulcer treatment. It is unclear how often patients should be turned, although most guidelines recommend every 2 to 4 hours.[34] Little evidence exists for specific types of mattresses, although some general recommendations can be made.[39] Long-term care facilities should consider nonpowered specialized mattresses throughout their facility for prevention as well as treatment. For stage III and stage IV pressure ulcers, a facility can consider a powered overlay or mattress. These are costly, so a facility may begin with a trial of the powered device to see if aides in healing. The National Pressure Ulcer Advisory Panel and the European Pressure Ulcer Advisory Panel are clear that the support surface should match patients' needs rather than determining the type of surface based exclusively on wound stage.[34] Nursing and rehabilitative therapists should collaborate to determine that the support surface minimizes friction, shear, and moisture accumulation. The literature does not support that powered mattresses are superior to nonpowered mattresses either for prevention or treatement.[39,45] Guidelines are based on expert opinion. Support surfaces are important for offloading of pressure, but they do not address the other ulcer causes, such as friction, shear, moisture, and so forth. In short, nothing can replace good personal attendant care with frequent turning, lifting, and transfers that minimize friction and shear.

For those long-term care patients who are primarily wheelchair users or spend a predominant amount of time in a favorite chair, rehabilitative therapists should evaluate their wheelchairs and cushions. Any skin breakdown that can be attributed to sitting should also prompt an evaluation of the chair and cushion. As patients age in place in long-term care and become more debilitated, their ability to sit upright in a wheelchair unsupported may be compromised. Also, weight gain from being sedentary or weight loss from poor oral intake results in poor wheelchair fitting. Specialized wheelchair cushions—gel, gel foam, or air filled—can be implemented after a therapist has evaluated the wheelchair. Strict bed rest is not recommended, because this may lead to worsening failure to thrive, depression, deconditioning, social isolation, pneumonia, deep venous thrombosis, and more pressure ulcers.[46,47] Providers may want to consider periods of bed rest for those patients with ischial and coccyx ulcers.[34]

LOCAL WOUND CARE: THE WOUND BED PARADIGM

Good wound care begins with reversing underlying conditions wherever possible and addressing patients' goals of care. Once those measures are taken, local wound care can be directed via the wound bed paradigm. The wound bed paradigm is the cornerstone of chronic wound healing treatment plans. It was initially described in the early 2000s when wound care experts unified years-old principles into a formal framework, and it is constantly being clarified.[48–50] Three principles comprise the wound bed preparation paradigm: moisture balance, bacterial balance, and débridement. When composing a local wound care treatment plan, providers must apply these principles in the context of patient concerns, whether the wound has the potential to heal, wound characteristics, and cost. This last consideration is particularly important when caring for patients in long-term care facilities where budgets may be restrictive.

There are more than 1000 products on the market, and staying up to date on the latest products can be daunting. Usually long-term care facilities negotiate optimal pricing for their wound care products. Providers should familiarize themselves with their facility's products of choice and the products' functions. Providers can then collaborate with nursing staff on using the optimal dressing for moisture balance, bacterial balance, and débridement.

Moisture Balance

Moisture balance is crucial to pressure ulcer management. Since the 1960s, the wound care community has known that moist wound healing is essential and that occlusive dressings do not increase the risk of infection.[51] If the wound is too dry, fibroblasts, keratinocytes, and other cell proliferators are unable to migrate across the wound bed. A wound that is too wet may lead to wound edge degradation. As described previously, chronic pressure ulcers exude wound fluid that retards wound healing.[21,22] Exudate must be controlled and balanced while maintaining a moist environment in a healable pressure ulcer.

There are a variety of products to maintain moisture balance. A dressing is considered moisture retentive when its moisture vapor transmission rate (MVTR) is less than 840 g/m^2 per 24 hours.[52] For instance, gauze has an MVTR of more than 1200 g/m^2 per 24 hours whereas hydrocolloids are less than 300 g/m^2 per 24 hours. The provider must determine whether moisture retention or exudate control is the primary goal and choose a product accordingly. Hydrocolloids, because of their low MVTR, have no absorptive capacity and are primarily used to hydrate a dry pressure ulcer. Hydrogels, calcium alginates, and foams have MVTRs that range from 800 g/m^2 to 5000 g/m^2.[53] Hydrogels are primarily used for dry pressure ulcers; calcium alginates are used for moderately exudative ulcers and are excellent for tunneling and undermining areas. Foams are best for highly exudative ulcers.

Proper management of exudate also protects the periulcer skin, and attention must be paid to the wound edge to prevent pressure ulcer progressing. Barriers, such as 40% zinc oxide or window dressings with hydrocolloid, are simple methods to protect the surrounding edge.

Bacterial Balance and Infection Management

All wounds, including pressure ulcers, contain some amount of bacteria. There are 4 recognized levels of bacteria in chronic wounds: contamination, colonization, critical colonization, and infection.[54]

- Contamination—Bacteria are present but not replicating or causing an immune response.

- Colonization—Bacteria are replicating but not causing host injury.
- Critical colonization—Replicating bacteria cause delayed wound healing and other evidence of host injury. The bacteria may be entering the superficial compartment of the wound. Signs of critical colonization include a red or bleeding pressure ulcer, increased exudate, increased necrotic tissue, increased smell, or an ulcer that is not healing despite adequate treatment.[54] It is at this point that a provider should consider topical antimicrobials.
- Infection—Replicating bacteria are in the deeper wound compartment and evoking an immune response locally and possibly systemically. Signs of infection include increasing size, increasing temperature near or at the wound bed, probe to bone or exposure to bone, new areas of breakdown, and worsening smell, erythema, exudate, and edema.[54] Increasing pain and new breakdown have been correlated with 100% specificity for chronic wound infection.[55] When only looking at wound culture results, a cell count of more than 10^5 organisms is considered an infected wound. Infection occurs when the host's immune system becomes overwhelmed with the level of microbial burden and/or virulence of the organism.[54] For long-term care patients whose immune system is compromised by chronic disease, the bacteria may not be exceedingly burdensome or virulent to cause infection.

Biofilms have recently come under close scrutiny with regard to their influence on delayed wound healing. Biofilms are communities of bacteria that attach to one another and interact synergistically. Via quorum sensing, the different species of bacteria genetically modify to encase themselves in the wound and invade blood vessels.[56] One study suggested that as many as 60% of chronic wounds contain biofilm (as opposed to only 6% in acute wounds).[57] Biofilms do not always show up on a wound culture. This observation may falsely reassure clinicians who are over-reliant on a culture to determine if a pressure ulcer is infected. The formation of biofilm in the wound bed leads to antibiotic resistance and delayed wound healing. Thus far, mechanical débridement is the débridement of choice for removing biofilm.[56]

For critical colonization, or superficial infection, of the pressure ulcer, a provider must choose a product that brings down the bacterial burden but does not increase the risk of resistance. An ideal product is one that is not used systemically (thus not associated with bacterial resistance), is nontoxic to the wound, and does not induce allergy.[54] Topical antibiotics have fallen out of favor in the wound care community because they are associated with increased resistance. Topical gentamycin and tobramycin are examples of topical antibiotics with increasing resistance. Bacitracin and neomycin—products often used in long-term care and other settings for minor wounds—are not recommended either because they induce skin sensitivity and increase bacterial resistance.[58,59] Silver compounds and cadexomer iodine are the products of choice for topical bacterial balance management.[54] Providers should choose the vehicle based on the other wound bed preparation tenets of moisture balance and débridement.

Once bacterial balance has been established, the provider must consider stopping the antimicrobial product because there is low-level toxicity to the pressure ulcer that may occur. If a patient is at high risk of infection (eg, immunocompromised state) then the provider may decide to continue the topical antimicrobial treatment. Careful re-evaluation of bacterial balance is necessary to determine if the product should be restarted.

Providers must use both clinical acumen and objective data to help assess for pressure ulcer infection. Because patients with pressure ulcers or other chronic wounds may have subtle signs of a wound infection, a wound culture can help direct management. More credence is being given to the validity of the Levine technique for wound cultures.[60,61] The ulcer is cleansed of debris. The swab is inserted into the cleanest, deepest part of the wound—care should be taken to avoid any necrotic tissue or purulent drainage. The swab is rotated in a 1-cm^2 area in a 360° motion. The swab should press against the ulcer bed such that wound fluid is expressed.[37] The culture is placed on a Petri dish in quadrants, and results range from 1+ (ie, scant) to 4+ (ie, heavy); 4+ (heavy) growth is usually correlated with a cell count of 10^5 organisms. Providers should be familiar with the standards of their local laboratory. It is important not to treat patients systemically with antimicrobials simply because a swab shows bacterial growth. The entire clinical situation has to be considered.

If a pressure ulcer is infected, then broad-spectrum oral or intravenous antibiotics should be considered. Chronic wounds, in particular pressure ulcers, have polymicrobial bacterial colonization. The antibiotic of choice covers gram-positive, gram-negative, and anaerobic bacteria. Long-term care facilities are considered reservoirs for methicillin-resistant *Staphylococcus aureus* (MRSA).[62] Empiric treatment plans should include MRSA coverage. A wound culture using the Levine technique can assist providers in narrowing the antibiotic choice.

Duration of antibiotics depends on the depth of infection. Soft tissue infections are often treated for 2 weeks, whereas osteomyelitis may require at least 6 weeks of intravenous therapy. Providers must weigh the risks, for example *Clostridium difficile* infection, kidney failure, need for frequent blood draws, and monitoring, when advising patients and families on this type of treatment.

The majority of evidence in determining the presence of osteomyelitis is from diabetic foot ulcers; this evidence has been extrapolated to pressure ulcer management. Plain radiographs may detect osteomyelitis if an infection has been present for a minimum of 3 weeks.[63] If duration of infection is not known, as is commonly the case in chronic pressure ulcers, then a more sensitive test may be required. MRI is the imaging modality of choice for the diagnosis of osteomyelitis, but this may not be an option for older patients living in long-term care. Challenges, such as dementia with agitation, immobility with contractures, and escort requirement, all make an MRI study problematic. CT scan, although less sensitive then MRI, is a reasonable alternative for these patients. CT can describe both osseous and soft tissue involvement.[63]

Pressure Ulcer Débridement

The importance of wound débridement in pressure ulcer management cannot be overemphasized. Débridement removes the slough and necrosis that, when in place, inhibits healing, supports bacterial growth, and masks signs of infection.[49] Almost any chronic wound needs débridement, the one exception being some heel wounds with a dry eschar. Débridement is needed not only to remove visible devitalized tissue but also to remove biofilm. Although there is limited experimental trial evidence to support or refute the need for débridement in pressure ulcers, there is strong expert consensus.[34]

Débridement strategies vary and include autolytic, enzymatic, mechanical, and sharp surgical. Autolytic débridement is the use of the body's naturally occurring enzymes to loosen and remove necrotic tissue with each dressing change. Occlusive dressings promote autolytic débridement. Enzymatic débridement is the use of a topical enzyme to augment the body's autolytic débridement. Providers should stay current with what products remain on the market. For example, papain urea, a commonly used enzymatic débrider, was removed from the US market in 2009.[64]

This was due to the Food and Drug Administration's concerns over adverse reactions to this product. Mechanical débridement primarily refers to wet-to-dry dressings. These dressings are nursing intensive (require changing more than twice a day), provide no bacterial balance, are painful, and nonselectively débride healthy tissue.[34,65] Wet-to-dry dressings are discouraged among expert wound care practitioners.[34] Surgical débridement is the fastest form of débridement but can also cause pain and bleeding. Providers should review patients' medication lists for anticoagulants and advise premedication for pain management for any débridement procedure.

If a pressure ulcer is in the extremities, adequate vascular supply must be determined prior to any débridement strategy. Ankle-brachial indices may not be specific among older adults or those with diabetes due to vessel calcification. In these cases, toe photoplethysmography, also known as toe pressure, may be indicated.[66] Toe pressures of 50 mm Hg or more are considered adequate for healing, 30 to 50 mm Hg are considered borderline for healing, and 30 mm Hg or below likely inadequate for healing to take place. Palpable pedal pulses usually indicate a toe pressure of 80 mm Hg.[67] Toe pressures can be obtained at most major tertiary care centers and are usually ordered with ankle-brachial indices.

PRESSURE ULCER MANAGEMENT AND PALLIATIVE CARE

As patients age in place in long-term care, they become more debilitated. Immobility often worsens, resulting in contractures, and oral intake decreases, especially in the setting of dementia. Patients and/or their families may opt for care plans that optimize quality of life rather than extended life. In those settings, reversing the conditions underlying pressure ulcers may not be consistent with the goals of care, and patients and families must be told that the pressure ulcer does not have the potential to heal. In cases where comfort and infection control are the goals, thorough, consistent documentation should be done by all members of the interdisciplinary team.

In cases of wounds that do not have the potential to heal, the wound bed paradigm is truncated to bacterial balance only. Moist interactive dressings and débridement may increase bacterial burden and infection risks.[54,68] In these situations, antiseptics may be necessary to prevent wound worsening. Because antiseptics have fallen out of favor by many wound practitioners and have been prohibited altogether in some facilities, it is important to document the potential healability of the wound. If a wound does not have the potential to heal, then this should be clearly stated, including the reasons for poor healability. This documentation supports the use of an antiseptic and protects facilities from citation by state surveyors.

Pain management for pressure ulcers is challenging. A palliative care specialist can facilitate communication with the family on natural progression of disease, assess nonpharmacologic modalities for comfort, and offer advice on oral and topical medications.

Collaboration between a palliative care specialist, wound care team, nurses, personal care attendants, and rehabilitative staff are instrumental in improving the quality of life for someone with nonhealable pressure ulcers. A palliative care specialist focuses on symptom management for the end-of-life disease process. The wound care team focuses on less frequent dressing changes (if possible) as well as any wound pain during and in-between dressing changes. Rehabilitative specialists collaborate with the patient and team on optimal positioning, including wheelchair usage, so that the patient can participate in activities. The nurses and personal care attendants coordinate medication management and self-care that minimizes discomfort.

QUALITY INDICATORS AND LITIGATION

Enter "pressure ulcer" in a search engine and the search returns a list of law firm Web sites. Because pressure ulcers are considered preventable, their development is used as a quality indicator for long-term care facilities, hospitals, and effectiveness of physician care.[69] The Omnibus Budget Reconciliation Act (OBRA) of 1987[70] established federal standards of care for long-term care facilities. This made it easier for a claimant to prove that a long-term care facility had been negligent after a pressure ulcer developed. Although case mix can dramatically affect rates of pressure ulcer development, it is now common for patients and families to choose a facility by looking at its published incidence and prevalence rates of pressure ulcers.[27]

Over the past 2 decades, many long-term care facilities have decreased their rates of incidence and prevalence of pressure ulcers through quality-improvement efforts and collaboratives.[71–74] Quality-improvement collaboratives are groups of health care organizations that address a particular problem by agreeing on a common strategy, implementing the same approaches across systems, and sharing results. Implementation of such strategies has been shown to lead to improvements in a majority of quality indicators as well as decreased pressure ulcer incidence.

Despite advances in pressure ulcer care, litigation over pressure ulcers in the United States continues to grow. A review of pressure ulcer lawsuits brought against long-term care facilities showed that the number of cases increased 2.6 times from 1984 to 2002; at the same time, there was 10.6% decrease in the number of pressure ulcer patients—87% of plaintiffs received some type of financial recovery from the facility.[75] The mean recovery for the period 1984 to 1999 was $3,359,259 compared with a mean of $13,554,168 for the period 1999 to 2002. The highest award was $312 million. In United Kingdom, there is usually little payable compensation, so little is gained by litigation. The National Health Service has a statutory procedure for handling pressure ulcer complaints in coordination with the Patient Advice and Liaison Service.[76]

Since the implementation of OBRA in 1987, long-term care facilities have implemented pressure ulcer protocols aimed at reducing incidence. It is believed that such interventions can decrease litigation or reduce damages if a case is taken to court. As should be clear from the previous discussion, development and worsening of some pressure ulcers can be unavoidable in gravely disabled patients when a family and care team make a conscious, coordinated decision to prioritize palliative care over standard practice of pressure ulcer prevention and management. In such cases, the facility must document assessment of risk, how the patient's medical condition (cachexia, metastatic cancer, severe peripheral vascular disease, or terminal illness) promotes development of ulcers and impedes healing, and why standard interventions are or are not appropriate for the patient's care.[77] Not only should all staff be trained in pressure ulcer risk modifications and appropriate documentation but also families should be taught to help with pressure reduction. Additionally, families should be warned that skin failure can occur especially in actively dying patients or patients who are difficult to turn due to their medical condition.[78]

Today, when a family arrives to photograph a pressure ulcer, the long-term care facility must be prepared for future litigation. When it seems that a family is contemplating legal action, the entire health care team should work with the patient and family. Levine and colleagues[79] recommend several actions to minimize pressure ulcer litigation. First, to avoid appearing defensive, administration should help the family document the pressure ulcer if they request assistance. Second, providers should maintain professionalism by involving the entire team, including facility administration in meetings with the family to improve trust, provide education, and set realistic expectations. Third, after a pressure ulcer develops, the team should review the history, re-evaluate the treatment plan, and review the facility's pressure ulcer policies. Finally, if a patient or family behaves in ways that put the patient at risk, such as family interference with the care plan or an extended absence by the resident, providers should objectively document the behaviors and counseling about the risks of such behaviors in the chart.

SUMMARY

Pressure ulcers are common in long-term care and costly to patients, facilities, and society. Although there is a dearth of high-quality evidence on pressure ulcer prevention and treatment, national and international guidelines based on best available data and expert opinion should direct care. Optimal management of pressure ulcers requires understanding of the differential diagnosis of chronic wounds, use of standardized assessment metrics, and treatment following the wound bed preparation model. A patient-centered approach incorporating consideration of individual patients' comorbidities, preferences, and goals of care is the cornerstone of good pressure ulcer care.

REFERENCES

1. Reddy M, Gill SS, Rochon PA. Preventing pressure ulcers: a systematic review. JAMA 2006;296:974–84.
2. Horn SD, Bender SA, Ferguson ML, et al. The national pressure ulcer long-term care study: pressure ulcer development in long-term care residents. J Am Geriatr Soc 2004;52(3):359–67.
3. Berlowitz DR, Brandeis GH, Anderson J, et al. Effect of pressure ulcers on the survival of long-term care residents. J Gerontol A Biol Sci Med Sci 1997;52A:106–10.
4. Wysocki AB. Decubitus ulcers. In: Freedberg IM, Eisen AZ, editors. Fitzpatrick's dermatology in general medicine. 5th edition. New York (NY): McGraw-Hill; 1999. p. 1538–54.
5. Lyder CH. Pressure ulcer prevention and management. JAMA 2003;289(2):223–6.
6. Park-Lee E, Caffrey C. Pressure ulcers among nursing home residents: United States—2004. NCHS Data Brief 2009;14:1–6.
7. Thomas DR. Issues and dilemmas in the prevention and treatment of pressure ulcers. J Gerontol 2001;56A:M328–40.
8. Centers for Medicare and Medicaid Services. Federal Register Part II 42 CFR Parts 411, 412, 413, and 489: changes to the hospital inpatient prospective payment systems and fiscal year 2008 rates; Final Rule. Federal Register 2007; 72(162):47201–5.
9. Brem H, Maggi J, Nierman D, et al. High cost of stage IV pressure ulcers. Am J Surg 2010;200(4):473–7.
10. Health Council of the Netherlands. Pressure ulcers. The Hague (The Netherlands): Health Council of the Netherlands; 1999. Publication 1999/23.
11. Bennet G, Dealey C, Posnett J. The cost of pressure ulcers in the UK. Age Ageing 2004;33(3):230–5.

12. Allman RM. Pressure ulcer prevalence, incidence, risk factors, and impact. Clin Geriatr Med 1997;13(3):421–36.
13. Cullum N, Clark M. Intrinsic factors associated with pressure sores in elderly people. J Adv Nurs 1992;17:427–31.
14. Agency for Health Care Policy and Prevention. Pressure ulcers in adults: prediction and prevention. Clinical Practice Guideline Number 3. Rockville (MD): US Department of Health and Human Sciences; 1992.
15. Horn SD, Bender SA, Bergstrom N. Description of the National Pressure Ulcer Long-Term Care Study. J Am Geriatr Soc 2002;50(11):1816–25.
16. Garcia AD, Thomas DR. Assessment and management of chronic pressure ulcers in the elderly. Med Clin North Am 2006;90(5):925–44.
17. Bergstrom N, Braden BJ, Kemp M, et al. Reliability and validity of the Braden Scale: a multi-site study. Nurs Res 1998;47(5):261–9.
18. Norton D, McLaren R, Exton-Smith AN. An investigation of geriatric nursing problems in hospital. London: National Corporation for the Care of Old People (now Centre for Policy on Ageing); 1962.
19. Waterlow J. Pressure sores: a risk assessment card. Nurs Times 1985;81: 49–55.
20. Goldberg SR, Dieglemann RF. Wound healing primer. Surg Clin North Am 2010; 90(6):1133–46.
21. Eming SA, Krieg T, Davidson JM. Inflammation in wound repair: molecular and cellular mechanisms. J Invest Dermatol 2007;127(3):514–25.
22. Bucalo B, Eaglstein WH, Falanga V. Inhibition of cell proliferation by chronic wound fluid. Wound Repair Regen 1993;1(3):181–6.
23. Clark M. Repositioning to prevent pressure sores—what is the evidence? Nurs Stand 1998;13(3):58–64.
24. Thompson P, Langemo D, Anderson J, et al. Skin care protocols for pressure ulcers and incontinence in long-term care: a quasi-experimental study. Adv Skin Wound Care 2005;18(8):422–9.
25. Hampton S, Collins F. Reducing pressure ulcer incidence in a long-term setting. Br J Nurs 2005;14(15):S6–12.
26. Cullum N, Deeks J, Sheldon TA, et al. Beds, mattresses and cushions for preventing and treating pressure sores [Cochrane Review]. Cochrane Database Syst Rev 2000;1:CD001159. Oxford: Update Software.
27. Berlowitz DR, Ash AS, Brandeis GH, et al. Rating long-term care facilities on pressure ulcer development: importance of case-mix adjustment. Ann Intern Med 1996;124:557–63.
28. Theodosat A. Skin diseases of the lower extremities in the elderly. Dermatol Clin 2004;22:13–21.
29. Wipke-Tevis DD. Caring for vascular leg ulcers: essential knowledge for the home health nurse. Home Healthc Nurse 1999;17(2):87–94.
30. Holloway GA. Arterial ulcers: assessment, classification, and management. In: Krasner DL, Rodeheaver GT, Sibbald RG, editors. Chronic wound care: a clinical source book for healthcare professionals. 4th edition. Wayne (PA): HMP Communications; 2007. p. 443–9.
31. Steed DL. Wounds in people with diabetes: assessment, classification, and management. In: Krasner DL, Rodeheaver GT, Sibbald RG, editors. Chronic wound care: a clinical source book for healthcare professionals. 4th edition. Wayne (PA): HMP Communications; 2007. p. 537–42.
32. Collier M. The assessment of patients with malignant fungating wounds—a holistic approach: Part 1. Nurs Times 1997;93(44):S1–4.

33. Available at: http://www.medicare.gov/default.aspx. Accessed December 30, 2010.
34. National Pressure Ulcer Advisory Panel and European Pressure Ulcer Advisory Panel. Prevention and treatment of pressure ulcers: clinical practice guideline. Washington, DC: National Pressure Ulcer Advisory Panel; 2009.
35. Levine JA, Roberson S, Ayello EA. Essentials of MDS 3.0 section M: skin conditions. Adv Skin Wound Care 2010;23:273–84.
36. Keast DH, Bowering CK, Evans AW. MEASURE: a proposed assessment framework for developing best practice recommendations for wound assessment. Wound Repair Regen 2004;12:S1–17.
37. Landis S, Ryan S, Woo K, et al. Infections in chronic wounds. In: Krasner DL, Rodeheaver GT, Sibbald RG, editors. Chronic wound care: a clinical source book for healthcare professionals. 4th edition. Wayne (PA): HMP Communications; 2007. p. 299–321.
38. Available at: http://npuap.org/tools.htm. Accessed December 30, 2010.
39. Reddy M, Gill SS, Kalkar SR. Treatment of pressure ulcers: a systematic review. JAMA 2008;300(22):2647–62.
40. Sibbald RG, Williamson D, Orsted HL, et al. Preparing the wound bed—debridement, bacterial balance, and moisture balance. Ostomy Wound Manage 2000;46:14–37.
41. Centers for Medicare and Medicaid Services. State operations manual appendix PP—guidance to surveyors for long care facilities 483.25 (d). P. 246. Available at: http://cms.hhs.gov/manuals/Downloads/som107ap_pp_guidelines_ltcf.pdf. Accessed December 30, 2010.
42. Desai H. Ageing and wounds. Part 2: healing in old age. J Wound Care 1997;6(5):237–9.
43. Thomas DR. The role of nutrition in prevention and healing of pressure ulcers. Med Clin North Am 1997;13:497–511.
44. Lown D. Wound healing. In: Matarese LE, Gottschlich MM, editors. Contemporary nutrition support practice, a clinical guide. Philadelphia: W.B. Saunders; 1998. p. 583–9.
45. Cullum N, McInnes E, Bell-Syer SEM, et al. Support surfaces for pressure ulcer prevention. Cochrane Database Syst Rev 1998;1:CD001735.
46. Corcoran PJ. Use it or lost it—the hazards of bed rest and inactivity. West J Med 1991;154(5):219–23.
47. Allen C, Glasziou P, Del Mar C. Bed rest: a potentially harmful treatment needing more careful evaluation. Lancet 1999;354:1229–33.
48. Falanga V. Classification for wound preparation and stimulation of chronic wounds. Wound Repair Regen 2000;8:347–52.
49. Schultz GS, Sibbald RG, Falanga V, et al. Wound bed preparation: a systemic approach to wound management. Wound Repair Regen 2003;11:1–28.
50. Panuncialman J, Falanga V. The science of wound bed preparation. Clin Plast Surg 2007;34:621–32.
51. Hinman CD, Maibach H. Effect of air explosure and occlusion on experimental human skin. Nature 1963;200:377–8.
52. Bolton LL, Johnson CL, Van Rijswijk L. Occlusive dressings: therapeutic agents and effects on drug delivery. Clin Dermatol 1991;9(4):573–83.
53. Seaman S. Dressing selection in chronic wound management. J Am Podiatr Med Assoc 2002;92(1):24–33.

54. Sibbald RG, Woo K, Ayello EA. Increased bacterial burden and infection: the story of NERDS and STONES. Adv Skin Wound Care 2006;19:447–61.
55. Gardner SE, Frantz RA, Doebbeling BN, et al. The validity of clinical signs and symptoms used to identify localized chronic wound infection. Wound Repair Regen 2001;9(3):178–86.
56. James GA, Swogger E, Wolcott R, et al. Biofilms in chronic wounds. Wound Repair Regen 2008;16(1):37–44.
57. Black CE, Costerton JW. Current concepts regarding the effect of wound microbial ecology and biofilms on wound healing. Surg Clin North Am 2010;90:1147–60.
58. Jankicevic J, Vesić S, Vukićević J, et al. Contact sensitivity in patients with venous leg ulcers in Serbia: comparison with contact dermatitis patients and relationship to ulcer duration. Contact Dermatitis 2008;58(1):32–6.
59. Saap L, Fahim S, Arsenault E, et al. Contact sensitivity in patients with leg ulcerations: a North American study. Arch Dermatol 2004;140(10):1241–6.
60. National Guideline Clearinghouse (NGC). Guideline synthesis: management and treatment of pressure ulcers. In: National Guideline Clearinghouse (NGC) [website]. Rockville (MD); 2006 (revised 2008 July). Available at: http://www.guideline.gov. Accessed January 10, 2011.
61. Gardner SE, Frantz RA, Saltzman CL, et al. Diagnostic validity of three swab techniques for identifying chronic wound infection. Wound Repair Regen 2006;14:548–57.
62. Gastmeier P. Healthcare-associated versus community-acquired infections: a new challenge for science and society. Int J Med Microbiol 2010;300(6):342–5.
63. Pineda C, Vargas A, Rodriguez AV. Imaging of osteomyelitis: current concepts. Infect Dis Clin North Am 2006;20(4):789–825.
64. Available at: http://www.fda.gov/Drugs/GuidanceComplianceRegulatoryInformation/EnforcementActivitiesbyFDA/SelectedEnforcementActionsonUnapprovedDrugs/ucm119646.htm. Website Accessed December 30, 2010.
65. Longe RL. Current concepts in clinical therapeutics: pressure sores. Clin Pharm 1986;5(8):669–81.
66. Reddy M, Sibbald G. Management of diabetic foot ulcers. Geriatr Aging 2005;8:33–7.
67. Second European Consensus Document on chronic critical leg ischemia. Circulation 1991;84(Suppl 4):IV1–26.
68. Drosou A, Falabella A, Kirsner RS. Antiseptics on wounds: an area of controversy. Wounds 2003;15(5):149–66.
69. Kapoor A, Kader B, Cabral H, et al. Using the case mix of pressure ulcer healing to evaluate nursing home performance. Am J Med Qual 2008;23:342–9.
70. Nursing Home Reform Amendments. US Code of Federal Regulations Title 42, Chapter 7, Subchapter XIX, Subpart 483.
71. Xakellis GC, Frantz RA. The cost-effectiveness of interventions for preventing pressure ulcers. J Am Board Fam Pract 1996;9:79.
72. Baier RR, Gifford DR, Lyder CH, et al. Quality improvement for pressure ulcer care in the nursing home setting: the northeast pressure ulcer project. J Am Med Dir Assoc 2003;4:291.
73. Makai P, Koopmanschap M, Bal R, et al. Cost-effectiveness of a pressure ulcer quality collaborative. Cost Eff Resour Alloc 2010;8:11.

74. Abel RL, Warren K, Bean G, et al. Quality improvement in nursing homes in Texas: results from a pressure ulcer prevention project. J Am Med Dir Assoc 2005;6(3): 181–8.
75. Voss CA, Bender SA, Ferguson ML, et al. Long-term care liability for pressure ulcers. J Am Geriatr Soc 2005;53(9):1587–92.
76. Dimond B. Pressure ulcer care: making and handling a complaint in the NHS. Br J Nurs 2006;15(22):1242–3.
77. American Medical Directors Association. Pressure ulcers in long-term care setting: clinical practice guideline. Columbia (MD): AMDA; 2008.
78. Langemo D, Brown G. Skin fails too: acute, chronic, and end-stage skin failure. Adv Skin Wound Care 2006;19(4):206–11.
79. Levine JM, Savino F, Peterson M, et al. Risk management for pressure ulcers: when a family shows up with a camera. J Am Med Dir Assoc 2008;9(5):360–3.

Transitional Care of the Long-Term Care Patient

S. Liliana Oakes, MD, CMD[a,*], Suzanne M. Gillespie, MD, CMD[b], Yanping Ye, MD[a], Margaret Finley, MD, CMD[a], Mathew Russell, MD[c], Neela K. Patel, MD, MPH[a], David Espino, MD[a]

KEYWORDS

- Long-term care • Transition • Acute care hospital
- Emergency department

Transitional care is a major part of long-term care (LTC) patient management. Patients may transition within one health care location, such as transitioning from an intensive care setting to a subacute care unit. Transitions also occur between different health care settings, such as a hospital discharge to a skilled nursing setting for rehabilitative care. Transitional care may vary depending on the location. Transitional care can therefore be defined as a set of actions designed to ensure the coordination and continuity of health care as patients transfer between different locations or different levels of care within the same location. A variety of individuals are involved in transitional care, including the patient, the patient's primary and specialty care providers, nurses, social workers, and informal and family caregivers. Successful transitional care involves the development of a comprehensive care plan and the availability of experienced LTC health practitioners who are provided relevant medical information about the patient's goals, preferences, and clinical status.[1]

LTC has been defined as a comprehensive, longitudinal, patient-centered system of formal and informal health and support services that are intended to improve, maximize, or stabilize, when possible, the function of patients with chronic disease across various settings over an extended period of time, including the provision of palliative care/hospice services.[2] The most common transitional LTC sites are nursing homes,

This article is supported by the funding from HRSA, Health Resources and Service Administration. GACA, Geriatric Academic Career Award. Title VII.
[a] Division of Community Geriatrics, Department of Family and Community Medicine, University of Texas Health Science Center at San Antonio, 7703 Floyd Curl Drive MC 7795, San Antonio, TX 78229, USA
[b] Division of Geriatrics and Aging, School of Medicine and Dentistry, University of Rochester, 601 Elmwood Avenue, Rochester, NY 14642, USA
[c] Section of Geriatrics, Boston University Medical Center, 88 East Newton Street Robinson 2, Boston, MA 02118, USA
* Corresponding author.
E-mail address: oakes@uthscsa.edu

skilled nursing facilities, assisted living facilities, and hospice care. Transitional care commonly involved patients from these settings. Most nursing home admissions are derived from acute care hospitals.[3]

Nursing home residents frequently use emergency department (ED) services, with more than 25% of nursing home residents receiving ED care annually.[4–6] These residents are also frequently admitted to acute care hospitals as part of their ED experience. Many patients are also admitted to LTC settings for postacute care and after a period of recovery and rehabilitation, are discharged from the LTC setting, transitioning to community-based homes. This high frequency of transition was also seen in a study using postacute and skilled nursing facility settings by a nationally representative cohort of elders. During a 2-year period, almost 5 million patients aged over 65 made more than 15 million transitions. Of note, 1.1 million of these patients had subsequent health care use, such as emergency room visits, potentially avoidable hospital stays, and returns to an institutional setting after discharge to the community.[7] This pattern of frequent subsequent health care use suggests a widespread problem with transitional care in older adults.

LTC patients, by virtue of their population's high degree of medical complexity, prevalent cognitive and functional impairments, and underlying psychiatric illnesses, are at high risk for complicated transitions of care.[8] Poor transitions may result in significant morbidity and mortality, stemming from issues such as medication errors, adverse drug events, lack of timely follow-up care, and potentially avoidable rehospitalizations.[9–12] This article reviews the literature on transitional care to and from the LTC environment, highlighting strategies to improve the quality of care transitions. Several factors are vital in the improvement of systems of care dealing with transitions. Key factors include communication with and among health care providers, effective medication reconciliation, advanced discharge planning, and timely use of palliative care.[13–15]

READMISSION FROM LTC TO THE ACUTE CARE HOSPITAL

Most admissions to LTC facilities come from acute care hospitals, of which most are placed in skilled nursing care.[3] However, almost one-fourth of the Medicare beneficiaries who were discharged from an acute care hospital to a skilled nursing facility were readmitted within 30 days.[16] Of those patients readmitted, half never saw an LTC health care provider during their LTC stay. Common diagnoses associated with potentially avoidable LTC to hospital readmissions are heart failure, renal failure, urinary tract infections, pneumonia, and chronic obstructive pulmonary disease.[17] Significantly, of those patients under LTC who are readmitted, 67.3% have multiple hospital readmissions. The 2-year mortality rate for these patients with multiple readmission doubles from approximately 15% to 30%. Also of concern is that 68.9% of these patients were rehospitalized or died within 1 year after discharge, with those discharged after surgery having a mortality rate of 53%.[18]

LTC to hospital readmissions are costly and hence disruptive to patients/families and providers and interrupt the rehabilitation process. Also, rehospitalization of these patients under LTC increases the risk for a variety of complications, including delirium, iatrogenic illness, deconditioning, polypharmacy, and pressure ulcers.[19] Identifying and decreasing LTC to hospital readmissions should decrease patient morbidity and mortality, lower health care cost, and improve rehabilitative potential.

Risk factors that have been identified as leading to an increase in LTC to hospital readmissions are included in the following sections.

Fiscal Pressures to Decrease Hospital Length of Stay and LTC Reimbursement

Just as diagnosis-related groups led to acute care health care practice changes, reimbursement policies have led to changes in LTC health care practices. In particular, there has been an increase in the LTC short-stay admissions, with a corresponding increase in clinical acuity.[20] The clinical status of the patient on admission to the LTC continues to affect performance improvement initiatives related to readmissions and other readmission prevention strategies in the foreseeable future.

Lack of Health Care Provider Continuity

Historically, primary care physicians provided patient care continuity during the transitional care period, following up individuals from the outpatient setting to the acute care hospital and then after hospital discharge, including LTC settings. However US health care has become more fragmented with most elders having multiple providers at each site of care, whether it is a primary care provider, hospitalist, specialist, or LTC provider. These patient care silos create barriers to obtaining comprehensive timely patient care information and enhance the possibility of having conflicting information shared with patients and families. Multiple health care provider care also creates an environment in which conflicting clinical care approaches and patient education messages are commonplace. Low salaries and high rates of LTC worker turnover also increase the risk of rehospitalization.[21]

Communication

Lack of communication between health care providers has been shown to adversely affect post–hospital discharge care transitions. The availability of a discharge summary at the first LTC after discharge provider visit is low (12%–34%) and has been shown to directly affect care quality in approximately 25% of subsequent LTC visits.[18] Furthermore, hospital discharge summaries often lack important information such as diagnostic test results, the treatment or hospital course, discharge medications, test results pending at discharge, and follow-up plans. An ideal transition record should include (1) principal admission diagnosis, (2) medical problem list, (3) medication list, (4) allergies, (5) treatment plan, (6) goals of care, (7) test results, (8) pending test results, (9) cognitive status, (10) advance directives, and (11) further planned interventions.[15]

Communication about changes in patient status often occurs after hours or on weekends. The challenges of providing optimum care under these conditions are influenced by the expertise of the after-hours nursing staff and the on-call health care provider team. Personnel turnover in both groups further complicate care.

Cultural Competence

Health care professionals increasingly recognize the crucial role that culture plays in a patients' health care. Differing cultural orientations and expectations may influence the success of transitional care. Similarly, differences in patient cognitive function, language fluency, and health literacy levels can have a significant effect on care planning issues, which is particularly true in the LTC population. Cultural competence is essential for successful client- or patient-centered transitions of care. Additional training for health care professionals that targets expanded cross-culture knowledge and skills, increased respect and values of different cultures, and improved self-awareness about patient-centered need in care is warranted.[22]

Medication Errors

Medication errors include inappropriate medications or inappropriate monitoring of high-risk medicines and adverse drug events. More than 1.5 million Americans are injured every year by drug errors in various settings, including nursing homes. The Institute of Medicine states that at least one-quarter of all medication-related injuries are preventable. It is estimated that 800,000 preventable medication-related injuries occur annually in nursing homes across the country. These injuries include inappropriate medications or inappropriate monitoring of high-risk medicines and adverse drug events.[23] Medication errors during transitional care remain common as long as LTC medication reconciliation remains a dynamic process. Transfers are common, and information provided back to the LTC care facility is often incomplete. Medication reconciliation also often occurs after hours and/or on weekends, increasing the possibility that the LTC health care provider for that patient may not be promptly involved in or made aware of changes in the medication regimen. Pharmacist consultants have greatly improved care, but a more expanded role, especially in directly managing high-risk medications, could greatly decrease morbidity and mortality. Effective medication reconciliation depends on the cooperative efforts of pharmacy, nursing, clerical, and medical staff. Processes that have improved medication reconciliation are based on the different disciplines working together to develop a process to keep the health care providers informed on key medication changes. The development of information technology solutions have proven to be of benefit in the hospital setting, but the costs for individual LTC institutions to implement similar systems are beyond the reach of most facilities at this time. A medical therapy management (MTM) program is developed by the American Pharmacist Association. This program is designed to improve the communication among pharmacists, physicians, and patients to optimize the medication use and improve patient outcomes.

The MTM services are focused on a patient-centered process of care. The pharmacists work collaboratively with physicians and patients. This model is being implemented in outpatient clinics, LTC facilities, and hospitals.[24]

Coleman and colleagues[9] have described 4 pillars necessary to improve transitional care; these pillars were derived from patient and caregiver feedback obtained from earlier qualitative investigations regarding those factors that are most valuable to patients and caregivers during care transitions. The 4 pillars included (1): assistance with medication self-management, (2) a patient-centered record owned by and maintained by the patient to facilitate cross-site information transfer, (3) timely follow-up with primary or specialty care, and (4) a list of red flags indicating a worsening condition and instruction on how to respond to them. The 4 pillars were operationalized through 2 mechanisms designed to encourage older patients and their caregivers to assert a more active role during care transitions and to foster care coordination and continuity across settings: (1) a personal health record and (2) a series of visits and telephone calls with a transitional care coach. Although this care transitions intervention has been best described when applied to acute hospital to community discharges, it has also been used to improve discharges from postacute rehabilitation settings in LTC. This application of the care transitions intervention supports the premise that person-centered care transition concepts can be successfully applied to both transitions from hospitals to LTC settings and from LTC settings to community homes.

TRANSITIONAL CARE BETWEEN LTC AND EDs

With more rapid transfers between LTC and hospital, the patient acuity level in most LTC facilities has increased significantly over the past 2 decades.[25] It is therefore not surprising to find that patients under LTC frequently use ED services. The data from the National Nursing Home Survey showed that 8% of patients under LTC had an ED visit in the 90 days before the survey.[26] For many, the ED is the primary site for a health care provider evaluation before a necessary acute hospitalization. Of concern, however, is that 40% or more of the patients under LTC who are treated in the ED are treated for ambulatory-type conditions. Also, the rates of transfer from LTC-skilled nursing facilities to the ED vary widely between LTC facilities.[27] Therefore, a significant number of LTC initiated ED visits may be potentially avoidable.[26,28] The rate of potentially avoidable LTC to ED transitions in the United States has been calculated to exceed those seen in the United Kingdom (36%), Canada (7%), or Australia (<1%).[29] Therefore, quality initiatives should strive to incentivize LTC facilities to both reduce unnecessary ED transfers and optimize LTC to ED patient transitions for those requiring ED evaluation.[30]

However, the decision to initiate an LTC to ED transfer is complex and depends on a variety of factors. Preexisting advanced directives, family preferences, health care provider experience, medical malpractice environment, LTC staffing levels, LTC staff comfort level, and the quality of LTC staff to provider communication all affect the transfer decision. Many of these factors have been shown to vary regionally as well as over time.[31] In addition, because patient status changes often occur after hours, the patient's regular health care providers often are not available for consultation, leaving the on-call provider, who is unfamiliar with the patient, to make the decision. LTC staffing challenges often result in the use of temporary nursing placement services, resulting in having an LTC nurse who has had no experience with the patients before their change in status. This scenario often results in having the key clinical decision makers with no prior knowledge of the patient. This unavoidable ED transfer demonstrates that an optimal outcome for the inexperienced providers may not be best for the patient.

Once the decision for the LTC to ED transfer has been made, information provided to the ED provider team becomes critical. Not surprisingly, poor communication has been cited as the main cause of poor transitions between LTC and EDs.[32] There is often a lack of a designated person to take responsibility for coordinating transitional care, either in the LTC or ED setting.[33] This lack of a responsible person can lead to communication lapses and suboptimal patient outcomes and adverse events. Significant variability in the quality and volume of LTC information provided has been noted with as many as 10% of patients under LTC arriving to the ED without any accompanying documentation, with the remaining LTC transfers have significant information gaps.[34–38] A recent Canadian study of LTC to ED transfers demonstrated that important informational gaps were noted in 85.5% of these transfers. Specific clinically relevant information gaps included reason for transfer, baseline cognitive function, communication ability, vital signs, advanced directives, medication changes, activities of daily living, and mobility issues.[39] Often, these gaps are not because of a paucity of information but rather because of the transfer of large amounts of largely clinically irrelevant LTC information. In one study, the average amount of LTC to ED transfer information sent was 24 pages.[40] Defining a standard format, content and structure, and manageable length for transitional communications between the LTC and the ED can likely improve care. Efforts to date have been limited by poor adoption rates for template forms. For example, a standardized transfer form implemented as part of the earlier-mentioned Canadian study was used in only 42.7% of transfers.

Many ED providers express a desire for verbal report of patient information between LTC and ED health care providers.[41] Although verbal communication may provide the opportunity for information clarification, critical clinical information may not reach the ED health care provider because of a variety of factors, such as patient assessment delays, shift changes, and LTC-ED provider changes.[34] Also, many patients under LTC are unable to provide key historical elements because of cognitive impairment. Mental status impairment is highly prevalent in older patients in the ED. One study documented a rate of 27% of cognitive impairment. Moreover, this finding was recognized by ED physicians in only 38% of cases.[42] For cognitively impaired patients, health care proxies or next of kin are often not immediately known or accessible. Moreover, these bystanders may not be present at an initial assessment in the ED. In addition, a significant percentage of patients under LTC presenting to the ED have some degree of sensory impairment, such as hearing or visual impairment,[43] that impedes effective communication between the patient and ED providers.

The Society for Academic Emergency Medicine Geriatric Emergency Medicine Task Force made a recommendation that all older patients in the ED receive some type of cognitive status assessment. Although the mini–mental state examination may be cumbersome for the busy ED health care provider, use of briefer alternatives, such as the Six-Item Screener and the Mini-Cog, have demonstrated promise as practical tools for use in the emergency setting.[44]

Also, LTC to ED transfers could be significantly improved through a basic succinct transfer of key patient information, including functional and cognitive status; plan of care and advanced care directives; current problem list; current treatment regimen, including all necessary equipment needed; allergies; meal consistencies; and recent laboratory, consultations, and diagnostic testing results.[45]

In addition, because key LTC health care providers may not be available, there is a need for clear delineation of advance directives. Furthermore, there is a need for improved assessment of the patient under LTC and nurse-provider communication. One study reported success with the use of communication and clinical practice tools and strategies designed to assist in reducing potentially avoidable hospitalizations.[46]

Moving forward, efforts to reduce avoidable ED use likely gathers more attention as a means to reduce patient burden, potential adverse events, and health care costs. One model of care, the Medical Assessment Team (MAT), was developed at the University of Texas Health Science Center at San Antonio to reduce unnecessary ED transfers from nursing facilities. In the MAT team model, participating facilities contact the MAT nurse when patients exhibit a short-term change in their medical status between 6 PM to 8 AM, 7 days a week. MAT nurses are registered nurses with experience in either emergency care or LTC. The MAT nurse then in person goes to the LTC facility and assesses the patient using preset protocols. As part of that assessment, the MAT nurse then gathers information to determine whether the patient benefits from a direct hospital admission and ED visit or from remaining at the facility. MAT nurses communicate with LTC on-call physicians to determine the final patient care recommendations and disposition. Over a 2-year period, the MAT program found that most patients under the LTC could be treated in place at the facility, thereby avoiding an ED transfer. Ninety percent of patients who required hospital admission were able to be admitted directly to the hospital floor, eliminating a transition of care through the ED.

TRANSITIONAL CARE AND ASSISTED LIVING FACILITIES

Assisted living (AL) represents one of the fastest growing trends in long-term residential care for older people. Elders who live according to AL frequently have cognitive and functional impairments. Eight percent of those residing according to AL have at least 1 activity of daily living deficiency, and more than 25% of AL patients have 4 or more deficiencies.[47] Patients in AL settings have high use rates of acute care services and comprise 8.6% of admissions to LTC nursing facilities.[48–50] However, information on transitions of care from AL settings to settings within the health care continuum is lacking. With continued growth in the AL market, understanding of transitional care issues for older adults coming to and from AL settings is an important part of future research.

TRANSITIONAL CARE AND HOSPICE AND PALLIATIVE CARE

The ability of the palliative care or hospice team to assist both nursing home and hospital staff during transitions of care is a unique contribution to patients and their families. Palliative care and hospice interdisciplinary team members can facilitate smooth transition to and from the hospital and to different sites for hospice care in hospital, nursing home, and community-based environments. Barriers to care transitions include goal differences, such as maintaining function versus providing palliative care; disagreement on curative versus palliative care, inconsistent pain management, limitations in patient-family communication time, and lack of point of service education; interhospice management differences and unclear LTC health care provider role; and the lack of joint plan of care collaboration between the LTC and the hospice.[51] In addition, the lack of and inconsistency of medical prognostication and diagnosis and review of comorbidities complicate and interfere with the smooth transition of patients between locations. And, the ineffective use of a comprehensive cross-cultural ethics approach to communicating with patients and families leads to ineffective and less favorable transitions of care.

Many hospitals have general inpatient (GIP) hospice units that allow the patient to stay in the hospital and avoid transfer of care, when the patient is expected to live only a few days and/or has unstable pain and symptoms related to their hospice diagnosis. GIP hospice services are also provided within the nursing home, either as GIP-certified beds or small GIP units located within the nursing home. The inpatient hospice beds allow receipt of the inpatient level of Medicare hospice care without requiring a transition to another facility, which is undesirable to nursing homes and burdensome for residents.

The hospice Medicare benefit allows nursing homes to work with the hospice team in providing end-of-life care. Nursing home interdisciplinary team and the hospice team collaboration decreases miscommunication and risk of avoidable transitions in care. If the patient faces a significant condition change, the hospice team is able to provide more hours of care, thus supporting the patient and their family while minimizing the pressures that lead to avoidable transfers. Another transition of care service provided by hospice programs in the nursing home is the level of care known as continuous or crisis care. In this type of care, hospice staff provides care for patients with a short-term change in condition associated with unstable pain or symptoms or end-of-life plan of care support for patients and their families.

A recent study examined the use of nonhospice palliative care and/or had on-site inpatient hospice beds to nursing home residents. Palliative care services included pain management consultation and allowed nursing home residents to receive specialized palliative care without waiving Medicare reimbursement for nursing home skilled care and/or when their prognoses are longer than 6 months.[51] The results indicated that the nursing home staff valued both the formal and informal education provided to staff.

Also, do-not-hospitalize (DNH) orders can be used to indicate that nursing home residents or their designated proxies desire to forego hospitalization in the event of clinical decline. Culberson and colleagues[52] found that after the implementation of the Patient Self Determination Act, the number of do-not-resuscitate orders increased, yet the DNH and the "no artificial hydration and nutrition" orders remained the same.

Increased use of these orders, no antibiotic orders, and family education regarding the benefits of the DNH order contribute to decreasing avoidable transfers.

In response to a desire to improve traditional practices of communicating patients' end-of life wishes during transitions, a program called the Physicians Orders for Life-Sustaining Treatment (POLST) has been developed. The POLST program includes a comprehensive approach to end-of-life planning to include cardiopulmonary resuscitation orders, medical intervention orders, antibiotic orders, medically administered nutrition or hydration orders, and a summary of medical conditions and the basis for the orders that can be used during the transition of patients across treatment settings.[53] Research has shown that the use of the POLST program facilitates documentation of a range of treatment preferences and improves transitional care communication.[54,55]

In a recent study conducted by Hickman and colleagues[56] comparing the use of the POLST program with traditional practice indicated that the use of POLST forms improved life-sustaining treatment preferences and nursing home residents were less likely to undergo undesired hospitalizations and medical interventions than other residents in the same facilities. It was hypothesized that the use of POLST-specific orders for a range of treatments during transitions among multiple settings may explain these findings.

MEASURING THE LTC QUALITY OF TRANSITIONAL CARE

The traditional lack of attention to transitional care issues is the result of multiple factors: poorly defined accountability; misaligned financial incentives, information systems that are not connected across LTC and acute care settings, the universality facility–based unique databases and documentation requirements, and minimal health care provider training in cross-site collaboration.[1,35,57–59] At present, there exists an array of promising measures that, if implemented nationally, could bring the requisite attention needed to stimulate quality improvement in transitional care, define accountability, realign financial incentives, and foster interoperable electronic health information systems.

The American Geriatrics Society recently released a position statement describing ways to improve transitional care. The recommendations included (1) actively involving patients and caregivers in transitional care decisions and preparing them for care issues in the next setting; (2) insuring good bidirectional communication between sending and receiving health care providers; (3) developing policies that promote high-quality transitional care, including reimbursement incentives; (4) providing education to all professionals involved in transitional care; and (5) conducting research to improve transitional care processes, focusing on enhancing patient/family involvement and training of health care professionals.[60]

Present US health care policy targets include focus on health, improvement of quality of life, and reduction of health care cost. The model of the patient-centered medical home has been a centerpiece of LTC in which the LTC facility truly is the patients "home."[61] Expanding the medical home model further in the LTC provides patients with better interdisciplinary team communications, which extends into transitional care, be it to the acute care hospital, home, or hospice. The challenge is to develop measures that can quantify the improvement of transitional care under the medical home model with the goal of minimizing unnecessary hospital/ED transfers.

The LTC culture change model is a transition from outcome-based measurements to quality-of-life and quality-of-care measurements within the "home" environment. One of the primary impediments to conducting a national dialog on the quality of life and quality of LTC transitional care is the ongoing uncertainty about the feasibility, costs, and outcomes that might be achieved through reorienting LTC culture to emphasize patient quality of life, staffing support, and the interconnectedness of the LTC to the acute care environment.

The Intervention to Reduce Acute Care Transfer (INTERACT II, www.interact2.net) has been successfully implemented in many nursing homes. The key components of this project are a communication form, a care pathway algorithm, and an advance directive form. The INTERACT II is an effective tool for educating the LTC interdisciplinary team to recognize condition changes early and to report to the on-call health care provider effectively.[46]

The health reform law has 5 pilot projects and 30 demonstrations in the bill, and many of them could be an opportunity to improve the transitional care. The Bundled Payment Pilot (section 3023) and the Hospital Readmission Reduction (section 3025) are 2 demonstration projects that potentially address the issue of improving care and reducing the cost in care transitions from one setting to the other.

One of the most popular tools of the Interact II tool is the SBAR.

SBAR COMMUNICATION TOOL

Situation	What is the current clinical situation?
Background	What is the relevant information about this patient?
Assessment	What is your clinical assessment?
Recommendation	What are you recommending as next course of action?

Training staff to use the SBAR has been shown to improve nursing care satisfaction as well as improving the provider-nurse communication.[62,63]

NEXT STEPS IN TRANSITIONAL CARE FOR LTC

It is clear that pieces of the transitional care puzzle are in need of further study. Assisted living facilities, senior housing, adult day care, intermediate care for the mentally disabled, and boarding home care are areas in which greater understanding is needed into how decisions on health care transitions occur. We have yet to have a clear picture on how and to what extent individual family decision making and the community malpractice environment drive transitional care. Likewise, the effect of changes in health care financing have the potential to significantly improve successful transitions, but how this will develop has yet to be determined.

ACKNOWLEDGMENTS

The authors would like to thank Inez I. Cruz, MSW, for her editorial assistance.

REFERENCES

1. Coleman E, Boult C. Improving the quality of transitional care for persons with complex care needs. J Am Geriatr Soc 2003;51(4):556–7.
2. American Medical Director's Association. Transitions of care in the long-term care continuum: practice guideline. Columbia (MD); 2010. Available at: http://www.amda.com/tools/clinical/TOCCPG/index.html. Accessed October 27, 2010.

3. Kasper J, O'Malley M. Changes in characteristics, needs and payment for care of elderly nursing home residents: 1999 to 2004. Washington, DC; 2007. Available at: http://www.kff.org/medicaid/index.cfm. Accessed October 27, 2010.
4. Jones AL, Dwyer LL, Bercovitz AR, et al. National Center for Health Statistics. The National Nursing Home survey: 2004 overview. Vital Health Stat 13 2009; 13(167):1–155. Available at: http://www.cdc.gov/nchs/nnhs/nnhs_products.htm. Accessed July 23, 2009.
5. Bergman H, Clarfield AM. Appropriateness of patient transfer from a nursing home to an acute-care hospital: a study of emergency room visits and hospital admissions. J Am Geriatr Soc 1991;39(12):1164–8.
6. Nawar EW, Niska RW, Xu J. National hospital ambulatory medical care survey: 2005 emergency department summary. Adv Data 2007;386:1–32.
7. Murtaugh CM, Litke A. Transitions through postacute and long-term care settings: patterns of use and outcomes for a national cohort of elders. Med Care 2002; 40(3):227–36.
8. Brown-Williams H, Neuhauser L, Ivey S, et al. From hospital to home: Improving transitional care for older adults. Berkeley (CA): University of California. Health Research for Action; 2006. p. 1–34. Available at: http://healthresearchforaction.org/research/hospital-to-home-summary-report.pdf. Accessed July 23, 2009.
9. Coleman EA, Parry C, Chalmers S, et al. The care transitions intervention: results of a randomized controlled trial. Arch Intern Med 2006;166:1822–8.
10. Boockvar K, Fishman E, Kyriacou CK, et al. Adverse events due to discontinuations in drug use and dose changes in patients transferred between acute and long-term care facilities. Arch Intern Med 2004;164(5):545–50.
11. American Medical Director's Association. Improving care transitions from the nursing facility to a community based setting. Columbia (MD); 2010. Available at: http://www.amda.com/governance/whitepapers/transitions_of_care.cfm. Accessed April 22, 2009.
12. Foster AJ, Murff HJ, Peterson JF, et al. The incidence and severity of adverse drug events affecting patients after discharge from the hospital. Ann Intern Med 2003;138(3):161–7.
13. Parker SG, Fadayevatan R, Lee SD. Acute hospital care for frail older people. Age Ageing 2006;35(6):551–2.
14. National Transitions of Care Coalition. Improving transitions of care: the vision of the national transitions of care coalition. Little Rock (AR) 2008. Available at: http://www.ntocc.org/Portals/0/PolicyPaper.pdf. Accessed January 4, 2011.
15. Kripalani S, Lefevre F, Phillips CO, et al. Deficits in communication and information transfer between hospitals-based and primary care physicians: implications for patients' safety and continuity of care. JAMA 2007;297(8):831–41.
16. Mor V, Intrator O, Feng Z, et al. The revolving door of rehospitalization from skilled nursing facilities. Health Aff (Millwood) 2010;29(1):57–64.
17. Donelan-McCall N, Eilersten T, Fish R, et al. Small patient population and low frequency event effects on the stability of SNK quality measures. Washington, DC: Medicare Payment Advisory Commission; 2006. Available at: http://permanent.access.gpo.gov/lps78983/Sep06_SNF_CONTRACTOR.pdf. Accessed October 27, 2010.
18. Jenks SF, Williams MV, Coleman EA. Rehospitalization among patients in the Medicare fee-for service program. N Engl J Med 2009;360(14):1418–28.
19. Ouslander JG, Lamb G, Perloe M. Potentially avoidable hospitalizations of nursing home residents: frequency, causes, and costs. J Am Geriatr Soc 2010; 58(4):627–35.

20. Carey K. Hospital cost containment and length of stay: an econometric analysis. South Econ J 2000;67(2):363–80.
21. Farnsworth TA, Waine S, McEvoy A. Subjective perception of additional support requirements of elderly patients discharged from accident and emergency departments. J Accid Emerg Med 1995;12:107–10.
22. National Transitions of Care Coalition. Cultural competence: essential ingredient for successful transitions of care. Little Rock (AR): ND. Available at: http://www.ntocc.org/Portals/0/CulturalCompetence.pdf. Accessed October 27, 2010.
23. Kripalani S, Jackson AT, Schnipper JL, et al. Promoting effective transitions of care at hospital discharge: a review of key issues for hospitalists. J Hosp Med 2007;2(5):314–23.
24. American Pharmacists Association and the National Association of Chain Drug Stores Foundation. Medication therapy management in pharmacy practice: core elements of an MTM service model. Washington, DC 2008. Available at: http://www.pharmacist.com/AM/Template.cfm?Section=Home2&TEMPLATE=/CM/ContentDisplay.cfm&CONTENTID=15496. Accessed July 23, 2009.
25. Shaughnessy P, Kramer A. The increased needs of patients in nursing homes and patients receiving home health care. N Engl J Med 1990;322:21–7.
26. CAffrey C. Potentially preventable emergency department visits by nursing home residents: United States 2004. Hyattsville (MD): Division of Health Care Statistics; 2010. Available at: http://www.cdc.gov/nchs/data/databriefs/db33.pdf. Accessed October 27, 2010.
27. Teresi J, Holmes D, Bloom H, et al. Factors differentiating hospital transfers from long-term care facilities with high and low transfer rates. Gerontologist 1991;31: 795–806.
28. Bowman CE, Elford J, Dovey J, et al. Acute hospital admissions from nursing homes: some may be avoidable. Postgrad Med J 2001;77(903):40–2.
29. Finucane P, Wundke R, Whitehead C, et al. Use of in-patient hospital beds by people living in residential care. Gerontology 2000;46(3):133–8.
30. AMDA White Paper H10. Improving care transitions between the nursing facility and the acute care hospital settings. Columbia (MD): Policy Resolution; 2010. Available at: http://www.amda.com/governance/whitepapers/H10.cfm. Accessed January 4, 2011.
31. Grabowski DC, Stewart KA, Broderick SM, et al. Predictors of nursing home hospitalization: a review of the literature. Med Care Res Rev 2008;65(3):3–39.
32. Hustey FM. Care transitions between nursing homes and emergency departments: a failure to communicate. Ann Long Term Care 2010;18(4):17–9.
33. Coleman EA, Berenson RA. Lost in transition: challenges and opportunities for improving the quality of transitional care. Ann Intern Med 2004;141(7):533–6.
34. Davis MN, Brumfield VC, Smith ST, et al. A one-page nursing home to emergency room transfer form: what a difference it can make in an emergency! Ann Long Term Care 2005;13(11):34–8.
35. Jones JS, Dwyer PR, White LJ, et al. Patient transfer from nursing home to emergency department: outcomes and policy implications. Acad Emerg Med 1997;4: 908–15.
36. Terrell KM, Brizendine EJ, Bean WF, et al. An extended care facility to emergency department transfer form improves communication. Acad Emerg Med 2005; 12(2):114–8.
37. Boockvar KS, Fridman B, Marturano C. Ineffective communication of mental status information during care transfer of older adults. J Gen Intern Med 2005; 20:1146–50.

38. Stier PA, Biles BK, Olinger ML, et al. Do transfer records for extended care facility patients sent to the emergency department contain essential information? Ann Emerg Med 2001;38:S102.
39. Cwinn MA, Forster AJ, Cwin AA, et al. Prevalence of information gaps for seniors transferred from nursing homes to the emergency department. CJEM 2009; 11(5):462–71.
40. Hustey F, Palmer R. The use of a computerized system to improve information transfer during patient transition from a skilled nursing facility to the emergency department. J Am Geriatr Soc 2009;57(4):S1.
41. Gillespie SM, Gleason LJ, Karuza J, et al. Healthcare providers' opinions on communication between nursing homes and emergency departments. J Am Med Dir Assoc 2010;11(3):204–10.
42. Hustey FM, Meldon SW, Smith MD, et al. The effect of mental status screening on the care of elderly emergency department patients. Ann Emerg Med 2003;41(5): 678–84.
43. Krauss NA, Altman BM. Research findings #5: characteristics of nursing home residents, 1996. Rockville (MD): Agency for Healthcare Research and Quality; 2004. Available at: http://www.meps.ahrq.gov/data_files/publications/rf5/rf5.shtml. Accessed January 4, 2011.
44. Wilber ST, Lofgren SD, Mager TG, et al. An evaluation of two screening tools for cognitive impairment in older emergency department patients. Acad Emerg Med 2005;12(7):612–6.
45. American Medical Drector's Association. Acute change of condition in the long term care setting: clinical practice guideline. Columbia (MD): AMDA; 2003.
46. Ouslander JG, Perloe M, Givens JH, et al. Reducing potentially avoidable hospitalizations of nursing home residents: results of a pilot quality improvement project. J Am Med Dir Assoc 2009;10(9):644–52.
47. National Center for Assisted Living. Fact and trends: the assisted living source book. Washington, DC: National Center for Assisted Living; 2001.
48. Hawes C, Rose M, Phillips CD. A national study of assisted living for the frail elderly. Washington, DC: Department of Health and Human Services; 1999. Available at: http://aspe.hhs.gov/daltcp/reports/facres.htm. Accessed May 15, 2009.
49. Phillips CD, Holan S, Sherman M, et al. Medicare expenditures for residents in assisted living: data from a national study. Health Serv Res 2005;40:373–88.
50. Zimmerman S, Sloane PD, Eckert JK, et al. How good is assisted living? J Gerontol B Psychol Sci Soc Sci 2005;60:S195–204.
51. Miller SC. A model for successful nursing home-hospice partnerships. J Palliat Med 2010;13(5):525–33.
52. Culberson J, Levy C, Lawhorne L. Do not hospitalize orders in nursing homes: a pilot study. J Am Med Dir Assoc 2005;6:22–6.
53. Center for Ethics in Health Care: Oregon Health & Science University. Physician orders for life-sustaining treatment paradigm. Portland (OR): 2008. Available at: http://www.ohsu.edu/polst/index.htm. Accessed October 27, 2010.
54. Hickman SE, Hammes BJ, Moss AH, et al. Hope for the future: achieving the original intent of advance directives. Hastings Cent Rep 2005;35:S26–30.
55. National Quality Forum. A national framework and preferred practices for palliative care and hospice care quality: a consensus report [on-line resource]. Washington, DC: National Quality Forum; 2006. p. 43–4.
56. Hickman SE, Nelson CA, Perrin NA, et al. A comparison of methods to communicate treatment preferences in nursing facilities: traditional practices versus

the physician orders for life-sustaining treatment program. J Am Geriatr Soc 2010;58(7):1241–8.
57. Coleman EA, Fox PD. One patient, many places: managing health caretransitions, part I: introduction, accountability, information for patients. Ann Long Term Care 2004;12(9):25–35.
58. Coleman EA, Fox PD. One patient, many places: managing health caretransitions, part II: practitioner skills and patient and caregiver preparation. Ann Long Term Care 2004;12(10):34–9.
59. Coleman EA, Fox PD. One patient, many places: managing health caretransitions, part III: financial incentives and getting started. Ann Long Term Care 2004;12(11):14–6.
60. Quinn CC, Port CL, Zimmerman S. Short-stay nursing home rehabilitation patients: transitional care problems pose research challenges. J Am Geriatr Soc 2008;56(10):1940–5.
61. Transform-Med- Transforming Medical Practices. Patient centered medical home. Leawood (KS) ND. Available at: http://www.transformed.com/resources/PCMH.cfm. Accessed July 23, 2009.
62. Leonard M, Bonacum D, Graham S. SBAR technique for communication: a situational briefing model. Kaiser Permanente of Colorado. Evergreen (CO) ND. Available at: http://www.ihi.org/IHI/Topics/PatientSafety/SafetyGeneral/Tools/SBARTechniqueforCommunicationASituationalBriefingModel.htm. Accessed July 23, 2009.
63. Whitson HE, Hastings SN, Lekan DA, et al. A quality improvement program to enhance after-hours telephone communication between nurses and physicians in a long-term care facility. J Am Geriatr Soc 2008;56(6):1080–6.

Doing Dementia Better: Anthropological Insights

Elizabeth Herskovits Castillo, MD, PhD[a,b,c,*]

KEYWORDS

- Anthropology of dementia • Agism • Personhood
- Embodiment

THE CULTURAL MEANING OF PERSONHOOD AND DEMENTIA: I AM NOT DEAD YET

I'm not sure the doctor knew how to deal with Alzheimer's. It was just diagnosed and that's it. "It looks like she may have Alzheimer's and we'll just have to wait and see." ...I felt like the doctors were really not much help to me. They didn't know what to do... It seems that once a person has been diagnosed with dementia, many doctors just ignore them. ...I would ask the doctors how he was doing and they would say fine, but when I went to see him I found him sitting with his head in his lap.[1]

"I was terrified the entire time [I took care of my mother. And after I dropped her off at a nursing facility], when I got home, I took the nightgown she had worn, the one I lent her, and put it in the trash. Just in case Alzheimer's was contagious."[2]

This article reveals the deleterious impact that cultural assumptions about dementia have on the care provided, and, through an exploration of anthropological theories of personhood, suggests a model of Personhood-Centered Care, comprised of strategies for preserving personhood in the face of dementia, to improve quality of life. As health care professionals, we live and work within a broader cultural context, and while medical training and practice engage us in a specific subcultural view of aging and dementia, we are also of a piece with the broader cultural fabric. Attitudes and preconceptions about aging, personhood, and the valued goals of life shape us and our disposition in clinical practice.

This work was supported by a Geriatric Academic Career Award (GACA) awarded by HRSA, 2008–2010.

[a] Geriatric Medicine Program, MAHEC (Mountain AHEC), 118 WT Weaver Boulevard, Asheville, NC 28804, USA

[b] Department of Family Medicine, UNC Chapel Hill School of Medicine, 590 Manning Drive, Chapel Hill, NC 27599, USA

[c] Givens Estates (CCRC), 2360 Sweeten Creek Road, Asheville, NC 28803, USA

* Geriatric Medicine Program, MAHEC (Mountain AHEC), 118 WT Weaver Boulevard, Asheville, NC 28804.

E-mail address: Liz.castillo@mahec.net

Clin Geriatr Med 27 (2011) 273–289
doi:10.1016/j.cger.2011.02.002 geriatric.theclinics.com
0749-0690/11/$ – see front matter

Patients with dementia and their families frequently report that they are less than pleased with their clinical encounters.[3,4] Trainees regularly suggest to me that they do not think they are well prepared to care for patients with dementia, and the literature supports their impression[5–7]; by second-year residency, they have well-developed clinical responses to shortness of breath and chest pain but are often unsure what to do when facing a confused older patient. Within the context of aging demography, evidence suggests that medical education may actually decrease one's interest in working with elders,[8] and agism within medical practice is increasingly noted.[9–11] Adelson has coined the term dementia-ism to refer to the distaste regarding working with patients who have dementia.[12] Indeed, many of us as doctors and nurses share the widespread cultural horror and fear about dementia.[13,14]

Dementia, or neurodegenerative disease, is a disease category, and yet it is widely described in popular and professional media as a horror story. Alzheimer disease "eradicates the essence of the person"[15] and causes the "unbecoming" of the self[16]; "the victim of Alzheimer's is one whose mind has been dissolved, leaving only a body from which the person has been removed"[17]; and "the victim of Alzheimer's must eventually come to terms with…the complete loss of self."[18] Are we describing a disease, or the plotline of a horror movie? One family caregiver captures the essence of our social imaginary by describing that Alzheimer disease is a brain-eating monster: "We started to get a good idea of the size and shape of the beast called Alzheimer's… To it, brain tissue is brain tissue, all of it equally tasty."[19]

Once in my geriatric consultation clinic, a patient's adult son said, "When we first got the verdict…wait–I don't mean Verdict–what's the word, I cannot think of it?" "Diagnosis?" I asked. "Yes: Diagnosis, well it felt more like a verdict." I hear similar comments when several times each year I lead interactive workshops on dementia; participants, including medical trainees, allied health professions, or individuals in the lay community, reenact the stereotypes and assumptions of cultural approach to aging and dementia. And not infrequently, the belief that people with dementia are not really alive penetrates the clinical setting:

> *Glenn was a patient with dementia, who lived in a nursing home. He conversed in simple sentences, flirted and laughed frequently with female staff, participated with apparent enjoyment in all musical recreational activities, and ate with gusto. His daughter Glenda requested a hospice referral, and as the attending physician, I requested a Family Meeting to better understand her thoughts and feelings. When invited to open the meeting, Glenda, who was seated next to her father, did not hesitate to tell us why she requested hospice: "My father is dead!" "This man is not my father!" Hospice, she felt, would be a method to help the physical body die and to match more accurately with what she perceived as her already-dead father. Although the social worker, nurse, and physician shared information about how Glenn was enjoying activities, relationships, and food, the daughter was not buying it. "My father is dead! This man is not my father!" Each time she said this with strong negative affect, her father seated next to her shrunk further into his wheelchair, a stricken look on his face intensifying.*

This case vividly depicts how the cultural perception of people with dementia as the walking undead increases suffering. But why do we perceive people with dementia as the already-dead and the not-truly-human? And what can we do to change course?

The first step to treating patients with dementia differently is to begin to recognize how cultural notions of personhood, of what makes a person a person, shape the meaning and experience of dementia. This article explores diverse models of personhood (**Table 1**) and their impact on the meaning and experience of dementia. Anthropological insights can help us as physicians and nurses to better understand

Table 1
Models of personhood and associated forms of excess disability[a]

Model of Personhood	Central Features	Related Forms of Excess Disability	Case-Based Illustrations
Cognitive/ Achievement	Cognitive ability and achievement are the essence of personhood	Cognitive deficits threaten personhood and valued identity	A tale of 2 readers
Independence/ Autonomy vs the Relational Self	Individual autonomy and independence is the essence of healthy adulthood	Interdependence leads to loss of personhood and valued identity	How do you solve a problem like Maria?
Social Interactionism	Social interactions make and unmake identity/ personhood	Malignant social interaction causes social death	Glenda's role in Glenn's social death
Spiritual Aspects of Personhood and Identity	Many individuals experience spirituality as central to their lifeways and their self-identity	Failure to recognize or emphasize spiritual personhood at worst erases the self and at best is a lost opportunity for preserved self-identity	—
Embodied Personhood	Daily physical practices may constitute personhood and self-identity	Failure to recognize or emphasize embodied personhood at worst erases the self and at best is a lost opportunity for preserved self-identity	The case of Dr Case
Creative Self-Expression; Man as Meaning Maker	Intrinsic drive toward making meaning and creative self-expression is essential to being human	Failure to recognize and provide opportunities for meaning making threatens personhood	Dementia story circles

[a] Excess disability.[82]

how contemporary US concepts of personhood lead to decreased function and increased suffering in dementia. By revealing these phenomena, such anthropological insights can point toward potential improvements in dementia care and quality of life. My hope is that as physicians and nurses, we can move from fearing patients with dementia to appreciating them as struggling individuals with varying functions and challenges:

> *As tired as I am when the shift is done, I look forward to work the next day. When I'm not there for a few days, I miss the place…mostly I miss the residents. They are collectively and individually, a handful, but they are also endearing and in their own ways, spirited. I enjoy their company. Their dementias and delusions, their personalities, are fascinating and distinct. Figuring out who they are and what makes them tick is intellectually and emotionally challenging. It is also deeply satisfying.*[2]

COGNITIVE/ACHIEVEMENT-ORIENTED PERSONHOOD: A TALE OF 2 READERS

Many have suggested that the dominant model of personhood in US culture hinges on the individual's ability for achievement and mastery. When people meet, they inquire

"What do you do?," searching for markers of employment and ability as indicators of valued personhood. Post[20] has suggested that we live in a hypercognitive society, taking Descartes at his word, "I think therefore I am." If our culture is oriented toward achievement and mastery rather than toward interpersonal relationship—that is, toward Do-ing rather than toward Be-ing—then one can argue that the subculture of medicine is even more action oriented. Many an experienced clinician admonishes young practitioners to be wary of this bias when they counsel: Don't just DO something, stand there.

In cultures and communities that subscribe heavily to a model of cognitive personhood, when people are no longer able to achieve, do they lose their value as people? Do they lose even their identity as people?

I was fortunate in my first year out of training to have a clinical experience that vividly illustrated this phenomenon. Two patients scheduled to see me in the same afternoon clinic had evidence of similar cognitive deficits, but very different personal experiences with those deficits. Both patients had been lifelong avid readers who now described difficulty remembering what their book was about and trouble holding onto the linear threads of the characters and the plot. The first patient, a retired business executive, now hated to read because he could not master the information he was reading. He also energetically described his anger and refusal to participate in recreational activities because he could no longer "win the candy bar" when there was any type of competition. The second patient, a retired homemaker who had raised 4 children, still loved to read because she relished sitting in a soft chair with a cup of tea, a book, and a sense of leisure, aware that she did not have to rush off to do something. Thus, the first patient's focus on mastery and achievement-oriented reading as integral to his self-identity increased his suffering, whereas the second patient found pleasure in reading despite cognitive deficits. Like Ralph Waldo Emerson, who in the face of dementia assured his friends, "I have lost my mental faculties but am perfectly well," my second patient felt well despite the loss of some cognitive capacity.

The recognition of cognitive/achievement-oriented personhood as deleterious in the context of dementia can be leveraged to improve quality of care and quality of life. A first essential strategy for improving quality of life in dementia is to openly acknowledge the American cultural priority on achievement and mastery, to make it visible to patients and their families, and then to offer alternatives. The noted geriatrician Philip Sloane reminds medical trainees that many, perhaps most, of the activities they enjoy on their day off are not cognitively contingent (Philip D. Sloane, personal communication, 2008); caregiver manuals listing enjoyable activities that do not rely on achievement or mastery are similar tools to redirect focus. Koenig Coste[21] coined the term habilitation to suggest that we should meet the person with dementia where they are rather than try and rehabilitate them to approach where we function. In educational workshops and in clinical interactions, I suggest that participants write down "five things that make me *me*," and then as we look over the lists together, we discover that seldom are more than 1 to 2 of the entries cognitive or achievement-oriented in character (eg, lawyer); most of the entries were described as relational (eg, husband), spiritual (worshiper), or physical/embodied (play the piano).

RELATIONAL PERSONHOOD: AUTONOMY VERSUS INTERDEPENDENCE

To be an adult healthy person in American culture, one must demonstrate autonomy and independence. When asked what they fear most, elders in the United States respond in surveys that they fear their loss of independence. The American value placed on individual autonomy, independence, and separation from others is a characteristic quite different than what is considered a normal and healthy personhood in most other communities and cultures. The ethics committee director of a major regional hospital in the southeast was surprised to discover at the 2010 International Conference on Medical Ethics that the US focus on autonomy and independence was considered an aberration, as evidenced by several paper sessions discussing the "pathology of US-based notions of patient autonomy and independence" (Mary Caldwell, PhD, MDiv, Director, Mission Hospital Ethics Committee, Asheville, North Carolina, personal communication, 2010).

In the United States, if cognitive or functional losses preclude independent autonomy, then full personhood is threatened, but medical and cultural anthropologists have reported that social interdependence and a relational model of personhood is more commonly evidenced throughout the world.[22] In communities that ascribe to a relational model of personhood, deep interpersonal relationships and their associated interdependency is seen as desirable and normal,[23,24] and autonomous independence is not normal nor desirable. Hence, grandma may have significant cognitive deficits, but she is, by definition, still and always, grandma. The cultural meaning of dementia in communities with a relational model of personhood does not entail the loss of the self. For example, Ikels[25,26] notes that in contemporary China, although dementia is recognized, it is not regarded with particular horror, given the Chinese concept of a relational self and filial piety. In his ethnography of aging in Benares, India, Cohen[27] reports that elders with cognitive deficits who have ample *seva* (family and community relationships and interdependence) are considered healthy and well, whereas those elders who have *seva* deficits may be seen as "going sixtyish." In this cultural frame, going sixtyish, or dementia, is not a result of cognitive losses but an ailment of the modern family and the modern urban setting in which healthy interdependency has broken down. Traphagan[28] reports that elders in Japan who lack interdependence are felt to be at risk of dementia-like conditions, whereas those who stay busy and engaged in social networks are recognized as healthy, even if they develop some cognitive dysfunction.

As a medical anthropologist who is aware of these different cultural models in which elder independence and autonomy are seen as signs of ill health rather than as wellness, I was struck by a recent patient case that I have taken to calling "How Do you solve a problem like Maria?"

Maria lived alone in an apartment in a Continuing Care Retirement Community (CCRC), and social workers and other staff repeatedly asked me to move her to higher-level care. On 4 successive house calls, I found Maria to have mild dementia: she was ambulatory without assistive device, independent with activities of daily living (ADL), and communicated appropriately with moderately complex sentences in linear conversation. She seemed to greatly enjoy social interaction, laughing and joking frequently, and consistently reported that she was enjoying her days, although she felt a bit lonely at times. But she was having trouble with instrumental ADL, and instead of doing laundry, she simply bought more bed linens and clothing, piling them up throughout her dwelling. She was a widow and had no family to help her out. And although she lived in a community setting, there were no friends or community members stepping in to help her with the laundry or with other functions she could not manage on her own. I could see no reason that Miss Maria needed to live in a nursing home, and she strongly wished to stay in her home; her legal guardian supported this choice and we attempted to find appropriate supportive services. The CCRC staff remained fairly distressed that she was living in her apartment independently, despite our consistent clinical evaluation regarding the relatively mild degree of her deficits. She required social interdependence, which was perceived by the staff as a marker of debility rather than as a sign of her healthiness. When eventually the patient required hospitalization and post-acute rehabilitation in the SNF, the CCRC staff vigorously advocated for her to stay permanently in that setting.

Such a case challenges us to reconsider what constitutes dementia requiring placement? In the case of Maria, her specific cognitive and functional deficits seemed quite mild, but the American cultural emphasis on independence and autonomy created increased suffering because her mild deficits threatened her ability to live in her apartment without interdependency. Because a failure of independence is considered pathologic in American culture, many staff felt that Maria's dementia warranted nursing home placement.

It can be strategic clinically to openly acknowledge the US cultural emphasis on independence and autonomy as essential to personhood, in order to improve quality of care and quality of life. In my clinical experience, active reframing of interdependence as healthier than individualistic independence is often welcomed by families and patients. The burgeoning medical literature on health risks related to social isolation provides convincing examples as well as the legitimacy of scientific authority. Beyond the clinical setting, community programming (such as Seattle's successful Elder Friends program) can be harnessed to increase social interaction and interdependence. Also, intergenerational programming in the long-term care (LTC) setting could be expanded and should be vigorously extended to other senior congregate residences and social settings (churches/synagogues/mosques, community centers, public schools).

SOCIAL INTERACTIONISM AND PERSONHOOD

Social interaction therapy posits that personhood is the result of social interactions rather than emanating from the individual alone.[29] Thus, we "make and unmake" each other through social interactions. When a medical student dons stethoscope and white jacket, others treat the student like a doctor, and this recognition contributes to the student's identity as a physician. Even if the student develops effective medical knowledge and perceives herself to be a doctor, if others do not treat the student like a doctor, the student will not be a doctor. The role of social interactionism in identity is depicted in the popular film Catch Me If You Can, in which a bright young con-man functions as a physician in part because others interact socially with him as a physician.

Kitwood, a geriatrician in the United Kingdom, coined the term malignant social interaction and developed a clinical model[30,31] describing how social actors, including doctors and nurses, contributed to the "social death"[32] of the person with dementia. In other words, Kitwood and those who have researched with his theoretic model as a framework, argue that loss of self in dementia arises not solely from the disease but rather from the way other people treat the person with dementia.[33,34] Much as Kitwood described in the United Kingdom, when contemporary North Americans encounter a person with cognitive deficits, it is the apparently normal person who behaves inappropriately socially: avoiding eye contact, studiously not talking to the impaired individual, and generally engaging in behaviors that disregard the impaired individual. The anthropologist Janelle Thompson describes these sociocultural processes, which she witnessed as her mother, a person with dementia, was gradually socially dislocated[35]; friends severed their relationships and stopped visiting and calling, and strangers asked repeatedly, "Does she still recognize you?" The driving force for social isolation (and hence social death) did not arise from the person with dementia but from those in the community who actively withdrew. Although the person with dementia may not recognize her husband, daughter, or friend, she certainly recognizes them as loving companions, and interact accordingly. It is the community that does not recognize the person with dementia–as a person.

Numerous accounts of dementia, both lay and professional, describe the persistence of social interpersonal functions.[36,37] Indeed, the clinical literature suggests that family and physician often fail to identify the person with dementia precisely because they maintain their ability to interact socially and thereby cover for their deficits.[38] Frontotemporal dementia is described as unique among dementias in its deleterious impact on social behavior, specifically because the ability to interact socially is a well-preserved function in most dementias. Similarly, emotional function seems to be generally preserved in most dementias, and one can find written accounts of the person with moderate or severe dementia who demonstrates emotional sensitivity to others.[39]

Given the relative sparing of social and emotional abilities in dementia, it is not surprising that the experience of dementia is less feared in cultural settings that focus on social relationships as central to personhood than it is in cultural settings where the phenomena of social death appears to be linked to a cultural emphasis on cognitive ability and independence as central to personhood.[22,40,41]

A WORD ABOUT HUMAN COMMUNICATION

Communication is an essential building block of meaningful social interaction and relationships. Perhaps, dementia's progressive impairment in verbal communication contributes to the social death of people with dementia. As clinicians, we test verbal function during formal cognitive assessment through confrontation naming, word generation, and assays of reading and writing. But we do not test the function of communication with these instruments. What constitutes communication, and how does dementia seem to affect it?

Communication is defined as a process by which information is exchanged between individuals through a common system of symbols, signs, or behavior (also, exchange of information).[42] Psychological and anthropological linguists agree that nonverbal communication comprises the greater part of human communication. Tone, rhythm, prosody, facial expression, bodily gestures, and touch are all essential nonverbal aspects of communication. Meaningful human communication is contingent on social and emotional interconnectedness.

Given the preservation of potential for social and emotional function, individuals with dementia can be expected to manifest significant potential for enduring communication. In fact, in both research and clinical settings, patients with dementia have been increasingly described as capable of communication but not in conventional linear verbal modalities. Even when unable to converse traditionally, people with dementia retain the urge to communicate and use eye contact or mutual gaze, and gesture to do so.[43,44] When unable to form recognizable words, people with dementia can often be observed participating in back-and-forth dialogue with fairly sophisticated rhythm and social cueing.[45]

> *We continue to be deeply connected…When I arrive, he smiles, runs up to me, and gives me a big hug. He's very affectionate and tender. We share lots of loving eye contact. We hold hands. He strokes my hair and kisses me. We still communicate with looks, and caresses, and smiles, and laughter. It's taken a while, but I've gotten used to it. Odd as it may sound, we still have fun together.*[46]

The psychologist Sabat[47] suggests that the method of indirect repair provides opportunities for clinicians and family members to communicate effectively with people with dementia. Indeed, research in the arena of communication potential and communication strategies in dementia is burgeoning, with attention to pragmatic training skills for family and health care professionals.[48,49] There is increasing recognition that improved forms of communication with people with dementia lead to improved function and behavior,[50,51] and hence, improved quality of life. Transcripts of conversations such as those published by Sabat[52] can encourage medical and nursing trainees to build meaningful and therapeutic relationships with patients who have advanced dementia.

The recognition of relational personhood is critical to improving quality of care and quality of life in dementia. Clinicians, LTC staff, and the general community need to be educated on the critical role each person plays in preserving or destroying the personhood of those with dementia. Clear examples appropriate to each setting not only facilitate this education but also foster a sense of responsibility for recognizing the person with dementia as a person. We must determine to be leaders in how people with dementia are treated socially in the community as well as in the clinical setting.

Similarly, renewed focus on the forms of communication in mid-stage and late-stage dementias will enhance the clinical care provided by physicians and nurses, as well as by LTC staff. Sabat's[47] practical concept of indirect repair is essential for professional and lay care providers and is a focus for training fellows and residents. Attention to re-learning communication skills indirectly provides support to families and caregivers, simultaneously enhancing the personhood of those with dementia.

THE PERSON IN THE BODY: EMBODIED IDENTITY

How can the body be recognized as an essential site of personhood? A growing literature on the experience of embodiment grapples with this question. Physicians and nurses are trained to perceive the body as a purely biologic phenomenon composed of anatomic structure and physiologic function. But for decades, anthropologists and sociologists have been trained to perceive and investigate how the biologic basis of the body is only the beginning of the human experience of the body and its functions.[53–55] Sociocultural work explores how the body serves as a type of raw material through which collective and individual human identities are worked and reworked, how the body makes cultural meanings and social mores concrete, and how the body provides a field on which human power-struggles unfold.

The complex phenomenon of the body is most readily approached through specific examples, such as human nutrition. The panda bear can eat only bamboo because biology hardwires its behavior. But *Homo sapiens* can, and do, feast on a surprising variety of foodstuffs. What and how people eat is a consequence of sociocultural and political-economic processes. Douglas[55] suggested that Jewish orthodox community rules about what is kosher or acceptable to eat were mechanisms that functioned to differentiate social communities with strict boundaries. Elias[56] identified the processes through which power struggles and social class correlated with the adoption of civilized dining customs in which the knife became domesticated. Bourdieu[57] demonstrated how the so-called personal taste in food can be recognized as social class embodied. Clearly, what it means to be human, to be a person, involves bodily perceptions and practices.

The human body in the context of dementia is a similarly complex phenomenon. It is generally accepted that procedural memory, such as the ability to dance, to play instruments, to sculpt or artistically manipulate a paintbrush, can be preserved in late-stage dementia. So, people who are unable to walk may be able to march[58] or dance,[59,60] and those unable to use a telephone or tie their shoelaces may be able to play the violin or piano (of course, only if they could previously do so!).[61,62] Individuals with severe dementia continue to paint exuberantly; de Kooning is simply one of the most famous such examples.

Sociocultural studies of embodied identity have focused on the daily physical practices of artists, athletes, and musicians as integral to their sense of self. In dementia, the preservation of such daily physical practices suggests that the embodied sense of self, at least for some individuals, may be meaningfully preserved. One patient with dementia reminded me of my embodied identity as a physician:

Dr Case, a retired obstetrician with fairly advanced dementia who lived in a nursing home, seemed to be most at ease in the company of the nurses and other health care professionals. He was generally seen carrying a clipboard and standing alongside the central nursing station. Vocalizing without recognizable words, in apparent dialogue with the nurses and aides, he would shuffle his walker alongside them, in an embodiment of his memories and self-identity as a physician performing daily rounds.

In this way, the daily physical practices of the physician, the embodied identity of the doctor, endured despite advanced Alzheimer dementia.

The recognition of embodied personhood in dementia can be leveraged to improve the quality of care. When patients and lay people ask me how they can best prevent or resist the ravages of dementia, I encourage them to take up an artistic practice, to learn an instrument, or to begin dancing in order to develop personal pleasure and personal identity in resilient embodied practices; it has been suggested that dancing is the most protective hobby against dementia,[63] perhaps because it integrates cognitive and physical intelligence, as well as social interaction. Similarly, Kontos and Naglie[64] invite doctors and nurses in the LTC setting to revitalize person-centered care by recognizing the embodied nature of the self in patients with dementia. This strategic approach emphasizes the clinical importance of physical activities that potentially reflect embodied personhood and fosters staff recognition of the enduring personhood of their patients with dementia. Such a focus and awareness would resist cultural processes that lead to social death and malignant social interaction.

SPIRITUAL PERSONHOOD

Many individuals and cultural communities recognize personhood as spiritual. Some have suggested that in the setting of dementia, the capacity for spiritual life expands. Many of the chaplains who work alongside me in the LTC setting have made this assertion, and patients themselves have told me that their relationship with God remains at the center of their life. Studies of people with dementia indicate that the spiritual experience of prayer and worship is, in its essence, an embodied phenomenon.[65,66] As the baby boomers approach elder years, meditation and yoga should be considered as well. Further, the social relational aspect of spiritual fellowship in a faith community can be identified as enhancing the quality of life of persons with dementia. Medical anthropologists have recorded cultural notions of dementia that ascribe spiritual meaning to the condition. For example, Henderson and Henderson[67] indicate that in certain Native American settings, confusion experienced by elders may be viewed favorably as evidence of a person's transition from the mundane to the sacred or spiritual realms, and Barker[68] describes similar phenomena in New Guinea.

Recognizing the role that spirituality can play in the enduring personhood of those with dementia will provide yet another avenue for enhancing quality of life; many

LTC communities are increasing resources for spiritual life on-site. Medical and nursing trainees can be reinforced with the awareness that for those patients who have had spiritual practices or communities at the center of their life, it is imperative to support the patient and family to continue those spiritual activities. Many patients tell me they can no longer go to their church because of fears related to incontinence or mobility, because of transportation issues, or because their family is too busy to take them. This is not a small loss to the patient, and addressing these barriers effectively should be considered a form of essential medical care, just as exercise regimens are often now ordered on formal prescriptions.

MAKING MEANING: DEMENTIA AND THE CREATIVE IMPULSE

Man is an animal suspended in self-spun webs of significance.[69]

Anthropologists suggest that what makes man unique among all animals is the intrinsic drive to make meaning. Clifford Geertz described culture as the stories we tell ourselves about ourselves, in other words, the meanings we make and remake unceasingly. This morning, did I put on the bracelet that symbolically tells me the story about a close friend who died of diabetes in her 30s? Or did I put on the bracelet that symbolically tells me a story about the man who is now my husband? Both are bracelets, but also more than bracelets.

Do the bracelets of the person with advanced dementia similarly carry stories and meaning? Photographs and other personal relics populate the rooms of nursing home residents, which are artifacts from a life and concrete memories providing opportunities to interact meaningfully with individuals who have dementia. I have found that when I pick up these artifacts and ask the person with dementia about them, it is often possible to make a personal connection. Reminiscence therapy seems to harness an awareness of the importance of such stories we tell ourselves about ourselves[70]; one of my nursing home resident patients led a popular weekly recreational activity in which she recounted personal stories to other residents.

Making meaning does not end with the advent of dementia. Some individuals with dementia make meaning of the dementia experience in their written accounts. The experience of early dementia has been described as heightening the ability to live in the moment: "I've come to the conclusion that everything has a purpose," Peter says, "maybe this was to slow me down to enjoy life and to experience: "I had truly forgotten what a beautiful sight a soft gentle snowfall could be." Jan believes that God allowed her the gift of seeing the snowfall as a child does–a gift that came not in spite of her condition but because of it.[71] Enjoy my family and to enjoy what's out there. And right now, I can say that I'm a better person for it, in appreciation of other people's needs and illnesses, than I ever was when I was working that rat race back and forth day to day."[72] Jan is another person with dementia who makes meaning from her.[72] Autobiographic accounts of early dementia describe a change in sensory perception and sometimes a sense of wonder, which reflect another form of meaning-making in the face of dementia.[73] Others with early-stage dementia have described spiritual awakening or deepening that they credit to the dementia experience.[74,75] Campbell[72] implores, "we should not ignore the voices of dementia patients and their loved ones, who sense that something profound is happening just beneath the surface of Alzheimer's—a process of detachment and discovery that is central to the mystery and dignity of the human person."

But what of those who have mid-stage or late-stage dementia? Do they continue to tell stories of significance? Do they continue to make meaning? Although verbal losses have, in the past, seemed to suggest that individuals with mid-stage or late-stage dementia had nothing to express, it is now known that this is not the case. A wide range of creative self-expression has been demonstrated in the face of dementia. Enjoyment of music and art persist well into late-stage dementia. Arts-related recreational activities are long recognized as therapeutically beneficial.[76,77] More recently, people with dementia have been recognized to be creative producers of paintings, music, dance, and dramatic performances.[78–81] Basting[78] vividly describes dementia storytelling groups, which she initiated in the 1990s. Basting begins with a photograph as a trigger, asks the group "what's going on in this picture," and then tapes the stories that the group creates spontaneously. Transcripts indicate that many people with dementia apparently retain a sense of narrative meaning and a desire to communicate meaning through stories, with preserved capacities in humor and poetic sensibility.

If, as some have asserted, one of the characteristics that distinguishes humans from other animals is the creative impulse for self-expression, it does seem that this drive persists into late-stage dementia. Certainly, many lay and professional advocates in dementia care already focus on the importance of art and music as pleasurable activities for people with dementia. But by recognizing that many people with dementia continue to have a strong intrinsic drive for self-expression and making meaning, the quality of life and care can be further elevated. In this era of resource scarcity, geriatricians and elder health care professionals will likely need to take a firm stand regarding the essential need for elder programming that enables creative self-expression. This is often not expensive but does require significant staffing. LTC and community-based programming that harness the enthusiasm and energy of graduate and college students will be a valuable strategy. Annual Centers for Medicare & Medicaid Services evaluations that emphasize quality of life quality indicators can be leveraged to push for expanded resources and programming.

CULTURAL MEANINGS OF DEMENTIA AND PERSONHOOD: EXCESS DISABILITY AND PERSONHOOD-CENTERED CARE IN DEMENTIA

According to the disability literature, functional capacity does not emanate from the individual organism but is a result of the relationship between the person and the environment.[82] This concept of person-environment fit recognizes that not only physical but also interpersonal factors can enhance or diminish an individual's functional ability. For example, sidewalk cuts and ramps, as well as recent historical shifts in social perceptions, have had a dramatic beneficial impact on the functional capacity of persons who use wheelchairs. The growing field of geriatric geography focuses on how improving architectural and interior design can improve function and quality of life of elders with or without dementia.[83] Given the altered perceptions found in some dementias, adjustments to the environmental stimuli or color, light, and sound have been found to potentially enhance patient function and quality of life.[84,85] These efforts to optimize the person-environment fit increase functional capacity. But when the person-environment fit is not optimized, the individual experiences excess disability. The term excess disability refers to those deficits that arise from the physical or social environment rather than from extant organic damage.[86,87]

Throughout this article, I have suggested that **American cultural conceptions of personhood and dementia inadvertently create significant excess disability and that in the United States we do dementia particularly badly.** Deeper understanding of the diverse models of personhood permits analysis of the dynamic processes that lead to excess disability, and medical anthropological studies of dementia in other cultural communities have been reviewed in this article to clarify how American cultural conceptions create a uniquely American experience of

Table 2
Models of personhood and strategies for improving quality of care and quality of life

Model of Personhood	Central Features	Strategies to Improve Care and Quality of Life	
Cognitive/ Achievement	Cognitive ability and achievement are the essence of personhood	Proactive recognition that the essence of personhood is not limited to cognitive ability and achievement Interactive training of elder health professionals and lay community	Individual identity lists that recognize the many aspects of personhood LTC programming that prioritizes noncognitive activities recognized as pleasurable
Independence/ Autonomy vs the Relational Self	Individual autonomy and independence are the essence of healthy adulthood	Proactive reframing: wellness = interdependency Community-based programming that emphasizes social interdependency with a focus on intergenerational	Emphasis on the literature demonstrating health risks of social isolation Attention to other cultural models of social interdependency
Social Interactionism	Social interactions make and unmake identity/ personhood	Comprehensive patient evaluation that demonstrates the preservation of relational and emotional abilities to family and patient Training elder health professionals and lay community	Communication training in nonverbal forms and methods of indirect repair LTC programming that actively makes personhood, with attention to each individual's history and identity
Spiritual Aspects of Personhood and Identity	Many individuals experience spirituality as central to their lifeways and their self-identity	Spiritual history taking by elder health professionals Recognition of and emphasis on supporting patients to continue in their established spiritual lifeways and self-expression	LTC programming on-site for spiritual expression Community resources and emphasis on transportation, chaperones, and other strategies to increase access to spiritual activities
Embodied Personhood	Daily physical practices may constitute personhood and self-identity	Recognition that embodied personhood can be carried by daily physical practices Awareness that procedural memory (dance, sport, artistic, and musical practices) is often preserved in dementia	Increased emphasis and availability for healthy elders to initiate and develop embodied practices LTC and community-based programming that expand opportunities to engage in these embodied practices
Creative Self-Expression; Man as Meaning Maker	Intrinsic drive toward making meaning and creative self-expression are essential to being human	Recognition that people with dementia retain the drive for creative self-expression and meaning making Training elder health professionals, LTC staff, and lay community	Increased LTC and community-based programming in creative arts, music, and dance Storytelling circles in LTC and community settings with cross-generational staffing from colleges/ high schools

dementia. The value of this exploration lies in its lessons for improving quality of care and enhancing the quality of life of those with dementia.

When discussing person-centered care in dementia, perhaps one should be considering what care helps to support the personhood of the patient—in other words, perhaps we should focus our attention on ***personhood-centered care*** in dementia. In dementia, a disease category that specifically threatens personhood, supporting the personhood of the patient may well be the most effective strategy for improving quality of life. The models of personhood explored throughout this article are suggestive of practical strategies for supporting the personhood of the patient (**Table 2**). Models of cognitive personhood create excess disability by overvaluing achievement and cognitive function as essential to personhood; hence, the patient who can no longer "win the candy bar" no longer counts. Models of personhood that valorize independence and autonomy create threats to personhood when functional deficits create interdependency. Social interactionist models of personhood recognize that malignant social interactions that "unmake" the person with dementia lead to the excess disability of social death. Disturbingly, the literature reminds us that many of our clinical habits or practices result in excess disability in dementia: the physician who stands at a distance without acknowledging the patient with dementia,[88] the nursing aides who use infantilizing speech patterns,[89] or caregiving habits that demean.[90] Awareness of these insights of social interaction models of personhood can inform person-centered care[91] and point toward clinical strategies that support the personhood of those with dementia, such as learning skills to communicate effectively and participate in indirect repair. Models of embodied personhood also suggest strategies for personhood-centered care; many of the physical practices that embody personhood overlap with procedural memory and so can be proactively targeted in community-based and LTC programming, again to bolster the personhood of those with dementia. Models of personhood that recognize the potential for spiritual expression and experience imply that this transcendent aspect of being human may in fact be unleashed by dementias and that physical and social space for spiritual practices must be prioritized in LTC facilities and community settings. Finally, the model of personhood as meaning-making and story-telling is particularly powerful in supporting the personhood of those with dementia. By recognizing that the intrinsic drive toward creative self-expression and meaning-making is perhaps the essential characteristic distinguishing humans from animals and further recognizing that this intrinsic drive endures in the face of dementia, we are invited as clinicians, caregivers, and community members to provide opportunities for people with dementia to tell stories, to paint, and to dance. For to engage creatively is truly at the heart of person-hood centered care.

ACKNOWLEDGMENTS

With appreciation to Phil Sloane, MD; Sharon Kaufman, PhD; and Lawrence Cohen, MD, PhD for generous mentorship, and to Debbie Skolnik for tirelessly navigating the literature.

REFERENCES

1. Markut LA, Crane A. Dementia caregivers share their stories. Nashville (TN): Vanderbilt Univ Press; 2005.
2. Kessler L. Dancing with Rose: finding life in the land of Alzheimer's. New York Viking Press; 2007.
3. Young RF. Medical experiences and concerns of people with Alzheimer's disease. In: Harris PB, editor. The person with Alzheimer's disease: pathways

to understanding the experience. Baltimore (MD): Johns Hopkins Univ Press; 2002. p. 29–48.

4. Keady J, Gilliard J. Testing times: the experience of neuropsychological assessment for people with suspected Alzheimer's disease. In: Harris PB, editor. The person with Alzheimer's disease: pathways to understanding the experience. Baltimore (MD): Johns Hopkins Univ Press; 2002. p. 3–28.
5. Connell CM, Boise L, Stuckey JC, et al. Attitudes toward the diagnosis and disclosure of dementia among family caregivers and primary care physicians. Gerontologist 2004;44(4):500–7.
6. Pimlott NJG, Persaud M, Drummon N, et al. Family physicians and dementia in Canada: understanding the challenges of dementia care. Can Fam Physician 2009;55(5):508–9.
7. Blumenthal D, Gokhale M, Campbell EG, et al. Preparedness for clinical practice: reports of graduating residents at academic health centers. JAMA 2001;286(9): 1027–34.
8. West CP, Popkave C, Schultz JH, et al. Changes in career decisions of internal medicine residents during training. Ann Intern Med 2006;145:774–9.
9. Kane MN. Awareness of ageism, motivation, and countertransference in the care of elders with Alzheimer's disease. Am J Alzheimers Dis Other Demen 2002; 17(2):101–9.
10. Gunderson A, Tomkowiak J, Manachemi N, et al. Rural physicians' attitudes toward the elderly: evidence of ageism? Qual Manag Health Care 2005;14(3): 167–76.
11. Greene MG, Adelman RD, Charon R, et al. Concordance between physicians and their older and younger patients in the primary care medical encounter. Gerontologist 1989;29(6):808–13.
12. Adelman RD, Greene MG, Ory MG. Communication between older patients and their physicians. Clin Geriatr Med 2000;16:1.
13. Leung S, LoGiudice D, Schwarz J, et al. Hospital Doctors' attitudes towards older people. Intern Med J 2009. [Epub ahead of print].
14. Kane MN. Social work students' perceptions about incompetence in elders. J Gerontol Soc Work 2006;47(3–4):153–71.
15. Dalziel WB. Dementia: no longer the silent epidemic. CMAJ 1994;151(10):1407–9.
16. Fontana A, Smith RW. Alzheimer's disease victims: the 'unbecoming' of self and the normalization of competence. Socio Perspect 1989;32:35–46.
17. Keane WL. The patient's perspective: the Alzheimer's association. Alzheimer Dis Assoc Disord 1994;8(3):151–5.
18. Cohen A, Eisdorfer C. The loss of self: a family resource for the care of Alzheimer's disease and related disorders. New York: WW Norton & Co; 1986.
19. Cooney E. Death in slow motion: a memoir of a daughter, her mother, and the beast called Alzheimer's. New York: HarperCollins; 2004.
20. Post SG. The concept of Alzheimer disease in a hypercognitive society. In: Whitehouse PJ, Maurer K, Ballenger JF, editors. Concepts of Alzheimer disease: biological, clinical, and cultural perspectives. Baltimore (MD): Johns Hopkins Univ Press; 2000. p. 245–56.
21. Koenig Coste J. Learning to talk Alzheimers. New York: Houghton Mifflin; 2004.
22. Sokolovsky J. The cultural context of aging: worldwide perspectives. 3rd edition. Westport (CT): Praeger Publishers; 2009.
23. Shweder RA, Bourne EJ. Does the concept of the person vary cross-culturally. In: Marsella AJ, White GM, editors. Cultural conceptions of mental health and therapy. Boston: Kluwer; 1982. p. 97–138.

24. Deal WE, Whitehouse PJ. Concepts of personhood in Alzheimer's disease: considering Japanese notions of a relational self. In: Long SO, editor. Caring for the elderly in Japan and the US. New York: Routledge; 2000. p. 318–33.
25. Ikels C. The experience of dementia in China. Cult Med Psychiatry 1998;22(3): 257–83.
26. Ikels C. Constructing and deconstructing the self: dementia in China. J Cross Cult Gerontol 2002;17(3):233–51.
27. Cohen L. No aging in India: Alzheimer's, the bad family, and other modern things. Berkeley: UC Press; 2000.
28. Traphagan JW. Taming oblivion: aging bodies and the fear of senility in Japan. Albany: SUNY Press; 2000.
29. Bogdan R, Taylor SJ. Relationships with severely disabled people: the social construction of humanness. Soc Probl 1989;36:135–48.
30. Kitwood TM. Dementia reconsidered. Philadelphia: Open University Press; 1997.
31. Kitwood T. Towards a theory of dementia care: the interpersonal process. Ageing Soc 1993;13(1):51.
32. Sweeting H, Gilhooly M. Dementia and the phenomenon of social death. Sociol Health Illn 1997;19(1):93–117.
33. Sabat SR. Excess disability and malignant social psychology; a case study of Alzheimer's disease. J Community Appl Soc Psychol 1994;4(3):157–66.
34. Reifler BV, Larson E. Excess disability in dementia of the Alzheimer's type. In: Light E, Lebowitz B, editors. Alzheimer's disease and family stress. London: Taylor and Francis Press; 1990. p. 363 82.
35. Taylor JS. On recognition, caring, and dementia. Med Anthropol Q 2008;22(4): 313–35.
36. Magai M, Cohen C, Gomberg D, et al. Emotional expression during mid to late stage dementia. Int Psychogeriatr 1996;8:383–95.
37. Bosche-Domenech, Nagel R, Sánchez-Andrés JV, et al. Prosocial capabilities in Alzheimer's patients. J Gerontol B Psychol Sci Soc Sci 2010;65B:119–28.
38. Boise L, Carnicioli R, Morgan DL, et al. Diagnosing dementia: perspectives of primary care physicians. Gerontologist 1999;39(4):457–64.
39. Peterson B, editor. Voices of Alzheimer's. Cambridge (MA): Da Capo Life Long Books; 2004. p. 53–7.
40. Caddell LS, Clare L. The impact of dementia on self and identity: a systematic review. Clin Psychol Rev 2010;30(1):113–26.
41. Leibing A. Flexible hips? On Alzheimer's disease and aging in Brazil. J Cross Cult Gerontol 2002;17:213–32.
42. Merriam Webster Dictionary: definition of "communication".
43. Bartol MA. Dialogue with dementia: nonverbal communication in patients with Alzheimer's disease. J Gerontol Nurs 1979;5(4):21–31.
44. Hubbard G, Cook A, Tester S, et al. Beyond words: older people with dementia using and interpreting nonverbal behavior. J Aging Stud 2002;16(2):155–67.
45. Kontos PC, Nagie G. Bridging theory and practice: imagination, the body, and person-centred dementia care. Dementia 2007;6(4):549–69.
46. Davidson A. Alzheimer's disease: a love story: one year in my husband's journey. Secaucus (NJ): Birch Lane Press; 1997.
47. Sabat SR. Facilitating communication with an Alzheimer's disease sufferer through the use of indirect repair. In: Hamilton HE, editor. Language and communication in old age. New York: Garland Publishing; 1999. p. 115–31.
48. Vorthems RC. Clinically improving communication through touch. J Gerontol Nurs 1991;17(5):6–10.

49. Powell JA. Communication interventions in dementia. Rev Clin Gerontol 2000; 10(2):161–8.
50. Orange JB, Colton-Hudson A. Enhancing communication in dementia of the Alzheimer's type. Top Geriatr Rehabil 1998;14(2):56–75.
51. Bourgeois M. Adults with dementia. J Speech Hear Res 1991;34:831–44.
52. Sabat SR. The experience of Alzheimer's disease: life through a tangled veil. Oxford (UK): Wiley-Blackwell; 2001.
53. Featherstone M, Hepworth M, Turner BS. The body: social process and cultural theory. Newbury Park (CA): SAGE Publications; 1991.
54. Shilling C. The body and social theory. Newbury Park (CA): SAGE publications; 2003.
55. Douglas M. Purity and danger: an analysis of concepts of pollution and taboo. London: Routledge & Kegan Paul; 1996.
56. Elias N. The history of manners: the civilizing process. New York: Pantheon; 1978. [Jephcott E, Trans.]
57. Bourdeiu P. Distinction: a social critique of the judgement of taste. Cambridge (United Kingdom): Harvard UP; 1979. [Richard Nice, Trans.]
58. Alterra A. The caregiver: a life with Alzheimer's. South Royalton (VT): Steerforth Press; 1999. p. 148.
59. Beatty WW, Rogers CL, Rogers RL, et al. Piano playing in Alzheimer's disease: longitudinal study of a single case. Neurocase 1999;5(5):459–69.
60. Ridder HM. Singing dialogue: music therapy with persons in advanced stages of dementia [unpublished PhD thesis]. Esbjerg (Denmark): Aalborg University; 2003.
61. Kontos PA. "The painterly hand": embodied consciousness and Alzheimer's disease. J Aging Stud 2003;17(2):151–70.
62. Phinney A, Chesla CA. The lived body in dementia. J Aging Stud 2003;17(3): 283–99.
63. Verghese J, Lipton RB, Katz MJ, et al. Leisure activities and the risk of dementia in the elderly. N Engl J Med 2003;348:2508–16.
64. Kontos PC, Naglie G. Tacit knowledge of caring and embodied selfhood. Sociol Health Illn 2009;31(5):688–704.
65. Kontos PS. Ethnographic reflections on selfhood, embodiment and Alzheimer's disease. Ageing Soc 2004;24:829–49.
66. Weaver G. Embodied spirituality: experiences of identity and spiritual suffering among persons with Alzheimer's dementia. In: Jeeves M, editor. From cells to souls–and beyond: changing portraits of human nature. Grand Rapids (MI): Eerdmans; 2004. p. 77–101.
67. Henderson JN, Henderson LC. Cultural construction of disease: a 'supernormal' construct of dementia in an American Indian Tribe. J Cross Cult Gerontol 2002;17: 197–212.
68. Barker J. Between humans and ghosts: the decrepit elderly in a Polynesian society. In: Sokolovsky J, editor. The cultural context of aging: worldwide perspectives. Boston (MA): Bergin and Garvey Pub; 1997. p. 295–313.
69. Geertz C. The interpretation of cultures. New York: Basic Books; 1973.
70. Goldwasser AN, Auerbach SM, Harkins SW. Cognitive, affective, and behavioral effects of reminiscence group therapy on demented elderly. Int J Aging Hum Dev 1987;25(3):209–22.
71. Post S. People with dementia: a moral challenge. In: Thomasma DC, Kushner TK, editors. Birth to death: science and bioethics. Cambridge (United Kingdom): Cambridge University Press; 1996. p. 154–62.

72. Campbell CC. The human face of Alzheimer's. The New Atlantis 2004;6:3–17.
73. Friedell M. Awareness: a personal memoir on the declining quality of life in Alzheimer's. Dementia 2002;1(3):359–66.
74. McKim DK. God never forgets: faith, hope, and Alzheimer's disease. Louisville (KY): Westminster John Knox Press; 1997.
75. Davis R. My journey into Alzheimer's disease. Wheaton (IL): Tyndale House Publishers, Inc; 1989.
76. Kinney JM, Rentz CA. Observed well-being among individuals with dementia: memories in the making, an art program, versus other structured activity. Am J Alzheimers Dis Other Demen 2005;20(4):220–7.
77. Gottlieb-Tanaka D, Small JA, Yassi A. A program of creative expression activities for seniors with dementia. Dementia 2003:125–35.
78. Bastings AD. Forget memory: creating better lives for people with dementia. Baltimore (MD): Johns Hopkins Univ Press; 2009.
79. Jonas-Simpson C, Mitchell G. Giving voice to expressions of quality of life for persons living with dementia through story, music, and art. Alzheimers Care Q 2005;6(1):52–61.
80. Violets-Gibson M. Dance and movement therapy for people with severe dementia. In: Evans S, Garner J, editors. Talking over the years: a handbook of dynamic psychotherapy with older adults. New York (NY): Brunner-Rutledge; 2004. p. 194–214.
81. Lepp M, Ringsberg KC, Horn AK, et al. Dementia–involving patients and their caregivers in a drama programme: the caregivers'experiences. J Clin Nurs 2003;12(6):873–81.
82. Verbrugge LM, Jette AM. The disablement process. Soc Sci Med 1994;38(1): 1–14.
83. Kramer AF. Geographical gerontology: the constitution of a discipline. Soc Sci Med 2007;65:151–68.
84. Eriksson S, Gustafson Y, Lundin-Olsson L. Characteristics associated with falls in patients with dementia in a psychogeriatric ward. Aging Clin Exp Res 2007;19(2): 97–103.
85. McDaniel JH, Hunt A, Hackes B, et al. Impact of dining room environment on nutritional intake of Alzheimer's residents: a case study. Am J Alzheimers Dis Other Demen 2001;16(5):297–302.
86. Brody EM, Kleban MH, Lawron MP, et al. Excess disabilities of mentally impaired aged: impact of individualized treatment. Gerontologist 1971;11(2 part 1): 124–33.
87. Teri L, Uomoto JM. Reducing excess disability in dementia patients. Clin Gerontol 1991;10(4):49–63.
88. The Healing Project, editor. Voices of Alzheimer's: the healing companion: stories for courage, comfort and strength. New York: LaChance Publishing; 2007.
89. Williams KN, Herman R, Gajewski B, et al. Elderspeak communication: impact on dementia care. Am J Alzheimers Dis Other Demen 2009;24(1):11–20.
90. Rogers JC, Holm MB, Burgio LD, et al. Excess disability during morning care in nursing home residents with dementia. Int Psychogeriatr 2000;12:267–82.
91. Edvardsson D, Winblad B, Sandman P. Person-centred care of people with severe Alzheimer's disease: current status and ways forward. Lancet Neurol 2008;7(4):362–7.

Long-Term Care of the Aging Population with Intellectual and Developmental Disabilities

Nae-Hwa Kim, MD[a], Georges El Hoyek, MD[b,c], Diane Chau, MD[b,c,*]

KEYWORDS

- Developmental disability • Intellectual disability • Elderly
- Long-term care

INTELLECTUAL AND DEVELOPMENTAL DISABILITIES

The population with intellectual and developmental disabilities (I/DD) compose 1% to 3% of the general population.[1] This population requires specialized health care services and community support because of the inability to live independently and the tendency to have coexisting characteristic illnesses. Traditionally, long-term care (LTC) facilities, in the form of institutions, had played the central role in the livelihood of this population whose life expectancy had been shorter than that of the general population. However, the life expectancy of the population with I/DD has been rising. By 2030, the population older than 65 years is expected to reach at least 670,000, possibly 4 million.[2] The incorporation of the baby boomers of this population into geriatric care adds an additional impact on the current health care system. In 2003, there were 136.4 people with I/DD for every 100,000 people in the United States that used residential services and associated health care.[3]

Developmental disability refers to a variety of childhood conditions that are pervasive throughout the lifespan and is demonstrated before the 22 years of age. This terminology is used in policy making, clinical research, and government funding. In

The authors have nothing to disclose.

[a] Department of Internal Medicine, Resident PGY 2, University of Nevada School of Medicine, 1000 Locust Street (111), Reno, NV 89502, USA
[b] Division of Geriatric Medicine, Department of Medicine, University of Nevada School of Medicine, 1000 Locust Street (111), Reno, NV 89502-2597, USA
[c] VA Community Living Center, Reno, NV, USA
* Corresponding author. Division of Geriatric Medicine, Department of Medicine, University of Nevada School of Medicine, 1000 Locust Street (111), Reno, NV 89502-2597.
E-mail address: dchau@medicine.nevada.edu

Clin Geriatr Med 27 (2011) 291–300
doi:10.1016/j.cger.2011.02.003
0749-0690/11/$ – see front matter. Published by Elsevier Inc.
geriatric.theclinics.com

current clinical research, intellectual disability (ID) refers to the diagnosis of mental retardation (MR). MR presents before 18 years of age, characterized by significant limitations both in intellectual functioning, measured by the IQ scale, and in adaptive behavior (ie, self-care, social/interpersonal skills, functional academic skills, work, or leisure).[4] Based on the IQ scale, mental retardation is further divided into 4 groups: profound, severe, moderate, and mild. The American Association on Intellectual and Developmental Disabilities, established in 1876, is one of many valuable sources in research and public policy.

Key point: Developmental disability encompasses all childhood conditions that are pervasive throughout a lifetime. Intellectual disability is a subset of developmental disability, measured by the level of mental retardation (ie, mild, moderate, severe, or profound).

COMPARISON OF CURRENT LONG-TERM CARE PROGRAMS

Studies spanning the last 40 years chronicle the population shift from large state institutions to supervised community settings. Prior to the 1970s, state institutions cared for the population with I/DD regardless of age, IQ, activities of daily living (ADLs), or maladaptive behaviors. In 1977, approximately 150,000 lived in state-run facilities, which dramatically diminished to approximately 34,000 in 2008.[5] Although the total number of residents in institutions has decreased, the representation of residents more than 40 years of age using institutions increased from 22.0% in the 1970s to 67.4% in 2008. Furthermore, the representation of the elderly increased from 3.7% in the 1970s to 10.7% in 2008.[5] This increase may reflect the aging adults having been grandfathered in from a young age.

There is a subset of higher-functioning adults who live by themselves, with family, or with home assistance. Family caregivers, who are aging themselves, eventually use long-term care. These aging parents, who have devoted their entire lives to their children, will sometimes take on the responsibility for their own parents. There is a growing body of research regarding this compound caregiver: identifying their needs, including long-term care planning.[6]

Current literature focuses on the effects of deinstitutionalization. Better quality of life is the primary goal. In the past few decades, public policy funding has been allocated to community-based programs so that those with I/DD may live as independently as possible. In the 1990s, more than 450,000 were using community living centers.[2] This program has certainly addressed the needs of the younger adult population and there is generally high satisfaction among residents and families. However, results may vary widely. This program faces economic challenges to sustain current growth. Quality services are in high demand. Higher risk of mortality is attributed to the lack of access to medical care. Paradoxically, the general growth of the entire aging I/DD population has been attributed to better health care. Formal training to provide appropriate care in the community is lacking. Although the community setting offers more social opportunities, participation is, in part, dependent on the resident's adaptive abilities. More friendships are established, but can be limited by the staff turnover. Family contact is determined by distance, resident ability, and parent age. Staff practices are a huge determinant in autonomy. Gains in adaptive skills are more likely in the subpopulation with profound and severe I/DD. Challenging behavior is treated more informally, but more sedatives are used. Conversely, more restrictive practices and easier access to professional behavioral support were used in the institutional setting. There are many studies that confirm polypharmacy of psychotropics may be no worse in the institutional setting. Community settings may not necessarily improve challenging behavior, psychotropic medication, or mortality.[7]

Key point: The predominant community-based residential system fulfilled the goal of a better quality of life. However, challenging behaviors, use of psychotropic medications, or mortality may not be better than in the institutional setting.

EPIDEMIOLOGY AND LIFE EXPECTANCY

Historically, adults with I/DD have had lower life-expectancy rates. In the 1930s, female life expectancy was 14.9 years and male life expectancy was 22.0 years. By the 1970s, a woman was expected to live 58.3 years; whereas, a man was expected to live 59.8 years. In the 1980s, life expectancy was 65.5 years.[8] This improvement can be attributed to government mandates focused on improved health care; community programs; assistive technology; and improved sanitation in the institutions, as in the 1950s in Great Britain. Although only 40% of all people with I/DD are expected to live past 60 years, multiple studies in the last decade endorse the increased life expectancy in the entire I/DD population.

Multiple results indicate that in the population with mild MR, life expectancy has generally approached that of the general population (ie, 76.9 years).[9,10] However, data is conflicting regarding severity of MR correlating to mortality risk. Some studies indicate that premature death is greater in the population with severe disability[11] and other studies do not.[12] Regardless, it is common practice to separate the subpopulation with mild mental retardation from the more severely afflicted population. Many factors, such as the dynamic changes in health care, deinstitutionalization, or small sample sizes, may confound the results among studies. Some studies indicate that the higher number of comorbid conditions and advancing age are associated with mortality and not necessarily with a diagnosis of I/DD.[13] For example, higher mortality has been associated with having a diagnosis of epilepsy in the I/DD subpopulation with severe mental retardation.[14]

The most common causes of mortality in adults are cardiovascular disease, including acute coronary syndrome (33%), respiratory infection (20%), cancer, and seizures. Rare causes include accident, homicide, suicide, smoking, and alcohol. Cancer rates peaked in the population aged 50 to 70 years when compared with other age groups.[10] Top causes of mortality in the subset of adults *with* moderate to profound MR include congenital, neurologic, psychiatric (including dementia), and respiratory infection.[11] Mortality caused by respiratory infection occurs 6 times more in the I/DD population than the general population. Mortality caused by cerebrovascular accidents occurs 2.4 times more, and dementia is associated with a mortality risk of 4.5 times more in men with I/DD than the general population. Women with I/DD tend to have higher mortality rates because of congenital or accidental causes (**Table 1**).

The Down syndrome (DS) population is well studied, with live birth rates estimated to be 1 in 800 to 1000. Prevalence in 2003 was estimated at 717,000. The population with DS may constitute 18% of the total I/DD population. The young are susceptible to

Table 1
Mortality in aging adults with intellectual and developmental disabilities

Most Common Causes	Rare Causes
Cardiovascular disease	Accident
Respiratory infection	Homicide
Cancer	Suicide
Seizure	Smoking, alcohol

congenital heart disease; childhood cancers, including leukemia and testicular.[15] Those older than 60 years are susceptible to aspiration pneumonia, ischemic disease, dementia, malignancy, and congenital heart disease. In the 1980s, life expectancy of an adult with DS was 25 years. In the 1990s, it was 49 years. It is possible that the diagnosis of DS itself does not confer mortality risk, but that the comorbid diagnoses, including dementia, may. Once an adult with DS has reached 65 years of age, life expectancy is comparable to that of the general population.[16]

DIAGNOSIS OF COMORBID CONDITIONS

Multiple studies have evaluated the comorbid conditions in the I/DD population. Rates of some disease states are equivocal because of differences in study design, lack of power, and diagnostic difficulties. These studies encompass psychiatric and medical conditions, maladaptive behavior, and polypharmacy. Misdiagnoses can occur when attributing presenting health problems to another I/DD trait rather than to the underlying true condition. These misdiagnoses stem from communication barriers as well as the lack of staff, medical, or rehabilitation therapy training. The guidelines of the *International Classification of Diseases, Tenth Revision* indicate that establishing some diagnoses ought to be based over a period of time, to assess deterioration from a baseline. However, this is difficult to perform. Additionally, despite validated instruments, differential diagnoses of dementia, including depression, is difficult to identify in the ID population because symptoms overlap, including apathy, diminished ADLs, and loss of speech.[17]

Certain sub-I/DD populations, such as cerebral palsy, may have increased incidence of congestive heart failure, hypertension, and coronary disease. At baseline, many in the I/DD population have barriers, including language, mobility, hearing and vision, and bladder and bowel dysfunction, all of which cause functional impairment. Approximately 29% to 44% of adults with I/DD will have difficulties with ADLs, including eating, dressing, toileting, and bathing.[18]

Adults with I/DD are estimated to have 5.4 medical conditions, with 50% unrecognized or poorly managed.[1] Obesity is estimated to be 35% to 40%, compared with Framingham's 18.9%.[19] Gastroesophageal reflux disease (GERD) has been estimated to be 12%. Hypothyroidism is estimated to be 15%, but higher in the DS population (48%).[19] Neuropathy was associated with lower intellectual functioning and higher body mass index. Epilepsy is estimated to be 18.7% among general I/DD populations, but can be higher among subsets, such as cerebral palsy and autism, which carries an increased mortality risk.[19] Increased Alzheimer's dementia among DS populations is well recognized and discussed later.

Studies indicate that 8% to 20% of adults with I/DD smoke (ie, < the general population).[19] In Los Angeles, individuals who lived alone had smoking rates that were comparable to the general population.[19] Smoking may be a protective factor.[20] This finding may be attributed to less severity with MR. Alcohol use is estimated at 4% to 20% lower than the general population.[21]

The I/DD elderly population is subject to the same common age-related illnesses as the general elderly population, including cardiovascular disease, cancer, DM, visual impairment, hearing loss, or poor oral hygiene.[14] Hearing loss rate has been estimated to be 25% in the general population aged 65 to 75 years and 50% in those aged older than 75 years. In the DS population, 70% of 50 to 59 year olds had the deficit.[14] In the late 1980s and early 1990s, causes of mortality mirrored those found in the general community: cardiovascular, pulmonary, and neoplasm.[11] Severity of MR has been associated with the higher prevalence of visual impairment (eg, cataracts, refractive error, glaucoma, and retinopathy) and occurrences at earlier ages.[14] Osteoporosis rates were worse among I/DD compared with the Third National Health and Nutrition Examination Survey from the Center of Disease Control and Prevention population. An estimated 7% had fractures and 10% had falls requiring medical attention. There may be a higher rate of accidental injuries in the elderly with I/DD in the community compared with the general population, including falls and higher usage of the emergency room (**Box 1**; **Table 2**).

CHALLENGING BEHAVIOR

Maladaptive behaviors include self-injurious behaviors, temper tantrums or violence toward a roommate or staff, lack of impulse control, apathy, lethargy, agitation, noncompliance, elopement, stereotypy, and self-stimulation. Some challenging behaviors may correspond to the syndrome (ie, stereotypy in autistic spectrum disorder). Commonly, such behaviors are dismissed as a manifestation of I/DD and are not attributed to the discomfort from an acute medical condition. Gastrointestinal, genitourinary, respiratory, and neurologic diseases corresponded to the presence of aberrant behaviors, including aggression, passivity, and emotional lability in a New York State study of 60,752 individuals.[22] Cardiovascular disease and cancer did not correspond to challenging behaviors. Conversely, during an acute illness, patients can be weaker and less resistant to physical examination. Goals should include recognizing new onset or a deteriorating pattern and alert staff to the possibility of an acute medical condition or a progressive condition beyond the I/DD diagnosis and prompt further investigation.

Some maladaptive behaviors correspond to attention seeking, commonly seen in institutions where programs for social interactions and community participation have been historically lacking. An estimated 23% of maladaptive behaviors are caused by the desire for social interaction.[23] Challenging behaviors tend to be common in adolescents and young adults with I/DD. Some studies report that challenging behaviors decrease as the I/DD population ages.[18,24] However, others indicate that some of these behaviors persist throughout the lifespan.[19] In an 11-year study of those with challenging behaviors, including self injurious behaviors and assault, 63% to 90% continued to exhibit these behaviors later in life.[21]

Challenging behaviors should not reflexively trigger a sedative or an antipsychotic drug administration. Providers should recognize that they might represent an underlying medical problem that requires further evaluation, such as infection, fecal

Box 1
Comorbidities unrecognized or poorly managed in the aging I/DD population

Commonly overlooked diseases

Epilepsy

Dysphagia

GERD

Chronic constipation

Dental disease

Sensory impairment

Psychiatric disorders

Osteoporosis

Table 2
Comparison of comorbidities in aging adults with I/DD compared with the general aging adult

Diseases with Higher Rates	Diseases with Similar Rates
Anxiety	Diabetes mellitus
Depression	Ischemic heart disease
Fatal respiratory infection	Cerebrovascular accident
Dementia	
Thyroid conditions	
Cardiac arrhythmias	
Obesity	

impaction, premenstrual symptoms, hemorrhoids, or GERD. Attempts at behavioral modification, redirection, and intervention should be attempted before any medication initiation. There are no currently available drugs with an indication specific for behavioral treatment among I/DD populations.

COEXISTING PSYCHIATRIC DISORDERS

The prevalence of a comorbid mental disorder in the I/DD population ranges from 33% to 70%.[25] The prevalence of a concurrent psychiatric diagnosis in individuals aged 45 to 59 years is 32%, 30% in those aged 60 to 74 years, and 17% in those aged older than 74 years.[22] It is estimated that 68.7% of the elderly have a comorbid psychiatric disorder.[26] Depression is more common in the middle-aged Alzheimer population with I/DD than without, with a prevalence rate of 22% and among subsets of I/DD, such as cerebral palsy, there is a 4-fold risk for developing depression.[13] The aging I/DD population has a higher rate of anxiety (9.0%) and depression (6.0%) than the general population at 5.5% and 4.1%, respectively.[24] Schizophrenia and autistic spectrum disorder rates in young adulthood remained similar to rates in aging adults.[26] Many studies indicate that older individuals with I/DD are more likely to have psychiatric symptoms. In the adult DS population, aged older than 40 years, depression can manifest as less initiative and more apathy.

The I/DD population is vulnerable to neglect, physical trauma, and sexual abuse/assault.[25] It is common for patients with I/DD to be treated for posttraumatic stress disorder. Although collateral information would be difficult to establish in nonverbal patients, it is important to entertain the possibility of this abuse in the form of behavioral change, either new onset or caused by a seemingly random trigger.

POLYPHARMACY

Polypharmacy has been a frequently studied topic of interest. Statistics from pharmaceutical records consistently indicate that a disproportionally high number of the I/DD population are taking antipsychotics without a corresponding psychiatric condition, but likely correspond to controlling aberrant behaviors. Polypharmacy was noted with those receiving psychotropic medications. One study noted that of the one-third of the adults who were receiving psychotropic medications, only 36% had a diagnosis on chart review.[27] Mortality is associated with use of psychopharmacologic therapy for agitation in the elderly.

Although discomfort can be demonstrated in the form of a challenging behavior, some in the I/DD population may actually have a high tolerance for pain, as in the autistic spectrum disorder or in severe MR, or the highly medicated with a blunted sensation. Higher risk of injury has been associated with moderate to profound levels of MR and has been attributed to aggression and side effects from antipsychotics. Any possible traumatic injury, including the postictal time period, should be evaluated and may require multiple visits to the emergency room, because many injuries can be missed on initial examination.

Key point: Psychotropic polypharmacy for maladaptive behavior without a psychiatric diagnosis is common. Ruling out an underlying medical condition or determining an environmental cause should be attempted before medicating.

FOCUS ON DEMENTIA

US Census prevalence rates of dementia have been estimated to be 0.057 per 1000 in the general population older than 65 years.[20] Dementia afflicts 5% of individuals aged 65 to 74 years, 19% in those aged 75 to 84 years, and 50% in those aged more than 85 years.[28] The current 4.5 million with dementia will become at least 11 million within the next 50 years. In the general population, dementia is associated with higher mortality rates because of the risk of respiratory infection and congestive heart failure.

Rates of dementia have been reported to be 2% to 44% in the elderly I/DD population, and higher in the DS population (estimated 75%).[2,13] Some studies indicate that the prevalence of Alzheimer dementia and all types of dementia in the I/DD population without DS is comparable to that of the general population[20]; whereas, other studies indicate that the rate of dementia is higher: 21.6% in the I/DD population compared with 2.7% in the general population.[24] Some studies indicate that Alzheimer dimentia occurs 3 times more in the I/DD population without DS than the general population; Lewy body and frontotemporal occurs with similar rates.[29] Vascular dementia occurs at a lower rate, which is confirmed by a low likelihood of smoking in the I/DD population with moderate, severe, or profound mental retardation.[13] Whether or not there is or is not a higher rate of dementia in the I/DD population, it does appear that age is the strongest factor associated with the risk of dementia.[13] A greater number of physical disorders has been predictive of the dementia diagnosis.[26] Age-related functional decline in the I/DD population may be comparable to that of the general population.[30] Sex and severity of mental retardation do not appear to be risk factors.[13]

There is a level of diagnostic uncertainty in those with severe and profound mental retardation; consequently, implementation of the appropriate management of comorbid conditions may be delayed (**Table 3**).

DEMENTIA AND DOWN SYNDROME ID POPULATION

From 55 to 59 years of age, the dementia rate was estimated at 32.1%. After 60 years of age, prevalence was 25.7%. The lower prevalence rate in adults older than 60 years can be attributed to increased mortality in those with dementia, similar to the general population. From 50 to 55 years of age, the prevalence was 17.7%; whereas, it was 32.1% in those aged 56 to 59 years.[17] Approximately one-third are expected to develop Alzheimer dementia in middle age (ie, aged more than 40 years). Although there are multiple alleles associated with an increased rate of Alzheimer dementia, the DS population has a well-studied genetic predisposition for this subtype of

Table 3
Comparison of dementia in the aging I/DD population to the general aging population

Higher Rate	Similar Rate	Lower Rate
Alzheimer disease	Lewy body Frontotemporal	Vascular

dementia caused by the overexpression (ie, triplication of APP [β amyloid precursor protein]) gene on chromosome 21. The subsequent A-β levels and the deposition of extracellular beta-amyloid protein that will form neuritic plaques, appear to correspond to the age at which dementia onset occurs in patients with DS. Clinical presentation at 40 years of age has been well documented since the 1950s.[31] There does appear to be a shift toward a young DS population afflicted by Alzheimer disease. Although there is this predisposition, studies have shown that not all adults living beyond 70 years of age will develop dementia in the Down syndrome population.[17] Dementia is associated with increased mortality in I/DD, like in the general population. Although reports indicate that lifespan has increased in the DS population, it is still shorter than others in the I/DD population.[11] Prevalence of dementia for the DS population after 65 years of age is 50% to 75%.[24] Death is likely to occur 2 to 7 years after the onset of dementia in an individual with DS.[10]

Key point: Dementia afflicts the I/DD population. Alzheimer dementia occurs in the Down syndrome population earlier in life and at a higher rate than the general population.

ACKNOWLEDGMENTS

We appreciate the valuable input provided by Drs Alya Reeve and Christopher Abbott from the University of New Mexico's department of psychiatry and continuum of care.

SUMMARY

The aging population with I/DD is joining the general aging population in long-term care. Although better health care is attributed to this growing aging population, inequities and unique challenges still exist. Providers must recognize coexisting conditions that confer higher mortality, perform appropriate evaluations for challenging behaviors, and avoid a reflex to polypharmacy. The current dynamic residential system has benefited the younger population, however, LTC communities continue to be the care settings for the aging I/DD population. Successful aging should include adequate care for age-associated and comorbid diseases, promotion of adaptive skills, and autonomy. LTC needs of the I/DD population are growing and will expand into the general geriatric population. This subset of the aging population poses unique challenges, which will undoubtedly call for collaborative efforts between health care providers in the geriatrics and I/DD fields to create new strategies or modify established strategies in management.

REFERENCES

1. Sullivan WF, Heng J, Cameron D, et al. Consensus guidelines for primary health care of adults with developmental disabilities. Can Fam Physician 2006;52:1410–8.
2. Silverman W, Zigman W, Kim H, et al. Aging and dementia among adults with mental retardation and Down syndrome. Top Geriatr Rehabil 1998;13(3):49–64.
3. Stancliffe RJ, Lakin KC, Prouty RW. Growth in residential services in Australia and the United States:1997–2002. J Intellect Dev Disabil 2005;30(3):181–4.
4. American Psychiatric Association. Diagnostic and statistical manual of mental disorders. 4th edition. Text Revision. Washington, DC: APA Press; 2000. 41–9.
5. Larson SA, Scott N, Salmi P, et al. Changes in number and characteristics of people living in state institutions, 1977–2008. Intellect Dev Disabil 2009;47(4): 329–33.

6. Perkins EA. The compound caregiver: a case study of multiple caregiving roles. Clin Gerontol 2010;33(3):248–54.
7. Kozma A, Mansell J, Beadle-Brown J. Outcomes in different residential settings for people with intellectual disability: a systematic review. Am J Intellect Dev Disabil 2009;114(3):193–222.
8. Janicki MP, Daltonoe AJ, Henderson CM, et al. Mortality and morbidity among older adults with intellectual disability: health services considerations. Disabil Rehabil 1999;21(5/6):284–94.
9. Fisher K, Ketti P. Aging with mental retardation-Increasing population of older adults with MR require health interventions and prevention strategies. Geriatrics 2005;60(4):26–9.
10. Janicki MP, Dalton AJ. Prevalence of dementia and impact on intellectual disability services. Ment Retard 2000;38(3):276–88.
11. Tyrer F, McGrother C. Cause-specific mortality and death certificate reporting in adults with moderate to profound intellectual disability. J Intellect Disabil Res 2009;53(11):898–904.
12. Margallo-Lana ML, Moore PB, Kay DW, et al. Fifteen-year follow-up of 92 hospitalized adults with Down's syndrome: incidence of cognitive decline, its relationship to age and neuropathology. J Intellect Disabil Res 2007;51(6):463–77.
13. Strydom A, Hassiotis A, King M, et al. The relationship of dementia prevalence in older adults with intellectual disability (ID) to age and severity of ID. Psychol Med 2009;39:13–21.
14. Patja K, Iivanainen M, Vesala H, et al. Life expectancy of people with intellectual disability: a 35-year follow-up study. J Intellect Disabil Res 2000;44(5):591–9.
15. Yang Q, Rasmussen SA, Friedman JM. Mortality associated with Down's syndrome in the USA from 1983 to 1997: a population-based study. Lancet 2002;359:1019–25.
16. Haveman M. Disease epidemiology and aging people with intellectual disability. Journal of Policy and Practice in Intellectual Disabilities 2004;1(1):16–23.
17. Coppus A, Evenhuis H, Verberne GJ, et al. Dementia and mortality in persons with Down's syndrome. J Intellect Disabil Res 2006;50(10):768–77.
18. Janicki MP, Davidson PW, Henderson CM, et al. Health characteristics and health services utilization in older adults with intellectual disability living in community residences. J Intellect Disabil Res 2002;46(4):287–98.
19. Messinger-Rapport B, Rapport D. Primary care for the developmentally disabled adult. J Gen Intern Med 1997;12:628–36.
20. Zigman WB, Schupf N, Devenny DA, et al. Incidence and prevalence of dementia in elderly adults with mental retardation without down syndrome. Am J Ment Retard 2004;109(2):126–41.
21. Totsilka V, Toogood S, Hastings R, et al. Persistence of challenging behaviours in adults with intellectual disability over a period of 11 years. J Intellect Disabil Res 2008;52(5):446–57.
22. Davidson PW, Janicki MP, Ladrigan P, et al. Associations between behavior disorders and health status among older adults with intellectual disability. Aging Ment Health 2003;7(6):424–30.
23. Peine H, Darvish R, Adams K, et al. Medical problems, maladaptive behaviors, and the developmentally disabled. Behav Interv 1995;10(3):149–59.
24. Torr J, Davis R. Ageing and mental health problems in people with intellectual disability. Curr Opin Psychiatry 2007;20:467–71.
25. Griswold KS, Goldstein MZ. Issues affecting the lives of older persons with developmental disabilities. Psychiatr Serv 1999;50(3):315–7.

26. Cooper SA. The relationship between psychiatric and physical health in elderly people with intellectual disability. J Intellect Disabil Res 1999;43(1):54–60.
27. Lewis M, Lewis C, Leakk B, et al. The quality of health care for adults with developmental disabilities. Public Health Rep 2002;117:174–84.
28. Duthie EH, Katz PR, Malone M. Practice of geriatrics. 4th edition. Philadelphia: WB Saunders; 2007. p. 681.
29. Strydom A, Livingston G, King M. Prevalence of dementia in intellectual disability using different diagnostic criteria. Br J Psychiatry 2007;191:150–7.
30. Fraser WL. Three decades after Penrose. Br J Psychiatry 2000;176:10–1.
31. Schupf N. Genetic and host factors for dementia in Down's syndrome. Br J Psychiatry 2002;180:405–10.

Cancer in Long-Term Care

Beatriz Korc-Grodzicki, MD, PhD[a,*], James A. Wallace, MD[b], Miriam B. Rodin, MD, PhD[c], Rachelle E. Bernacki, MD, MS[d]

KEYWORDS

• Cancer • Long-term care • Nursing home • Geriatric

The purpose of this article is to describe the range of cancer patients in long-term care and to provide a framework for clinical decision making. The benefits and burdens of providing standard therapy to a vulnerable population are discussed as far as the data exist. The authors ask whether long-term care residents should be screened for cancer; the answer is probably already known. The burdens of screening exceed the benefit. These patients will likely die of something else before the cancer causes clinical disease or suffering. Perhaps, under some circumstances, cancer screening might be beneficial if we can confidently analyze individualized burdens and benefits. To give more specific guidelines for advocates of treatment, skeptics, and others, the authors present best estimates of the current burden of cancer in the long-term care population and current screening guidelines as they apply to elderly long-term care residents. Our decisions as clinicians depend on our ability to confidently estimate remaining life expectancy (RLE) for screening and our ability to extrapolate clinical trial data to a less fit population. Finally, the American public has had at least 50 years of rising expectations about cancer treatment and cancer screening despite egregious disparities in their application. Correctly identifying patients with limited life expectancy and recognizing onset of terminal decline in long-term care should also be accompanied by skill in explaining it to patients and families. This article offers experience-based suggestions for oncologists and clinicians involved in long-term care to help them respond to patient and family concerns about the limitations of cancer care.

The authors have nothing to disclose.
[a] Geriatrics Service, Department of Medicine, Memorial Sloan Kettering Cancer Center, 1275 York Avenue, New York, NY 10065, USA
[b] Specialized Oncologic Care and Research of the Elderly (SOCARE), University of Chicago–Ongology/Geriatrics, 5841 South Maryland Avenue, MC 6098, Chicago, IL 60637-1470, USA
[c] Division of Geriatrics, Department of Internal Medicine, St Louis University Medical School, 1402 South Grand Boulevard Room M238, St Louis, MO 63104, USA
[d] Pain and Palliative Care Program, Dana Farber Cancer Institute, Harvard Medical School, Southwest 411, 44 Binney Street, Boston, MA 02115, USA
* Corresponding author.
E-mail address: korcgrob@mskcc.org

Clin Geriatr Med 27 (2011) 301–327
doi:10.1016/j.cger.2011.03.011 **geriatric.theclinics.com**
0749-0690/11/$ – see front matter

CANCER IS AN AGE-ASSOCIATED DISEASE

Cancer occurs more commonly in older adults. It is projected that approximately 61% of patients diagnosed with cancer were older than 65 in the most recent Surveillance, Epidemiology, and End Results summary data through 2006[1–3] Age-specific rates of cancer continue to increase into the ninth decade of life. Cancer mortality in the elderly is also higher, and 71% of all cancer deaths occur in people of Medicare age. Nonetheless, there are 6.5 million cancer survivors older than 65, of whom 4.4 million are long-term (>5 years) survivors whose screening needs may be different from those of an unselected population. Therefore, population studies of cancer and cancer survivorship are studies of aging.[4,5]

As shown in **Table 1**, cancer is the leading cause of death for men and women aged 60 to 79 years, followed by heart disease.[6] This statistic is reversed among those aged 80 and older, with heart disease causing more deaths than cancer. Thus cancer as a cause of death declines in importance relative to cardiovascular diseases in advanced old age. As shown in **Table 2**, the most common cancers affecting adults are breast, prostate, lung, and colon cancer. More than half of all new diagnoses of breast, lung, and colorectal cancer are made in those aged 65 and older.[6] From **Table 3** it is clear that the common cancers have good prospects for prolonged survival. If detected at an early stage, all but lung cancer have better than 50% 5-year survival.[6] Incidence figures suggest that screening for early malignancy should be especially productive in the elderly at first glance, but the nature of screening is more complex.

Older adults with cancer trigger unique concerns. Frailty and decreased physiologic reserve may increase the risk of further functional decline and determine higher susceptibility to adverse outcomes such as institutionalization and/or mortality.[7,8] Increase in comorbidity may affect survival as well as treatment tolerance.[9] Cancer patients aged 70 years and older have on average 3 comorbidities that can affect detection, evolution, and treatment of cancer.[10] There is a larger incidence of cognitive dysfunction than in the younger cancer patients. A diagnosis of dementia is associated with shortened survival, and patients who have a diagnosis of dementia are likely to be diagnosed with cancer at a more advanced stage and less likely to receive curative therapy. At the same time, cancer therapy may worsen cognitive function in older adults.[11,12]

LONG-TERM CARE AND ITS RESIDENTS

Long-term care (LTC) is thought of as largely for the infirm elderly, but in fact covers a more heterogeneous population of children and adults with developmental

Table 1
Five leading causes of death: men and women age 60 years and older, United States, 2009

Age 60–79		Age 80 and Older	
Men	**Women**	**Men**	**Women**
Cancer	Cancer	Heart disease	Heart disease
Heart disease	Heart disease	Cancer	Cancer
COPD	COPD	Stroke	Stroke
Stroke	Stroke	COPD	Alzheimer disease
Diabetes	Diabetes	Alzheimer disease	COPD

Abbreviation: COPD, chronic obstructive pulmonary disease.
Data from Jemal A, Siegel R, Ward E, et al. Cancer statistics, 2009. CA Cancer J Clin 2009; 59(4):225–49.

Table 2
Five most common sites of cancer mortality: men and women age 60 years and older, United States, 2009

Age 60–79		Age 80 and Older	
Men	**Women**	**Men**	**Women**
Lung	Lung	Lung	Lung
Colon	Breast	Prostate	Colon
Prostate	Colon	Colon	Breast
Pancreas	Pancreas	Urinary bladder	Pancreas
Esophagus	Ovary	Pancreas	Hodgkin lymphoma

Data from Jemal A, Siegel R, Ward E, et al. Cancer statistics, 2009. CA Cancer J Clin 2009;59(4): 225–49.

diagnoses (DD) and the chronically mentally ill (CMI), all under the rubric of least-restrictive environment. The reasons for admission to a nursing home (NH) vary. In particular, an individual's access to entitlement programs, private financial resources, family and informal caregivers, and eligibility and availability of formal NH diversion programs strongly influence the likelihood of NH admission. There are considerable disparities and geographic variability in how people get into NHs. NH diversion programs include a panoply of nonresidential LTC including PACE (Program of All-inclusive Care for the Elderly) programs, hospital-at-home programs, the Veterans Administration hospital-based homecare, formal Medicare Part B home care, adult day care, and nonnursing residential care including small group homes for CMI patients, dementia patients, and physically and developmentally impaired adults. These programs are nearly all under some sort of regulatory control by federal, state, and local governments.

Centers for Medicare and Medicaid Services and other payors define eligibility for rehabilitation services by standardized documentation of a recent decline in function for which some recovery is possible. The guidelines define exactly which nursing

Table 3
Percentage 5+-year survival by cancer site, 1996 to 2004

All cancers	66
Prostate	99
Breast	89
Urinary bladder	81
Rectal	67
Colon	65
Non-Hodgkin lymphoma	65
Ovary	46
Esophagus	17
Lung and bronchus	16
Multiple myeloma	16
Pancreas	5

Data from Jemal A, Siegel R, Ward E, et al. Cancer statistics, 2009. CA Cancer J Clin 2009;59(4): 225–49.

procedures performed outside of a hospital qualify for reimbursement. Strict rules define eligibility for rehabilitation and skilled nursing as Part A, a restricted number of days of nursing care in a residential facility, or Part B, the same services provided to an outpatient, or someone living in their own home or other residence. Fewer than 5% of persons admitted to NHs will still be alive in 10 years,[13–15] and about 50% of persons admitted to NHs with a diagnosis of cancer will survive 1 year.[16]

Mor[17] and Intrator and colleagues[18] have described the multiple transitions of LTC populations. Hospitals send subacute patients to skilled nursing facilities (SNFs); some patients go home in a few weeks, some return to the hospital, some transition to "less restrictive" residential alternatives, some die, and some remain. Some patients encounter all of these transitions. In this mix, the patients in transit represent a medically unstable group for whom cancer screening is not appropriate. For residents who go home or to another stable long-term residence, there should be a primary care physician that can determine appropriateness of cancer screening. The data on the longevity of long-stay residents is only developing, but there are clearly two different groups. There are severely impaired patients with tracheostomy, feeding tube, and other high-skill care requirements. Few of these patients have decisional capacity, and cancer screening would be inappropriate. Some long-stay residents have chronic medical comorbidities and are expected to experience a slow downward course. Patients with dementia, oxygen-requiring chronic obstructive pulmonary disease (COPD), stage 3 and 4 congestive heart failure, multiple strokes, and Parkinson disease may all be eligible for hospice care because they have limited life expectancy. The second group consists of stable, frail, mainly female residents who require assistance with activities of daily living (ADL). A stable hemiparesis, an amputation, bad arthritis, and mild to moderate but stable cognitive impairment are common functional problems, but these patients are not ill; they take few medications and they do not decline over periods of a few years.

Cancer patients in NHs illustrate the complexity of managing transitions in care. With the aging population and increased number of older adults with cancer, more cancer patients are being admitted to NHs.[4,19] Some are admitted to NHs for SNF or subacute rehabilitation following a cancer-related or cancer-treatment–related hospitalization. Some are long-stay residents who are diagnosed in situ while living in the NH. The prevalence of patients with a documented cancer diagnosis living in NHs was estimated to be about 1 in 10, varying from 6.1% of patients in NHs in Texas to 12.5% in Maine.[20] Based on analysis of the data recorded in the Minimal Data Set (MDS) of more than 548,000 NH admissions during 2002, 11.3% of these residents had a diagnosis of cancer on admission.[16] This figure translates to more than 190,000 older adults living in nursing facilities with a known cancer diagnosis.

Johnson and colleagues[20] analyzed the national repository of MDS data, which includes individual-level data regarding diagnoses, functional status, drugs, and selected symptoms, notably pain and weight loss. 3.9% of NH residents were receiving chemotherapy and 14% were being treated with radiation within 14 days of their MDS assessment. Hospice services were used in 4.8% of persons. Eleven percent of NH cancer patients were assessed to be terminally ill but only 23% of the terminally ill were receiving hospice care. A study reporting patterns of cancer diagnosis, survival, hospice use, and treatment for a population-based sample of Medicaid-insured NH patients showed preponderance of late or upstaged disease. These patients experienced high mortality within a few months of diagnosis, low hospice use, and very little cancer-directed treatment. Among patients with early-stage cancer for which treatment can alleviate symptoms and possibly prolong life, very little cancer-directed treatment was recorded.[21] Diagnosis and treatment of cancer was highly dependent on NH characteristics.[22] For example, residents in NHs with lower staffing and in counties with fewer hospital beds were more likely to be diagnosed at death; further, NHs with a higher percentage of Medicaid residents were less likely to receive any pain medication in the month of or the month following the diagnosis of cancer.[22]

Research regarding cancer care in NHs is largely limited to studies of palliative or end-of-life care. Hospice care is closely associated with cancer care, and studying the quality of palliative care in NHs is reasonable considering that a cancer diagnosis is associated with more than 50% 1-year NH mortality.[23] However, the remaining cancer patients admitted to NHs do not die in the NH. Some may transition to hospice at home or simply be sent back to the hospital. A few are being treated with curative or life-prolonging intent, and many are admitted for rehabilitation after surgery or following a hospitalization for toxicity-related weakness and deconditioning. A small number receive outpatient cancer treatment while living in the NH, due to transportation problems. Cancer patients are complex, resource intensive, and challenging for NH physicians, nurses, and administrators. Transitions of care for cancer patients are more complicated than the average resident for many reasons. NH-hospital and hospital–NH transitions are associated with increased risk of adverse drug events, loss of diagnostic information, and lack of follow-up on test results.[24–26] Cancer patients admitted from acute oncology units often bring little documentation of disease status, advance directives, cancer treatment received or planned, response to treatment, prognosis, or what was disclosed to the patient and family.[27] Hospitalists often have incorrect expectations about transfusions, laboratory, radiology, pharmacy, and procedural services that cannot be provided by most NHs. If the medications are changed on the day of hospital discharge, the adverse drug events occur in the NH. Side effects of chemotherapeutic agents that develop days or weeks later may not be recognized as such by the untrained NH staff.[24] Expectations of patient and family may be unrealistic and are usually related to lack of information at discharge, leading to a perceived shortfall on the part of the LTC facility in meeting the needs of patients and relatives.[28]

If present trends continue, the largest number of cancer patients who enter LTC will be older, frailer, and more symptomatic than cancer patients at home.[27] In other words, cancer patients are admitted to LTC for the same reasons as noncancer patients: ADL dependency, functional decline, limited or no social support, and financial issues. Compared with end-stage dementia patients, advanced cancer patients admitted to New York NHs reported more pain, dyspnea, constipation, and weight loss than dementia patients.[29] Cancer patients were significantly more likely to be male and older compared with other residents at admission. A significantly larger proportion of NH residents with cancer experienced daily pain, greater ADL dependency, unstable health patterns, and acute episodes or flare-ups of chronic problems, and were expected to have 6 or fewer months to live. The difference in pain at admission was statistically significant; more than 37% of residents with cancer reported moderate or excruciating daily pain compared with 25% of other residents. More residents with cancer also had anemia and smoking-related COPD. However, residents with cancer were also significantly more likely to be cognitively intact than other residents at admission. Residents with cancer received less physical, occupational, speech, and psychological therapies, but a larger proportion received respiratory therapy and special procedures including intravenous medications, ostomy care, chemotherapy, radiation therapy, or hospice care. On the basis of this analysis of the MDS, NH residents with cancer require a higher level of skilled nursing care compared with NH residents without cancer.[16,29]

Key Points #1: Cancer patients in the NH

1. The number of cancer patients in NHs is increasing
2. Cancer patients in NHs are at increased risk for adverse events, due to the number and complexity of "hand-offs" in their care
3. NH residents with cancer require complex and resource-intensive care
4. Cancer patients in NH are older, frailer, and more symptomatic than cancer patients at home
5. One-year mortality for cancer patients admitted to NHs is about 50%
6. Research regarding cancer care in the NH is very limited.

ESTIMATING LIFE EXPECTANCY

Estimating prognosis based on functional status began in oncology populations; the Karnofsky Index (100 = normal; 0 = dead) and the Eastern Cooperative Oncology Group (ECOG) scale (0 = normal; 5 = dead) are the most commonly used scales. A median cancer survival of 3 months roughly correlates with a Karnofsky score of less than 40 or ECOG score greater than 3.[30] Newer prognostic scales tuned to different stages of disease have been developed to help provide prognostic information. The simplest method to assess functional ability is to ask patients: "How do you spend your time? How much time do you spend in bed or lying down?" If the response is greater than 50% of the time and is increasing, estimate the prognosis at 3 months or less.[30] An increasing number of physical symptoms, especially dyspnea, are also a good indication that time is short. Pain per se, interestingly, is not a good prognosticator of impending death. The Palliative Performance Scale (PPS) uses 5 observer-rated domains; it is a reliable and valid tool and correlates well with actual survival and median survival time for patients. It has been found useful for purposes of identifying and tracking potential care needs of palliative care patients, particularly as these needs change with disease progression.[31]

Estimating RLE when the end of life is approaching thus has several validated tools. Estimating RLE when a patient is not at the end of life requires different tools. One such tool was published by Walter and Covinsky,[32] who described the upper, middle, and lower quartiles of life expectancy for the United States population according to sex and age showing the substantial variability in life expectancy that exists at each age. Lubitz and colleagues[33] showed the interaction of functional status with survival for each of 3 functional states at age 70 (no limitations, instrumental ADL [IADL]/ADL limitations, or institutionalized) as extrapolated from observational cohorts. As the severity of functional impairment increases, life expectancy decreases. Persons with no limitations had the longest life expectancy (14.3 years on average) while institutionalized people's life expectancy was shortest (~5.2 years on average). Rozzini and colleagues[34] studied the association between 5-year survival and ADL dependency among a community-dwelling sample of elderly persons (**Table 4**). These investigators showed that even one ADL dependency is associated with a twofold increased adjusted mortality risk at 5 years; and 3 or more ADL dependencies is associated with a nearly threefold increased 5-year mortality. Extensive research has shown that comorbidities, functional impairment, and frailty phenotype markers (which include slowness, limited physical activity, subjective exhaustion, muscle weakness, poor nutrient intake, and gradual weight loss) may occur in the same people but that they are conceptually and demonstrably distinct.[35] This distinction has been also been shown in cancer patients.[10] Geriatric syndromes (ie, falls, dementia, failure to thrive, delirium, and so forth) are contributable to early mortality in elderly patients. Koroukian and colleagues,[36] while evaluating the mortality of

Table 4
Relationship between functional status and 5-year mortality

Functional Status	Deaths	Adjusted[a] Relative Risk[b]
Unimpaired in ADL (n = 406)	75	1.0 (reference)
Disabled in bathing (n = 67)	28	2.1 (1.3–3.4)
Disabled in dressing, toileting and transferring (n = 56)	30	2.6 (1.5–4.4)

Abbreviation: ADL, activities of daily living.
[a] Adjusted for age, sex, education, cognition, depression, number of comorbidities, social interaction, and living alone.
[b] 95% confidence interval in parentheses.
Data from Rozzini R, Sabatini T, Ranhoff AH, et al. Bathing disability in older patients. J Am Geriatr Soc 2007;55(4):635–6.

elderly colorectal cancer patients, identified a 25% reduction in 5-year overall survival if 2 or more geriatric syndromes were present (vs none identified).

Key points #2: Estimating life expectancy

1. Physical frailty, comorbidity, and functional impairment are independently associated with life expectancy
2. Any ADL dependency more than doubles the 5-year mortality risk
3. The presence of one geriatric syndrome increases mortality risk by 30%
4. Based on observational studies, these factors are probably additive.

CANCER SCREENING GUIDELINES AND THE ELDERLY

Screening does not prevent disease; it detects disease that is clinically silent. The rationale is that effective treatment is available and will cure the disease or at least improve the quality or quantity of life. Thus incidence rates reflect the sum of cancers that are detected clinically, or by "luck," as well as by intentional screening. For the population, benefits of screening should be seen in stage drift, that is, a trend over time to proportionately more early-stage malignancies; this should result as well in declining cancer site-specific mortality. If, however, treatment is not effective and the natural history of the disease is to progress slowly over time, earlier detection only gives the appearance of improved survival, the so-called Will Rogers effect.[37]

For individuals, however, screening is either positive or negative. Or is it? The rationale for screening is population based. The choice of screening modalities is based on measures that are derived from population experience. Screening populations is only cost effective if the screening test is balanced in terms of sensitivity and specificity. Sensitivity and specificity are not independent characteristics of the test, but are calculated from its population performance, so they can vary with the population being screened. For this reason, screening is only useful for relatively common diseases. A too sensitive test produces too many false positives and subjects many patients to increasingly invasive tests to be "ruled out." In a very low prevalence population nearly all the positive tests will be false positives. Conversely, a too specific test might miss clinically important cancers, even in a population with a comparatively high prevalence of disease.

Additional concerns about screening relate to lag time. In other words, if routine interval screening is begun in a population, how long will it be before routine screening demonstrates an advantage for screened over unscreened populations?[38] A related concept is lead time. How long does it take for a cancer that is detectable by screening to become clinically detectable (symptomatic)? Much of the controversy surrounding cancer screening for the elderly derives from these concepts. Are we screening people who may not live long enough to benefit from early detection? Are we able to detect cancerous or precancerous lesions that are unlikely to be clinically significant during the patient's lifetime? Should we search for asymptomatic diseases for which treatment may be ineffective or burdensome during the patient's lifetime? Essentially, the decision to screen should be preceded by a prior decision to go ahead with treatment if a cancer if found.

For the common cancers among elderly people, each has a different screening literature, different clinical behavior, and different treatment strategies. A review of current cancer screening guidelines can be summarized readily through the United States Preventive Services Task Force (USPSTF) recommendations on cancer screening in adults.[39] The USPSTF has concluded that there is insufficient evidence to recommend breast cancer screening for women aged 75 and older; the USPSTF recommends against screening men aged 75 and older for prostate cancer, against screening people older than 75 for colorectal cancer, and even more strongly recommends against screening those older than 85 years. The USPSTF recommends against screening Papanicolaou (Pap) smears for previously screened women older than 65 years. Lung cancer screening is deemed unproven, and screening for ovarian cancer is strongly advised against. By the same token, no recommendation as a result of insufficient evidence is not a recommendation against screening. The USPSTF further qualifies screening recommendations based on the previous screening history of the individual. Appendix 1 shows the current USPSTF guidelines with their strength of recommendation. However, specialty societies have identified specific risk factors that might raise the value of screening for selected individuals. The best studied are breast, prostate, and colorectal cancer.

The American Cancer Society (ACS) guidelines differ considerably from those of the USPSTF.[39] The ACS 2009 breast cancer screening guidelines recommend annual clinical breast examination (CBE) by a health professional and annual mammography from age 40 years, with no upper age limits. Analysis of the mammography trials, which largely excluded women older than 70, indicated that the population of benefit of screening mammography, the lag time, emerged after about 5 years of screening.[38] This finding has been interpreted to mean that women with less than a 5-year life expectancy would not benefit from mammography. There are several age-related differences in both the cancer and screening tests that bear on this. First, beyond the climacteric breast cancers are less likely to be biologically aggressive, so-called triple-negative, and are more likely to be low-grade and hormonally responsive.[40] Furthermore, with atrophy of the breast tissue mammograms are more sensitive and specific than in the dense breast tissue of younger perimenopausal women. Therefore the likelihood of false positives goes down and the yield of actual malignancies goes up.[41] But are these malignancies likely to metastasize early?

Walter and Covinsky[32] performed actuarial calculations to put this into perspective. There is a wide variation in survival among people within the same sex and 5-year age interval. Walter and Covinsky calculated the median survival within each quartile of survival by sex and 5-year age interval. The resulting tables have demonstrated how dramatically physicians may underestimate the survival of some elderly. Mandelblatt and colleagues[42] applied cost-benefit analysis under 3 scenarios including perfect treatment and imperfect treatment. These investigators concluded that mammographic screening was cost effective at least to age 80, and possibly beyond, for women in the upper quartile of life expectancy.[41]

ACS guidelines recommend annual screening with serum prostate-specific antigen (PSA) and digital rectal examination (DRE) in "average" risk men older than 50 with a life expectancy of 10 years or more. This recommendation is based on assumptions about the biological behavior of cancer, or the "dwell time" between malignant transformation and metastasis. The US Prostate, Lung, Colorectal and Ovarian (PLCO) randomized controlled trial of screening men in the community failed to find a benefit of screening when compared with the positive trials conducted in Europe.[43,44] However, examination of screening yield for potentially aggressive prostate cancers has not actually fulfilled the screening expectation that interval cancers detected in follow-up screening examinations are necessarily more aggressive than the mix of bland and aggressive tumors found in an initial screen.[45] The American Urological Association (AUA) acknowledges unproven benefit in men with life expectancies of less than 10 years, but recommends making individual patient decisions without formal timing for discontinuation with annual DRE with PSA (starting at age 40).[46] PSA and DRE are by default the screening gold standard, but they have limited sensitivity and specificity.[47] The estimated likelihood of detecting clinically insignificant disease in a 75-year-old man is 56%.[48] Consensus exists that if a patient has fewer than 10 years of life expectancy, they will be unlikely to benefit from screening.[49] This assumption is pertinent to the decision to screen an elderly man for prostate cancer who has previously been screened. Contrary to expectation, a Scandinavian trial reported it was less likely that a new aggressive cancer emerged in a screened group at follow-up. Thus for a previously screened man older than 75, routine screening does not appear to offer any survival advantage, and the treatment of asymptomatic or "PSA" disease may even be harmful.[50,51]

In the United States, 2008 estimates revealed that 67% of patients diagnosed with colorectal cancer were older than 65 years. One-third of mortality associated with colorectal cancer occurs in patients older than 65.[52] Recommendations differ among national organizations without a designated consensus in patients older than 65. The ACS recommends screening of average-risk individuals to start at age 50, and earlier for high-risk families. Testing may consist of colonoscopy (every 10 years), sigmoidoscopy (every 5 years), double-contrast barium enema (every 5 years), or computed tomographic (CT) colonography (every 5 years). Annual testing options in the absence of the above include fecal occult blood test or fecal immunochemical test.[39] The USPSTF recommends screening to include fecal occult blood testing, sigmoidoscopy, or colonoscopy beginning at age 50 and continuing until age 75 years. Screening in adults aged 76 to 85 is not recommended, although they suggest making "individual" decisions surrounding screening in this age group. No screening is recommended for adults older than 85 years. The USPSTF finds evidence supporting CT colonography and fecal DNA testing to be inconclusive.[53] The American College of Gastroenterology recommends colonoscopy every 10 years (beginning at age 50) as the preferred screening strategy. In settings where colonoscopy is not available, or patients are ineligible or unwilling, alternative methods include flexible sigmoidoscopy (every 5–10 years), CT colonography (every 5 years), or cancer detection test (fecal immunochemical test for blood).[54] Despite controversy regarding screening options, the general consensus is that screening will not benefit patients with a life expectancy of less than 5 years.[32]

Several studies have examined the population benefit of serial screening colonoscopy. These studies do not differentiate between "no disease" and various nonmalignant or premalignant polyp-forming conditions detected on screening. Only colonoscopy with clearance of premalignant or early noninvasive malignant polyps is associated with a demonstrable improvement in disease-specific survival. Overall survival has not been demonstrated. The 10-year interval is based on observational studies suggesting that it takes an average of 10 years for premalignant polyps to undergo transformation and invasion into healthy tissue. So a normal colonoscopy need not be repeated for 10 years. In previously screened healthy persons in their 70s or possibly even early 80s, a 5-year polyp or 10-year colonoscopy follow-up is not unreasonable if they have a 10-year life expectancy. The difficulty of the preparation, and the risk of endoscopic complications of perforation or anesthesia-related events remain small but increase with age. Cervical screening with Pap tests are recommended every 2 to 3 years and may be stopped for women who have had a total hysterectomy and women older than 70 who have had 3 normal smears in a row. The guidelines are on firmer ground here because the causal association between human papilloma virus (HPV) infection and cervical cancer has been established.

Surveillance data are clear that CMI and developmentally delayed populations receive poor-quality preventive care, are more likely to present with advanced cancers, and are less likely to receive standard-of-care therapy. Their risk factor profiles suggest a need for more aggressive preventive and screening services. For the purposes of this discussion, however, adherence to nationally promulgated screening guidelines is appropriate for younger long-stay NH residents. Given the invasiveness of the screenings for breast, colon, cervical, and prostate cancer, specialized providers sensitive to the needs of these populations should be used. Such is also true with regard to the elderly, particularly those with cognitive impairment, who may not be able give informed consent or participate comfortably with screening procedures.

SHOULD THIS PATIENT BE SCREENED FOR CANCER?

Screening recommendations should be based on the clinician's best estimate of RLE and an objective assessment of the magnitude of benefit expected from treatment if screening is positive. The calculations of Walter and Covinsky[32] give some realistic ideas about how long elderly people can live. Even in the lowest survival quartile, however, median survival for 80-year-olds was 5 years. The tables do not tell us how to estimate an individual's RLE. Functional status and comorbidity independently predict life expectancy. Further, newer indicators have emerged including various measures of gait speed.[55–59] The observational literature is quite clear that the onset of IADL dependence predicts further functional decline.[60] The onset of ADL dependence predicts intermediate-term mortality.[61,62] Frailty as a phenotype of weakness, slowness, and low body weight has less predictive power, as cohorts have shown that many patients, mainly women, may live a long time in this state.[61,63] However, several investigators have identified ways to categorize the elderly as long, average, or short life expectancy, based on various indices of comorbidity and on typical geriatric measures.[64,65]

Looking at a cohort of hospitalized elderly, Walter and colleagues[66] found that any preexisting ADL dependency associated with age greater than 80 years predicted shorter life expectancy. These investigators developed a scoring system: male sex (1 point); number of dependent ADL at discharge (1–4 ADL, 2 points; all 5 ADL, 5 points); symptomatic congestive heart failure (2 points); cancer (solitary, 3 points; metastatic, 8 points); creatinine level higher than 3.0 mg/dL (265 μmol/L) (2 points); and low albumin level (3.0–3.4 g/dL, 1 point; <3.0 g/dL, 2 points). Several variables associated with 1-year mortality in bivariable analyses, such as age and dementia, were not independently associated with mortality after adjustment for functional status. In the derivation cohort, 1-year mortality was 37% in the group with 4 to 6 points, and 68% in the highest-risk group (>6 points). Results were nearly identical in the validation cohort. A score of more than 5 predicted a greater than 50% probability of death at 1 year. Dementia rated as severe on a standard screening tool was associated with 50% 4-year mortality.[15] Balducci[67] proposed a cancer-specific check-list of geriatric impairments that would suggest appropriate limits for curative cancer therapy. Balducci added a history of geriatric syndromes including falls, fractures, delirium, failure to thrive, and living in an NH to preexisting conditions that might limit the treatment of cancers. He did not include urinary incontinence. However, if an NH resident meets Balducci's criteria of frailty, clearly screening would not be indicated. Moreover, for clinically advanced cancers, cancer-directed treatment would not be indicated.

So for these reasons, it is extremely important that screening decisions be based on individual patient assessments. Accurate data on the severity and rate of progression of disablement, the trajectory, is as important as the specific comorbidities in estimating remaining life expectancy. Flaherty and colleagues[68] developed the concept of functional glide paths to tailor primary care interventions such as vaccines and screening, to the rate of decline. Extensive epidemiologic data describe these trajectories. One clear conclusion is that it is complex; while functional impairment on a population level is associated with higher 2-, 5-, and 10- year mortality, there is considerable variability. So the rate of decline is critical for prognostication. If we can construct functional trajectories derived from those who know the patient well, the Walter actuarial tables, and what we know about survival associated with specific comorbid diseases, this gives us firm ground for advising LTC patients on cancer screening. If we then add what oncologists know about the survival curves of specific cancers, we can participate in the decisions on cancer-directed treatment.

CANCER SCREENING IN THE NURSING HOME

To the authors' knowledge, no specific policy addressing cancer screening in the NH population exists. Medicare has paid for screening mammograms since 1991, and dropped the co-pay in 1998. There is no rationing based on age, preexisting health, or residence. This situation has led to some abuses, with mass screenings provided "as a service" by for-profit providers. Strategies to navigate present policy while practically addressing concerns about medical necessity and individualized decision-making are outlined in this section, with a particular focus on the 3 most common cancers (excepting skin cancer) for which screening is widely advocated: breast, colorectal, and prostate cancer.

Breast Cancer

Breast cancer incidence peaks in the mid-70s and approximately two-thirds of breast cancer deaths occur in women older than 65 years.[69,70] Among the oldest women, breast cancer presents more commonly with advanced disease.[71] Mandelblatt[41] has shown that among older women, mammograms were often performed on women with multiple comorbidities including dementia, with higher income, and with living spouses. Despite the rising incidence, the majority of breast cancers in older women have favorable biological features and are less aggressive.[72–74] Therefore, a subpopulation of functionally stable long-stay NH residents with breast cancer may benefit from therapy and so might benefit from screening. The question remains whether biennial screening as currently advocated by the ACS makes sense. In this regard the woman's previous screening history is pertinent.

Walter and colleagues[75] tested this hypothesis by analyzing the results of breast cancer screening associated with the On Lok PACE program. Mandated by the California Department of Public Health, all PACE enrollees were screened. Two hundred and sixteen mammograms yielded 38 positives of whom 32 agreed to biopsy, yielding 4 low-grade malignancies. With treatment, all 4 women died of other causes in less than 5 years. There are 2 important points about this small study. First, the On Lok program served mainly the San Francisco Chinese community, a population with very low background incidence and little or no previous screening. Second, the PACE model is designed as an NH diversion program, it is long-term care at home. So for present purposes, it is less important that the screening appeared to do more harm in terms of cost and distress than good in terms of curing disease, than that it shows that in a frail population, screening and treatment of low-grade malignancies was irrelevant to survival. This study replicates the earliest inquiry about the interaction of comorbidity and breast cancer survival. Satariano and Ragland[76] followed a cohort of Detroit women screened in the late 1980s and found that those with comorbid congestive heart failure (CHF) were unlikely to die of breast cancer.

More recent controversy has arisen as USPSTF has revised their guidelines to specify biennial versus annual mammogram screening. Ultimately, it is suggested that if life expectancy is estimated at less than 5 years, older women do not benefit from screening. There is increased harm associated with screening, including complications from false-positive results, psychological distress, and treatment toxicity risk, with the added potential complications of treating clinically evident disease that would not have progressed within the patient's lifetime.[38,77] The following cases are derived from the authors' practices to illustrate how to apply the prognostication tools to clinical decision making about cancer in NHs.

Clinical scenario #1

A 74-year-old woman, Mrs A, had annual mammograms throughout most of her middle years. She was treated for hypertension, hyperlipidemia, and stage 3 renal insufficiency. She lived alone with no assistance. She suffered an acute cerebrovascular hemorrhage resulting in left-sided hemiparesis. She transferred to an SNF for subacute rehabilitation. After completing 90 days of Part A stroke rehabilitation, she remained dependent for dressing, bathing, and toileting. She could transfer independently and had a good appetite. The patient and her daughter decided she should stay at the NH and she was transferred to the long-stay hall. One day the daughter reminded the NH physician, not her previous primary care physician, that her mother was due for her annual mammogram. What questions should the physician ask?

Based on the Walter and Covinsky study,[32] the life expectancy of a 74-year-old woman with multiple stable comorbidities and functional dependence is estimated to be in the lower quartile of typical women within the 70- to 75-year-old category. Therefore, life expectancy is roughly estimated at between 6 and 10 years.[32] Referring to the hospitalized elders survival calculator, when she was discharged from the hospital she scored 4, estimating 37% 1-year mortality. Her previous mammogram about 2 years previously was entirely normal. As far as the patient and daughter recalled, she had never had an abnormal mammogram. There was no family history. The patient stated that if an abnormality suspicious for cancer was found, she wanted treatment. In this case the patient possibly had more than 5 years of life expectancy, a history of favoring screening, and a wish for treatment. The attending physician arranged for a wheelchair-adaptive mammogram.

The mammogram was read positive for a new 1.5-cm lesion on the right breast. The biopsy revealed ER/PR+ receptors, Her2/neu-negative infiltrating ductal carcinoma.

The standard therapy in this case at the time, since recommendations have recently changed, was lumpectomy with sentinel lymph node sampling, radiation, and adjuvant chemotherapy followed by hormone ablative therapy. Alternatively, modified radical mastectomy that includes axillary dissection, adjuvant chemotherapy, and hormone ablation could be offered. The relative value of adjuvant chemotherapy in this setting has been simulated by Extermann and colleagues.[78] For adjuvant chemotherapy to reduce the risk of death by 5% for an 85-year-old, the risk of recurrence should be 50% within 5 years and nearly 100% at 10 years. This patient is unlikely to have a 10-year life expectancy. Her risk of recurrence at 5 and 10 years is about 25% without chemotherapy. Without chemotherapy it is possible that cancer would recur, but it is unlikely to cause her death. Muss and colleagues[79] extrapolated data from pooled Cancer and Leukemia Group B trials and found that highly selected women older than 65 years, of whom fewer than 2% were older than 70, may have benefited more from adjuvant therapy than younger women. This conclusion has limited generalizability because the elderly trial participants were mostly healthy and had more to gain since they had more advanced nodal disease than the younger women. The trials data do not address the clinical decision points for the present patient. She is relatively immobile, so the increased risk for deep venous thrombosis caused by tamoxifen should be considered versus first-line use of aromatase inhibitors. The impact of the aromatase inhibitors on quality of life include accelerated osteoporosis, joint pain, and hot flushes. Her immobilized left side is already at risk for disuse demineralization. The risk of insufficiency fractures on her left side is increased by hormonal therapy. Modified radical surgery or axillary exploration may affect her ability to use her right arm, on which she is dependent.

In a comparison case, the authors were asked by the wound nurse to see Mrs B, a 79-year-old severely demented woman, for a nonhealing ulcer. The ulcer was a large fungating mass on the chest wall. Her son stated that when she was 72 and living at home, her primary care physician had found a mass but did not pursue it because "she will probably die of something else first." With the son's permission, an outpatient biopsy was performed, revealing triple negative histology. She was not able to be positioned for palliative radiation, and the surgical field was too large and contaminated to attempt toilet mastectomy. A metastatic workup was not pursued. At her son's request, the authors tried single-agent palliative chemotherapy. She tolerated a brief trial of oral chemotherapy without toxicity, but there was no regression in the visible tumor mass, and hospice care was initiated.

A study looking at NHs in the Midwest found that most lacked policies regarding cancer screening.[80] It is not clear why an NH needs a cancer screening policy because the decision-making process is between the physician and the patient, or the patient's representative in the case of decision-incapacitated residents. The benefit or intention for screening remains to find clinically silent early-stage cancers so that therapy can be undertaken to prevent morbidity and suffering attributable to advanced malignancy. Whereas routine mass screening is inappropriate in an NH, missing a treatable cancer diagnosis or ignoring an early cancer sign may result in future suffering among stable long-stay residents.[75] The second patient had clinical breast cancer for 7 years before any notice was taken. The first patient was doing well after 2 years under simple mastectomy, prophylactic intravenous bisphosphate, and aromatase inhibitors.

Colorectal Cancer

Clinical scenario #2

An 82-year-old man, Mr C, had mild to moderate vascular dementia, and a history of coronary artery disease, CHF (American Heart Association Class II), and type 2 diabetes. He was a long-stay resident in an NH because he required 24-hour supervision and assistance with 4 out 5 ADL including dressing, grooming, feeding, and toileting. His family that lived across the country supported him financially but rarely visited. One day his daughter notified the NH physician that they received a mail reminder from his local gastroenterologist to come in for his screening colonoscopy.

This represents an unambiguous case regarding the need for screening. An 82-year-old man, considered in the lower quartile of health for his age (80–84 years old), has an estimated life expectancy of 3.5 years. As his life expectancy is estimated less than 5 years, he should not be screened for "routine" indications.

For comparison, let us vary the scenario. Mr D is an 82-year-old man who leads an active life in his retirement community. Initially he moved there because his wife's dementia had progressed to the point that she needed 24-hour assistance, but he did not want her to go to an NH. The couple compromised by moving into an assisted living facility (ALF) where he could call staff at night if he needed help for his wife. She attended a dementia day-care program and he took his meals in the well-appointed dining room. After her death he stayed on, and although his arthritis bothered him increasingly he still played bridge, poker, and trivial pursuit. He enjoyed the Wii golf and bowling leagues. At age 77, before moving to the ALF he had undergone a screening colonoscopy, which took place at age 65 as well. Both showed polyps with hyperplastic changes. His gastroenterologist sent him a notice reminding him of his upcoming 5-year colonoscopy.

Life expectancy for patients with colorectal cancer varies by age, stage, and comorbidity. Detailed RLE estimates are available at http://www.annals.org/content/145/9/646.full.pdf±html.[81] **Table 5** shows the association between burden of preexisting comorbidities and colorectal cancer survival by age.[82] Patients who had CHF, dementia, chronic renal failure, or metastatic cancer, or were homebound had 5-year mortality greater than 50%.[82] Based on age alone, this patient's life expectancy is about 8 years. If screening reveals limited stage 1 or 2 colorectal cancer, his life expectancy is still 8 or more years. As shown by **Table 5**, age is a more powerful predictor of 5-year survival with early-stage colon cancer than comorbidities as measured by a standard scoring device. In this case, a man with no ADL impairments but a slow, orthopedic gait and some volitional IADL dependency lives in an ALF. It is not an NH, but it falls under long-term care. Endoscopy might reveal dysplastic changes unlikely to cause symptomatic disease during his lifetime or early-stage invasive disease requiring colorectal surgery. His perioperative risk for intra-abdominal surgery is low, his main risk factor being age over 75, so if surgical disease were found he would be fit for surgery. He is at slightly increased risk for colorectal cancer based on his history of benign polyps. He is able to give informed consent. It is appropriate to offer screening colonoscopy.

Table 5
Association between burden of preexisting comorbidities and colorectal cancer 5-year mortality (approximate percentage) by age

Age (Years)	No Comorbidities (%)	Average Comorbidities (%)	Severe Comorbidities (%)
70–74	13	25	47
75–79	18	32	54
≥80	31	48	66

Data from Walter LC, Lindquist K, Nugent S, et al. Impact of age and comorbidity on colorectal cancer screening among older veterans. [Summary for patients in Ann Intern Med 2009 Apr 7;150(7):I-42; PMID: 19349627]. Ann Intern Med 2009;150(7):465–73.

Prostate Cancer

Prostate cancer, other than skin cancer, is the most prevalent cancer among men, and age is the most significant risk factor for developing this cancer. In 2010 it is estimated that 217,730 new cases of prostate cancer will be diagnosed and 32,050 men will die of prostate cancer.[39] However, many if not most of these men will have lived many years with prostate cancer as a chronic disease. Prostate cancer accounts for nearly 10% of new cancer diagnoses in the NH, and screening persists (often by default) in men older than 75 years.[21,83] As with mammography among chronically ill older women,[84] chronically ill elderly men are screened for prostate cancer more often than healthier, younger men, as a side effect of the frequency of their contact with the medical profession.[85] Abnormal PSAs occur incidentally when men are assessed for lower urinary tract symptoms (LUTS).[46] The disparity is heightened by the fact that elderly men in NHs are frailer, sicker, and more cognitively impaired, and experience higher mortality than women in NHs.[23] Prostate cancer screening and indeed ordering PSA tests to evaluate LUTS in men living in NHs should be discouraged.

Clinical scenario #3

Mr E. is a 74-year-old man with a history of coronary artery disease, type 2 diabetes, peripheral vascular disease, and peripheral neuropathy who underwent below-knee amputation due to a nonhealing ischemic ulcer on his foot. After a long hospitalization (including nosocomial pneumonia, delirium, and urinary retention) he was transferred to an SNF for subacute rehabilitation. He was unable to return home after he completed his Part A rehabilitation because of persisting functional impairment. He was transferred to the long-stay unit. He again developed LUTS and nurses were not able to pass a Foley catheter. He was evaluated by a urologist as an outpatient. A Foley catheter was placed. As part of the evaluation, DRE revealed an enlarged, boggy prostate. A PSA was sent, which was returned as elevated (12.8 ng/μL).

The patient was not consistent in expressing his wishes about further evaluation. The family consented to ultrasound-guided transrectal biopsies of the prostate, which revealed adenocarcinoma (Gleason 3 + 3 = 6). Computed tomography of pelvis and abdomen was suggestive of right-sided inguinal and retroperitoneal lymphadenopathy (ie, not a candidate for either prostatectomy or radiation). The bone scan was negative for metastatic disease. The urologist initiated androgen ablation therapy, which quickly produced an undetectable PSA. However, the patient continued to experience functional decline, cognitive decline, depression, night sweats, immobility, and fatigue. He did not recover the ability to void independently. He died of pulmonary embolism 8 months after cancer diagnosis.

This case illustrates the danger of following "routine" workups. A 74-year-old man with significant underlying comorbidities demonstrated his vulnerability through a previous history of hospital-acquired delirium, poor functional reserve as shown by his poor tolerance of a low-risk surgery, his lack of progress in rehabilitation at the NH, and his inability to participate in his own decision making. Although he is not described as having active cardiac ischemia, significant renal failure, or dementia, he fits within the lower quartile for age, his life expectancy being 4.0 years.[32] Incidental DRE did not identify a discrete mass, and he had no bone pain, no hematuria, and other explanations for his LUTS. PSA should not have been measured. Once it had been measured, it would have been reasonable to observe and recheck it in a few months (active surveillance), or do nothing at all (watchful waiting). Once the biopsy revealed intermediate-grade prostate adenocarcinoma, a Gleason score of 6, and absence of pelvic nodes, surgery should not have been considered based on his poor tolerance of the amputation and based on the fact that his life expectancy was already less than that expected for an untreated similar stage and grade of prostate cancer. A healthier 75-year-old with his stage and grade of disease would expect a median survival of more than 8 years. Treatment options included androgen ablation or watchful waiting. Lu-Yao and colleagues[86] studied survival following primary androgen deprivation therapy (ADT) among men with localized (T1–T2) prostate cancer. ADT was not associated with improved survival among the majority of elderly men with T1 to T2 prostate cancer. The significant side effects and cost associated with ADT should trigger a very careful consideration of the rationale for initiating ADT in these patients.[86] A conservative but proactive approach would be pharmacologic therapy for symptomatic benign prostatic hyperplasia and watchful waiting regarding his prostate cancer.[87] ADT may have contributed to his functional decline, poor quality of life, and proximal cause of death. Parker[87] compares the concept of "active surveillance," which aims to individualize the management of early prostate cancer, with "watchful waiting," a policy of observation with the use of palliative treatment for symptomatic patients. **Table 6** presents a way to explain to patients and families how "not treating the prostate cancer" (watchful waiting) is not the same as not treating the patient.[87]

HOW TO DISCUSS CANCER IN THE NURSING HOME WITH PATIENTS AND FAMILIES

The aforementioned clinical scenarios present cases for patients, doctors, and families to make decisions based on best estimates about RLE, cancer behavior, and benefits of cancer treatment as measured in the usual cancer metrics: cancer death, total mortality, and cancer-free survival. For patients and families, and even sometimes the doctors, this objectivity is impossible and it is often more important to build a relationship based on trust, confidence, and concern than to get the facts straight. In this section the authors suggest ways to discuss forgoing futile screening and futile cancer treatment with patients who have little to gain. In the context of the NH, a major concern is that patients and families often regard NH placement as tantamount to abandonment. Conflating legitimately beneficial decisions to forgo medical interventions with medical abandonment has to be approached delicately. It is also true, however, in some cases where medical nihilism may deny an NH resident potentially beneficial palliative cancer care.

Table 6
Active surveillance versus watchful waiting

	Active Surveillance	Watchful Waiting
Patient characteristics	Fit for treatment; Age 50–80 y	Age >70 or life expectancy <15 y
Tumor characteristics	T1–T2, Gleason ≤7, Initial PSA <15	Any T stage, Gleason <7, any PSA
Monitoring	Frequent PSA testing and repeat biopsies	PSA testing not important. No repeat biopsies
Indications for treatment	Short PSA doubling time. Upgrading on biopsy	Symptomatic progression
Treatment timing	Early	Delayed
Treatment intent	Curative	Palliative

Abbreviation: PSA, prostate-specific antigen.

Data from Parker C. Active surveillance: towards a new paradigm in the management of early prostate cancer. Lancet Oncol 2004;5(2):101–6.

How to Talk About Prognosis

From the clinician's point of view, the treatment a patient receives depends on the patient's prognosis. From the patient's point of view the question is not what is the treatment, but "how long do I have?" Patients and families expect the physician to know. Communicating this information to patients and families when they are ready to hear it is crucial in helping them prioritize and plan for the future. These discussions should not focus narrowly on length of life but on how near or far death is from the horizon, what events can be expected, and how the patient can be assisted in the coming days, weeks, and months. Prognosis provides the foundation for discussing goals of care, especially for patients residing in NHs.[88,89] Many (but not all) patients want to discuss prognosis, and avoidance, inadequacy, or perceived distortion of the information is one the greatest complaints patients and families have about end-of-life care in retrospect.[90,91] It is also not a one-time discussion. As the clinical course evolves, families have questions, patients may change their minds about their care, and the negotiations often involve several people. In the NH, the staff become involved in the discussions as well and, depending on circumstances, their presence can facilitate or disrupt the dialogs.

Despite the importance of prognosis, physicians are often reluctant to reveal their prognostication. In a national survey of physicians, 90% felt they should avoid being specific about prognosis. Furthermore, 57% felt inadequately trained in prognostication.[92] In another study looking at the accuracy of physician prognostic skill, physicians were asked provide survival estimates of terminally ill patients at the time of hospice referral. Physicians were accurate 20% of the time and overestimated survival by factor of 5.3.[93] In addition, if the duration of the physician-patient relationship increased, prognostic accuracy decreased, suggesting that physician feelings toward patients impair their ability to prognosticate.

Not only is prognosis important for planning, but patients may change their minds based on perception of prognosis. In a study of older adults, subjects were asked about preferences for cardiopulmonary resuscitation (CPR). Before learning the true probability of survival, 41% of subjects wanted CPR. After learning the true probability of survival, 22% of subjects wanted CPR. If life expectancy was less than 1 year, 5% of subjects wanted CPR.[94] In NHs advance directives are often missing in action, due to either real or assumed cognitive impairment advance directives that may be taken from presumed well-meaning family members. These family members are frequently wrong in their idea of what the elder wants. Residing in an NH can be a dispiriting and disenfranchising experience. People may become enured to letting other people make their choices. It is the fortunate NH resident who has a staff, family, or publicly appointed advocate for their autonomy.

Discussing Life Expectancy

Discussing a patient's life expectancy or prognosis in regard of cancer treatment or screening should be considered as a "Breaking Bad News" conversation, and similar protocols should be followed.[95] SPIKES (Setting, Perception, Invitation, Knowledge, Empathy, and Strategic Summary) is a practical method for breaking bad news and is applicable to most situations, including cancer.[96] Imagine that you are a contractor and you must inform your client that the project will cost twice as much as you estimated and that it will take twice as long to complete. It is important to ensure the right time and setting are arranged, especially given the shared space most NH patients encounter. For discussing an active cancer diagnosis, all persons the patient wishes to be present should attend, even if some must participate via speaker phone, including the consultant physicians. For screening decisions the physician, the patient, and their chosen representative should be involved. The patient and family's current understanding of the illness (or the need for screening) should be elicited first. Then is it very useful to ask how much prognostic information is wanted and the degree of detail desired. It is always required to ask the patient who should be included (and excluded) from these discussions, and patients have even asked for themselves to be excused from these discussions: "I'll let my daughter handle that." Some patients desire exact information. It should be explained how a prognosis is estimated and that although that is your best estimate now, the situation may change with time. Whether or not a patient wishes to participate in these discussions, a health care proxy or surrogate must be named to participate in shared decision making. If the patient is unable to designate a proxy, and to avoid a legal proceeding or guardianship every effort should be made to have the family arrive at consensus on a lead person, a family spokesperson. The information should then be shared, allowing time for reaction without sharing additional information.

These discussions can become quite emotional. For physicians who are not comfortable with conflict and emotion, there are two useful strategies. First, identify a moderator or mediator ahead of the family council. Nursing and social work professionals, chaplains, and sometimes managers are often skilled and experienced. Second, have a repertoire of prepared responses so the patient's family can get continuous reassurance that you are present and attentive. Simple statements such as "I know that this is very difficult to hear" are effective.[97] Undoing the conflation of "hope" with "cure" is an important part of the work to be accomplished. Many physicians are concerned about "taking away hope" when discussing a poor prognosis. One common phrase, "hope for the best, prepare for the worst," acknowledges that hope can remain while simultaneously planning realistically. One way of dealing with this is to set realistic goals for the patient early in the discussion, which gives them a future on which to focus. Furthermore, communication of the prognosis is not a one-time occurrence, but a dynamic process that continues on an ongoing basis throughout the patient's life span and disease trajectory.

Informed Refusal and Requests to Withhold Information

Encounters between providers and patients of different backgrounds are common given the diversity in the United States, and therefore there are many opportunities for cross-cultural misunderstandings.[98] While autonomy is the legal basis for medical decision making in the United States, many families expect to make medical decisions as a unit. Some elderly people are comfortable handing over the reins to their children, while some resist fiercely. Adult children commonly wish to protect their parent from bad news and may ask the clinician not to tell the truth. Elderly persons may prefer to protect their "own business" and choose who they wish to tell what and when. Providers can address this issue directly, explaining to the family that information will not be imposed but will be offered, if the patient indicates an explicit desire to know. This is done by asking the patient, privately and with the family, if he or she is the kind of person who prefers all the details about the illness, or if he or she would rather hear a general outline and leave the details of decision making to a family member. Such communication demonstrates respect for the patients' wishes without making any assumptions or judgments about their culture, personality, or competence. It is better to assume little, because doctors do not appear to be very good at predicting the decision-making preferences of their patients.[99] The kinds of discussions suggested here can only happen once, so it is best to assume little in advance rather than have to backtrack and redirect.

Clinical scenario #4

A 79-year-old woman, Mrs F, is admitted to the NH after a brief hospital stay for pneumonia. She is expected to complete subacute Part A rehabilitation for deconditioning. After a few weeks it becomes evident that she will stay long term. She has moderately severe dementia with a little suspiciousness and an unsteady gait. She exhibits little carryover from therapy. Her type 2 diabetes and hypertension are easily controlled in the NH, although according to her daughter she never was controlled at home. At care plan she asks to have the physician send her for "good gyne exam" because she has never had one, and at the hospital they had offered a Pap smear but had not followed through. The physician was called for orders, and refused. The daughter was angry. She perceived the refusal to be dismissing her mother as "not worth the bother." The physician asked the patient whether she wanted a Pap smear and was told "I don't need no nasty poking around." The daughter did not feel her mother had the judgment to refuse. The task was to communicate admiration and appreciation of the daughter's advocacy for her mother and at the same how the mother would most likely experience the examination as an assault, especially because the gynecologic examination in elderly women is often difficult and requires some skill. The dwell time for HPV-related disease is approximately 10 years, so most likely if she had cervical cancer it would have been symptomatic by now. Because she had never been screened to the best of the daughter's memory, and because of the patient's long history of nonadherence to medical advice, she probably had not been screened, if at all, since the birth of her last child 40 years ago, so a one-time screening probably would not be wrong in a willing, cooperative patient. The USPSTF advises against intentional screening for endometrial cancer and for ovarian cancer, both of which might be detected on a pelvic examination motivated by symptoms. A compromise was reached.

PSYCHOLOGICAL ISSUES AND BEREAVEMENT

Timing of the end-of-life discussion is variable, and involving formal hospice in NH care for cancer patients is not straightforward. Some NHs are prepared to deliver palliative care and symptomatic care, but many are not. Sometimes the role of the hospice supplements the NH staff for care of the family. Sometimes however desirable, the patient's payor does not permit formal hospice. Specifically, Part A SNF can be used to pay for complex symptomatic management depending on how many days the patient has left and how the diagnosis is coded. However, Medicare hospice benefit does not pay the NH but rather pays an outside hospice organization to provide home hospice in the NH, and the patient is then responsible to pay the per diem rate at the NH. Some families can afford to pay these rates, while others have public payors for the per diem. Unfortunately, many families are placed in difficult situations where they have to choose to pay or take their loved ones home. Sometimes, hospice can be the key to letting the patient go home for their last days. However, every effort should be made to prevent futile, expensive, and burdensome hospital transfers of actively dying patients.

To this end physicians who have not had the personal experience should remember and acknowledge the stress and guilt experienced by families whose loved ones are declining in NHs. The stress on NH staff is little acknowledged and little intervened upon. Physicians and supervisors need to recognize when caregivers are stressed, and refer to social work and other community resources. When no further cancer treatment is to be offered, patients can feel abandoned by their oncologists. In the NH, physicians should ameliorate this as far as possible and demonstrate active involvement in care. Calling patients and families can reassure patients that a referral to hospice is not abandonment by the physician. It is important to express thanks and appreciation for the privilege of caring for the patient, and when appropriate, to say goodbye to the patient and their family members. Physicians must also be aware of normal and complicated grief, and screen and address those appropriately (see **Table 4**).[100,101] Hospice programs provide bereavement services and follow-up for 12 months after the death of the patient. Finally, all providers can discuss and offer coping strategies to determine the most constructive approach to dealing with loss based on individual family needs and temperament.

Key points #3: Disclosing life expectancy and prognosis

1. Ask what the patient and family knows and understands; this keys you into vocabulary
2. Assess how much information is desired about prognosis by the patient
3. Emphasize prognosis is an estimate. Use ranges: days to weeks, weeks to months, months to years (you may have to explain why your estimate is different from the hospital physician's)
4. Acknowledge individuals' emotions
5. Check understanding by asking them to summarize "so far," encourage questions
6. Schedule a follow-up to address outstanding questions; Assure nonabandonment
7. Document the discussion to ensure information communicated by providers is consistent
8. Respect a patient's hopes while encouraging realistic plans for the future
9. Designate a proxy decision-maker or spokesperson.

APPENDIX 1:

United States Preventive Services Task Force Recommendations for Cancer Screening (Most Recent Update.) Colorectal Cancer Screening Summary of Recommendations (2008)

- The USPSTF recommends screening for colorectal cancer (CRC) using fecal occult blood testing, sigmoidoscopy, or colonoscopy, in adults, beginning at age 50 years and continuing until age 75 years. The risks and benefits of these screening methods vary.
  Grade: A Recommendation.
- The USPSTF recommends against routine screening for colorectal cancer in adults age 76 to 85 years. There may be considerations that support colorectal cancer screening in an individual patient.
  Grade: C Recommendation.
- The USPSTF recommends against screening for colorectal cancer in adults older than age 85 years.
  Grade: D Recommendation.
- The USPSTF concludes that the evidence is insufficient to assess the benefits and harms of computed tomographic colonography and fecal DNA testing as screening modalities for colorectal cancer.
  Grade: I Statement.

Lung Cancer Screening Summary of Recommendations (2004)

- The U.S. Preventive Services Task Force (USPSTF) concludes that the evidence is insufficient to recommend for or against screening asymptomatic persons for lung cancer with either low dose computerized tomography (LDCT), chest x-ray (CXR), sputum cytology, or a combination of these tests.
  Grade: I Statement.

Ovarian Cancer Screening Summary of Recommendation (2004)

- The U.S. Preventive Services Task Force (USPSTF) recommends against routine screening for ovarian cancer.
  Grade: D Recommendation.

Prostate Cancer Screening Summary of Recommendations (2008)

- The USPSTF concludes that the current evidence is insufficient to assess the balance of benefits and harms of prostate cancer screening in men younger than age 75 years.
  Grade: I Statement.
- The USPSTF recommends against screening for prostate cancer In men age 75 years or older.
  Grade: D Recommendation.

Cervical Cancer Screening Summary of Recommendations (2003)

- The USPSTF strongly recommends screening for cervical cancer in women who have been sexually active and have a cervix.
  Grade: A Recommendation.
- The US PSTF recommends against routinely screening women older than age 65 for cervical cancer if they have had adequate recent screening with normal Pap smears and are not otherwise at high risk for cervical cancer (go to Clinical Considerations).
  Grade: D Recommendation.
- The USPSTF recommends against routine Pap smear screening in women who have had a total hysterectomy for benign disease.
  Grade: D Recommendation.
- The US PSTF concludes that the evidence is insufficient to recommend for or against the routine use of new technologies to screen for cervical cancer.
  Grade: I Statement.
- The USPSTF concludes that the evidence is insufficient to recommend for or against the routine use of *human papillomavirus* (HPV) testing as a primary screening test for cervical cancer.
  Grade: I Recommendation.

Breast Cancer Screening Summary of Recommendations (2009)

- The USPSTF recommends biennial screening mammography for women aged 50 to 74 years.
  Grade: B Recommendation.

- The decision to start regular, biennial screening mammography before the age of 50 years should be an individual one and take patient context into account, including the patient's values regarding specific benefits and harms.
  Grade: C Recommendation.
- The USPSTF concludes that the current evidence is insufficient to assess the additional benefits and harms of screening mammography in women 75 years or older.
  Grade: I Statement.
- The USPSTF recommends against teaching breast self-examination (BSE).
  Grade: D recommendation.
- The USPSTF concludes that the current evidence is insufficient to assess the additional benefits and harms of clinical breast examination (CBE) beyond screening mammography in women 40 years or older.
  Grade: I Statement.
- The USPSTF concludes that the current evidence is insufficient to assess the additional benefits and harms of either digital mammography or magnetic resonance imaging (MRI) instead of film mammography as screening modalities for breast cancer.
  Grade: I Statement.

REFERENCES

1. Greenlee RT, Hill-Harmon MB, Murray T, et al. Cancer statistics, 2001. CA Cancer J Clin 2001;51(1):15–36.
2. Yancik R, Ganz PA, Varricchio GC, et al. Perspectives on comorbidity and cancer in older patients: approaches to expand the knowledge base. J Clin Oncol 2001;19(4):1147–51.
3. Yancik R, Ries LA. Aging and cancer in America. Demographic and epidemiologic perspectives. Hematol Oncol Clin North Am 2000;14(1):17–23.
4. Smith BD, Smith GL, Hurria A, et al. Future of cancer incidence in the United States: burdens upon an aging, changing nation. J Clin Oncol 2009;27(17): 2758–65.
5. Yancik R. Population aging and cancer: a cross-national concern. Cancer J 2005;11(6):437–41.
6. Jemal A, Siegel R, Ward E, et al. Cancer statistics, 2009. CA Cancer J Clin 2009; 59(4):225–49.
7. Fried LP, Tangen CM, Walston J, et al. Frailty in older adults: evidence for a phenotype. J Gerontol A Biol Sci Med Sci 2001;56(3):M146–56.
8. Covinsky KE, Justice AC, Rosenthal GE, et al. Measuring prognosis and case mix in hospitalized elders. The importance of functional status. J Gen Intern Med 1997;12(4):203–8.
9. Klein BE, Klein R, Knudtson MD, et al. Frailty, morbidity and survival. Arch Gerontol Geriatr 2005;41(2):141–9.
10. Extermann M, Overcash J, Lyman GH, et al. Comorbidity and functional status are independent in older cancer patients. J Clin Oncol 1998;16(4):1582–7.
11. Gorin SS, Heck JE, Albert S, et al. Treatment for breast cancer in patients with Alzheimer's disease. J Am Geriatr Soc 2005;53(11):1897–904.

12. Gupta SK, Lamont EB. Patterns of presentation, diagnosis, and treatment in older patients with colon cancer and comorbid dementia. J Am Geriatr Soc 2004; 52(10):1681–7.
13. Kelly A, Conell-Price J, Covinsky K, et al. Length of stay for older adults residing in nursing homes at the end of life. J Am Geriatr Soc 2010;58(9):1701–6.
14. Levine SK, Sachs GA, Jin L, et al. A prognostic model for 1-year mortality in older adults after hospital discharge. Am J Med 2007;120(5):455–60.
15. Larson EB, Shadlen MF, Wang L, et al. Survival after initial diagnosis of Alzheimer disease. Ann Intern Med 2004;140(7):501–9.
16. Buchanan RJ, Barkley J, Wang S, et al. Analyses of nursing home residents with cancer at admission. Cancer Nurs 2005;28(5):406–14.
17. Mor V. Defining and measuring quality outcomes in long-term care. J Am Med Dir Assoc 2007;8(3 Suppl 2):e129–37.
18. Intrator O, Hiris J, Berg K, et al. The residential history file: studying nursing home residents' long-term care histories. Health Serv Res 2011;46(1 Pt 1):120–37.
19. Bourbonniere M, Van Cleave JH. Cancer care in nursing homes. Semin Oncol Nurs 2006;22(1):51–7.
20. Johnson VM, Teno JM, Bourbonniere M, et al. Palliative care needs of cancer patients in U.S. nursing homes. J Palliat Med 2005;8(2):273–9.
21. Bradley CJ, Clement JP, Lin C. Absence of cancer diagnosis and treatment in elderly Medicaid-insured nursing home residents. J Natl Cancer Inst 2008; 100(1):21–31.
22. Clement JP, Bradley CJ, Lin C. Organizational characteristics and cancer care for nursing home residents. Health Serv Res 2009;44(6):1983–2003.
23. van Dijk PT, Mehr DR, Ooms ME, et al. Comorbidity and 1-year mortality risks in nursing home residents. J Am Geriatr Soc 2005;53(4):660–5.
24. Boockvar K, Fishman E, Kyriacou CK, et al. Adverse events due to discontinuations in drug use and dose changes in patients transferred between acute and long-term care facilities. Arch Intern Med 2004;164(5):545–50.
25. Coleman EA, Berenson RA. Lost in transition: challenges and opportunities for improving the quality of transitional care. Ann Intern Med 2004;141(7):533–6.
26. Moore C, McGinn T, Halm E. Tying up loose ends: discharging patients with unresolved medical issues. Arch Intern Med 2007;167(12):1305–11.
27. Rodin MB. Cancer patients admitted to nursing homes: what do we know? J Am Med Dir Assoc 2008;9(3):149–56.
28. Maccabee J. The effect of transfer from a palliative care unit to nursing homes—are patients' and relatives' needs met? Palliat Med 1994;8(3):211–4.
29. Mitchell SL, Kiely DK, Hamel MB. Dying with advanced dementia in the nursing home. Arch Intern Med 2004;164(3):321–6.
30. Glare P, Virik K. Independent prospective validation of the PaP score in terminally ill patients referred to a hospital-based palliative medicine consultation service. J Pain Symptom Manage 2001;22(5):891–8.
31. Pirovano M, Maltoni M, Nanni O, et al. A new palliative prognostic score: a first step for the staging of terminally ill cancer patients. Italian Multicenter and Study Group on Palliative Care. J Pain Symptom Manage 1999;17(4):231–9.
32. Walter LC, Covinsky KE. Cancer screening in elderly patients: a framework for individualized decision making. JAMA 2001;285(21):2750–6.
33. Lubitz J, Cai L, Kramarow E, et al. Health, life expectancy, and health care spending among the elderly. N Engl J Med 2003;349(11):1048–55.
34. Rozzini R, Sabatini T, Ranhoff AH, et al. Bathing disability in older patients. J Am Geriatr Soc 2007;55(4):635–6.

35. Fried LP, Ferrucci L, Darer J, et al. Untangling the concepts of disability, frailty, and comorbidity: implications for improved targeting and care. J Gerontol A Biol Sci Med Sci 2004;59(3):255–63.
36. Koroukian SM, Xu F, Bakaki PM, et al. Comorbidities, functional limitations, and geriatric syndromes in relation to treatment and survival patterns among elders with colorectal cancer. J Gerontol A Biol Sci Med Sci 2010;65(3):322–9.
37. Feinstein AR, Sosin DM, Wells CK. The Will Rogers phenomenon. Stage migration and new diagnostic techniques as a source of misleading statistics for survival in cancer. N Engl J Med 1985;312(25):1604–8.
38. Nyström L, Andersson I, Bjurstam N, et al. Long-term effects of mammography screening: updated overview of the Swedish randomised trials. Lancet 2002; 359(9310):909–19.
39. American Cancer Society. 2010. Available at: http://www.cancer.org/Healthy/FindCancerEarly/CancerScreeningGuidelines/american-cancer-society-guidelines-for-the-early-detection-of-cancer. Accessed February 26, 2010.
40. Figueiredo MI, Cullen J, Hwang YT, et al. Breast cancer treatment in older women: does getting what you want improve your long-term body image and mental health? J Clin Oncol 2004;22(19):4002–9.
41. Mandelblatt J. To screen or not to screen older women for breast cancer: a new twist on an old question or will we ever invest in getting the answers? J Clin Oncol 2007;25(21):2991–2.
42. Mandelblatt JS, Sheppard VB, Hurria A, et al. Breast cancer adjuvant chemotherapy decisions in older women: the role of patient preference and interactions with physicians. J Clin Oncol 2010;28(19):3146–53.
43. La Rochelle J, Amling CL. Prostate cancer screening: what we have learned from the PLCO and ERSPC trials. Curr Urol Rep 2010;11(3):198–201.
44. Vis AN, Roemeling S, Reedijk AM, et al. Overall survival in the intervention arm of a randomized controlled screening trial for prostate cancer compared with a clinically diagnosed cohort. Eur Urol 2008;53(1):91–8.
45. Shen Y, Huang X. Nonparametric estimation of asymptomatic duration from a randomized prospective cancer screening trial. Biometrics 2005;61(4): 992–9.
46. Holmes HM, Goodwin JS. Screening for prostate cancer in long-term care. Ann Long Term Care 2009;17:22–8.
47. Thompson IM, Ankerst DP, Chi C, et al. Operating characteristics of prostate-specific antigen in men with an initial PSA level of 3.0 ng/ml or lower. JAMA 2005;294(1):66–70.
48. Draisma G, Boer R, Otto SJ, et al. Lead times and overdetection due to prostate-specific antigen screening: estimates from the European Randomized Study of Screening for Prostate Cancer. J Natl Cancer Inst 2003;95(12):868–78.
49. Mohile SG, Lachs M, Dale W. Management of prostate cancer in the older man. Semin Oncol 2008;35(6):597–617.
50. Mohile SG, Mustian K, Bylow K, et al. Management of complications of androgen deprivation therapy in the older man. Crit Rev Oncol Hematol 2009; 70(3):235–55.
51. Bylow K, Dale W, Mustian K, et al. Falls and physical performance deficits in older patients with prostate cancer undergoing androgen deprivation therapy. Urology 2008;72(2):422–7.
52. Raftery L, Sanoff HK, Goldberg R. Colon cancer in older adults. Semin Oncol 2008;35(6):561–8.

53. Whitlock EP, Lin JS, Liles E, et al. Screening for colorectal cancer: a targeted, updated systematic review for the U.S. Preventive Services Task Force. Ann Intern Med 2008;149(9):638–58.
54. Rex DK, Johnson DA, Anderson JC, et al. American College of Gastroenterology guidelines for colorectal cancer screening 2009 [corrected]. Am J Gastroenterol 2009;104(3):739–50.
55. Rosano C, Newman AB, Katz R, et al. Association between lower digit symbol substitution test score and slower gait and greater risk of mortality and of developing incident disability in well-functioning older adults. J Am Geriatr Soc 2008;56(9):1618–25.
56. Cesari M, Kritchevsky SB, Newman AB, et al. Added value of physical performance measures in predicting adverse health-related events: results from the Health, Aging And Body Composition Study. J Am Geriatr Soc 2009;57(2): 251–9.
57. Blain H, Carriere I, Sourial N, et al. Balance and walking speed predict subsequent 8-year mortality independently of current and intermediate events in well-functioning women aged 75 years and older. J Nutr Health Aging 2010;14(7): 595–600.
58. Abellan van Kan G, Rolland Y, Andrieu S, et al. Gait speed at usual pace as a predictor of adverse outcomes in community-dwelling older people an International Academy on Nutrition and Aging (IANA) Task Force. J Nutr Health Aging 2009;13(10):881–9.
59. Studenski S, Perera S, Patel K, et al. Gait speed and survival in older adults. JAMA 2011;305(1):50–8.
60. Gill TM, Baker DI, Gottschalk M, et al. A prehabilitation program for the prevention of functional decline: effect on higher-level physical function. Arch Phys Med Rehabil 2004;85(7):1043–9.
61. Chen JH, Chan DC, Kiely DK, et al. Terminal trajectories of functional decline in the long-term care setting. J Gerontol A Biol Sci Med Sci 2007;62(5):531–6.
62. Min L, Yoon W, Mariano J, et al. The vulnerable elders-13 survey predicts 5-year functional decline and mortality outcomes in older ambulatory care patients. J Am Geriatr Soc 2009;57(11):2070–6.
63. Karlamangla AS, Singer BH, McEwen BS, et al. Allostatic load as a predictor of functional decline. MacArthur studies of successful aging. J Clin Epidemiol 2002;55(7):696–710.
64. Carey EC, Covinsky KE, Lui LY, et al. Prediction of mortality in community-living frail elderly people with long-term care needs. J Am Geriatr Soc 2008;56(1): 68–75.
65. Carey EC, Walter LC, Lindquist K, et al. Development and validation of a functional morbidity index to predict mortality in community-dwelling elders. J Gen Intern Med 2004;19(10):1027–33.
66. Walter LC, Brand RJ, Counsell SR, et al. Development and validation of a prognostic index for 1-year mortality in older adults after hospitalization. JAMA 2001; 285(23):2987–94.
67. Balducci L. Aging, frailty, and chemotherapy. Cancer Control 2007;14(1):7–12.
68. Flaherty JH, Morley JE, Murphy DJ, et al. The development of outpatient clinical glidepaths. J Am Geriatr Soc 2002;50(11):1886–901.
69. Aapro M, Monfardini S, Jirillo A, et al. Management of primary and advanced breast cancer in older unfit patients (medical treatment). Cancer Treat Rev 2009;35(6):503–8.

70. Jemal A, Siegel R, Ward E, et al. Cancer statistics, 2008. CA Cancer J Clin 2008; 58(2):71–96.
71. Yancik R, Wesley MN, Ries LA, et al. Effect of age and comorbidity in postmenopausal breast cancer patients aged 55 years and older. JAMA 2001;285(7): 885–92.
72. Diab SG, Elledge RM, Clark GM. Tumor characteristics and clinical outcome of elderly women with breast cancer. J Natl Cancer Inst 2000;92(7):550–6.
73. Daidone MG, Coradini D, Martelli G, et al. Primary breast cancer in elderly women: biological profile and relation with clinical outcome. Crit Rev Oncol Hematol 2003;45(3):313–25.
74. Molino A, Giovannini M, Auriemma A, et al. Pathological, biological and clinical characteristics, and surgical management, of elderly women with breast cancer. Crit Rev Oncol Hematol 2006;59(3):226–33.
75. Walter LC, Eng C, Covinsky KE. Screening mammography for frail older women: what are the burdens? J Gen Intern Med 2001;16(11):779–84.
76. Satariano WA, Ragland DR. The effect of comorbidity on 3-year survival of women with primary breast cancer. Ann Intern Med 1994;120(2):104–10.
77. Walter LC, Lewis CL, Barton MB. Screening for colorectal, breast, and cervical cancer in the elderly: a review of the evidence. Am J Med 2005;118(10): 1078–86.
78. Extermann M, Balducci L, Lyman GH. What threshold for adjuvant therapy in older breast cancer patients? J Clin Oncol 2000;18(8):1709–17.
79. Muss HB, Woolf S, Berry D, et al. Adjuvant chemotherapy in older and younger women with lymph node-positive breast cancer. JAMA 2005;293(9):1073–81.
80. Basset SD, Smyer T. Health screening practices in rural long term care facilities. J Gerontol Nurs 2003;29:42–9.
81. Gross CP, McAvay GJ, Krumholz HM, et al. The effect of age and chronic illness on life expectancy after a diagnosis of colorectal cancer: implications for screening. Ann Intern Med 2006;145(9):646–53 [Summary for patients in Ann Intern Med 2006;145(9):I20.
82. Walter LC, Lindquist K, Nugent S, et al. Impact of age and comorbidity on colorectal cancer screening among older veterans. Ann Intern Med 2009;150(7): 465–73 [Summary for patients in Ann Intern Med 2009;150(7):I-42.
83. Konety BR, Sharp VJ, Verma M, et al. Practice patterns in screening and management of prostate cancer in elderly men. Urology 2006;68(5):1051–6.
84. Mehta KM, Fung KZ, Kistler CE, et al. Impact of cognitive impairment on screening mammography use in older US women. Am J Public Health 2010; 100(10):1917–23.
85. Walter LC, Bertenthal D, Lindquist K, et al. PSA screening among elderly men with limited life expectancies. JAMA 2006;296(19):2336–42.
86. Lu-Yao GL, Albertsen PC, Moore DF, et al. Survival following primary androgen deprivation therapy among men with localized prostate cancer. JAMA 2008; 300(2):173–81 [Erratum appears in JAMA 2009;301(1):38].
87. Parker C. Active surveillance: towards a new paradigm in the management of early prostate cancer. Lancet Oncol 2004;5(2):101–6.
88. Zerzan J, Stearns S, Hanson L. Access to palliative care and hospice in nursing homes. JAMA 2000;284(19):2489–94.
89. Saraiya B, Bodnar-Deren S, Leventhal E, et al. End-of-life planning and its relevance for patients' and oncologists' decisions in choosing cancer therapy. Cancer 2008;113(Suppl 12):3540–7.

90. Hanson LC, Danis M, Garrett J. What is wrong with end-of-life care? Opinions of bereaved family members. J Am Geriatr Soc 1997;45(11):1339–44.
91. Steinhauser KE, Christakis NA, Clipp EC, et al. Factors considered important at the end of life by patients, family, physicians, and other care providers. JAMA 2000;284(19):2476–82.
92. Iwashyna TJ, Christakis NA. Attitude and self-reported practice regarding hospice referral in a national sample of internists. J Palliat Med 1998;1(3):241–8.
93. Christakis NA, Lamont EB. Extent and determinants of error in doctors' prognoses in terminally ill patients: prospective cohort study. BMJ 2000;320(7233): 469–72.
94. Murphy DJ, Burrows D, Santilli S, et al. The influence of the probability of survival on patients' preferences regarding cardiopulmonary resuscitation. N Engl J Med 1994;330(8):545–9.
95. Back AL, Anderson WG, Bunch L, et al. Communication about cancer near the end of life. Cancer 2008;113(Suppl 7):1897–910.
96. Baile WF, Buckman R, Lenzi R, et al. SPIKES—A six-step protocol for delivering bad news: application to the patient with cancer. Oncologist 2000;5(4):302–11.
97. Pantilat SZ. Communicating with seriously ill patients: better words to say. JAMA 2009;301(12):1279–81.
98. Kagawa-Singer M, Blackhall LJ. Negotiating cross-cultural issues at the end of life: "You got to go where he lives". JAMA 2001;286(23):2993–3001.
99. Bruera E, Willey JS, Palmer JL, et al. Treatment decisions for breast carcinoma: patient preferences and physician perceptions. Cancer 2002;94(7):2076–80.
100. Stroebe M, Schut H, Stroebe W. Health outcomes of bereavement. Lancet 2007; 370:1960.
101. Prigerson HG, Maciejewski PK, Reynolds CF 3rd, et al. Inventory of complicated grief: a scale to measure maladaptive symptoms of loss. Psychiatry Res 1995; 59(1–2):65–79.

Index

Note: Page numbers of article titles are in **boldface** type.

A

Acetaminophen, 185–186
Acupuncture, in nausea, 218
Agitation, dementia and, 139–142
Alzheimer dementia, 165
Alzheimer stages of decline, FAST 7 in, 157, 166
American Cancer Society, guidelines for cancer screening, 308
Analgesics, 180–185
  opiate, 186–187
  topical, and local injections, 185
Antibiotics, adverse effects of, in elderly, 124–125
  for elderly, treatment duration in use of, 125
  in pressure ulcers, 251
  selection of, in pneumonia, 123
Anticonvulsants, antidepressants and, 187
Antidepressants, 180
  and anticonvulsants, 187
  choosing of, and removing inappropriate antidepressants, 182–185
Antiemetics, in nausea, 218
Antipsychotics, actions of, 175
  indications for, 176
  potential toxicity of, 176
  side effects of, 177
Aripiprazole, 176
Assessment in Advanced Dementia Scale, 163
Assisted living facilities, transitional care and, 264–265

B

Baclofen, 187
Bedside teaching, 207
Benzodiazepines, for short-term use, 179
  in dyspnea, 221
  risks of, 178
  uses of, 178
Bisphosphonates, 187
Breast cancer, clinical scenarios of, 311–313

C

Calcitonin, 187
Cancer, 5-year survival by site, 303

Clin Geriatr Med 27 (2011) 329–335
doi:10.1016/S0749-0690(11)00033-4

Cancer (*continued*)
as age-associated disease, 302
care in nursing homes, 305
clinical scenarios of, 311–316
discussion of, with patients and families, 316–319
in long-term care, **301–327**
informed refusal and requests to withhold information in, 318–319
life expectancy in, 306–307
discussion of, 317–318
prognosis in, discussion of, 317
psychological issues and bereavement in, 319–320
screening for, American Cancer Society guidelines for, 308
in nursing home, 311–316
recommendations in, 310–311
United States Preventive Services Task Force recommendations for, 320–322
screening guidelines, and elderly, 307–310
sites of mortality, 303
Cholinesterase inhibitors, for dementia, 135–137
Clozaril, 176–177
Cognitive/achievement-oriented personhood, 275
Colorectal cancer, clinical scenarios of, 313–314
Communication, human, 279–280
Constipation, evaluation of, 222
medications to treat, 222, 223
opioid-induced, 222
Corticosteroids, in nausea, 218
Creative impulse, dementia and, 282–283

D

Death, in long-term care facilities, 213
leading causes of, 302
Dementia, advanced, optimizing function and quality of life in, 164–165
Alzheimer, 165
and agitation, 139–142
and creative impulse, 282–283
and depression, 138–139, 140
and Down syndrome, 297–298
and intellectual and developmental disabilities, 297
and personhood, cultural meaning of, 273–275, 283–285
cholinesterase inhibitors and memantine for, 135–137
doing it better, anthropological insights into, **273–289**
eating problems associated with, 142–143, 161
evaluation of, 143
management options for, 143–146
goals of care in, discussing with families/surrogate decision makers, 161
in long-term care, palliative care for patients with, **153–170**
in long-term care patient, management of, **135–152**
infections and, 155–156
moderate, optimal environment for, 137–138
prognostication for, 156–158, 166

transitions of care in, 154–155
tube feeding in, 158–161
Depression, dementia and, 138–139, 140
Developmental disabilities, definition of, 292
Diphenhydramine, 179
Donepezil, 136–137
Down syndrome, 293–294
dementia and, 297–298
Dyspnea, benzodiazepines in, 221
evaluation of, 220
opioids in, 220–221
supplemental oxygen in, 221
treatment of cause of, 220

E

Eating problems, associated with dementia, 142–146, 161
Educational methods, for teaching, 207–208
Educational programs, barriers to, 208
Emergency departments, and long-term care, transitional care between, 262–264
Emphysema, senile, 119
End of life, symptoms at, 214, 215
management strategy in, 216–217
Evidence-based medicine, application in long-term care facilities, 195–197
concept of, 194–195
what long-term care providers need to know, **193–198**

F

FAST 7, Alzheimer stages of decline and, 157, 166
Fentanyl, 186

G

Geriatric competencies, teaching of, 204–206
Geriatrics, teaching of, in medical schools, 200

H

Health systems-based practice, 203
Hospice care, and palliative care, transitional care and, 265–266
Hospital, acute care, readmission to, from long-term care, 260–262
length of stay in, fiscal pressures to decrease, 260–261
Hydrocodone, 186
Hydromorphone, 186
Hydroxyzine, 179

I

Identity, embodied, 280–281
Infections, and dementia, 155–156

Infections (*continued*)
control issues in long-term care, 119
in long-term care, 117
multidrug-resistant, risk of, 119
urinary tract. See *Urinary tract infections*.
Intellectual and developmental disabilities, 291–292
aging population with, long-term care of, **291–300**
compared, 292–293
comorbid conditions in, 294–295
dementia and, 297
epidemiology and life expectancy in, 293
maladaptive behaviors in, 295–296
polypharmacy and, 296–297
psychiatric disorders in, 296
Intellectual disability, definition of, 292
Interprofessional teamwork and group dynamics, 203

L

Long-term care, definition of, 259

M

Medication errors, transitional care and, 261–262
Medications, in long-term care, when less is more, **171–191**
reductions of, history of, 171–172
why, when, how, and what, 174–175
Memantine, for dementia, 135–137
Mirtazapine, 146
Mortality Risk Index, 157, 158
risk estimate of death and, 157, 158

N

Nausea, and other nonpain symptoms, challenges in management of, 214–216
in long-term care, **213–228**
causes of, and treatment of, 218, 219
evaluation of, 217–218
screening for, 217
Neuropsychiatric illnesses, prevalence of, 172–174
NSAIDS, 186
Nursing Home Reform Act, 171

O

Opiate analgesics, 186–187
Opioids, for pain relief, 164, 165
in dyspnea, 220–221
Oral hygiene, pneumonia and, 125–126
Oxycodone, 186
Oxygen, supplemental, in dyspnea, 221

P

Pain, assessment and management of, 162–164
nonverbal indicators of, 163
treatment of, in long-term care facilities, 180–188
Palliative care programs, 161–162
Personhood, cognitive/achievement-oriented, 275
relational, autonomy versus interdependence, 276–278
social interactionism and, 278–279
spiritual, 281–282
Physicians Orders for Life-Sustaining Treatment, 266
Pneumonia, algorithm for management of, 122, 123
antimicrobial treatment of, 124
cause of, 118–119
clinical evaluation in, 121
diagnostic challenges in, 120
due to aspiration, 121, 125
epidemiology of, 118–120
in long-term care, **117–133**
laboratory evaluation in, 121
morbidity and mortality associated with, 118
oral hygiene and, 125–126
palliative and end-of-life care in, 126–127
pathophysiology of, 120
prevention of, 125
prognosis in, 125
treatment of, 121–122
in inpatient hospitals, 123–124
location of, 122–125
vaccines and, 126–127
Pressure ulcers, assessment of, 245–247
bacterial balance and infection management in, 249–251
débridement of, 251–252
diagnosis of, 244–245
in long-term care, **241–257**
incidence, prevalence, and costs of, 242
interdisciplinary management of, 247–248
local wound care in, 249–252
management of, and palliative care, 252–253
moisture balance and, 249
phases of healing of, 243
prevention of, 243–244
quality indicators and litigation in, 253–254
risk factors for, 242–243
staging of, 246
Prostate cancer, clinical scenarios of, 315–316
Psychologic medications, on inappropriate medications lists, 173

Q

Quality improvement methods, 202

R

Ramelteon, 179
Relational personhood, autonomy versus interdependence, 276–278
Residency programs, nursing home component in, 201
Respiratory system, aging, physiology of, 119–120
Risperidone, 176

S

SBAR communication tool, 267
Sedatives/hypnotics, 179–180
Skeletal muscle relaxants, 187
Social interactionism, and personhood, 278–279
Spiritual personhood, 281–282
Steroids, systemic, 187

T

Teaching, bedside, 207
  educational methods for, 207–208
  funding of, 199
  in long-term care setting, update on, **199–211**
  of educational domains, 202–207
  of geriatric competencies, 207–208
  of geriatrics, in medical schools, 200
  of transitional care, 203
  requirements and structure for physician trainees, 200–202
Transcutaneous electrical nerve stimulation, 181
Transitional care, and assisted living facilities, 264–265
  and hospice and palliative care, 265–266
  between long-term care and emergency departments, 262–264
  communication and, 261
  health care provider continuity and, 261
  measurement of quality of, 266
  of long-term care patient, **259–271**
  teaching of, 203
Trazodone, 179
Tube feeding, in dementia, 158–161

U

United States Preventive Services Task Force, 308
  recommendations for cancer screening, 320–322
Urinary tract infections, antimicrobial susceptibility testing in, 234
  areas of research in, 236
  diagnosis of, 231–233
  epidemiology of, 229–230
  in long-term care residents, **229–239**
  management of, 234–235
  microbiology of, 230

prevention of, 235–236
risk factors for, 230–231

V

Vaccines, pneumonia and, 126–127
Valium, 178

Z

Ziprasidone, 176

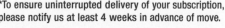

Printed and bound by CPI Group (UK) Ltd, Croydon, CR0 4YY
03/10/2024
01040447-0004